PEARSON ALWAYS LEARNING

Rebecca J. Donatelle

My Health

An Outcomes Approach

Second Custom Edition for Western New England University

Taken from:
My Health, The MasteringHealth Edition, by Rebecca J. Donatelle

Cover Art: Courtesy of Stockbyte/Getty Images and Corbis.

Taken from:

My Health
by Rebecca J. Donatelle

New York, New York 10013

This special edition published in cooperation with Pearson Learning Solutions.

Pearson Learning Solutions, 330 Hudson Street, New York, New York 10013
A Pearson Education Company
www.pearsoned.com

Printed in the United States of America

1 2 3 4 5 6 7 8 9 10 V0UD 19 18 17 16 15

000200010271970234

CW

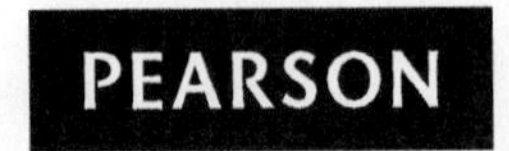

ISBN 10: 1-323-12555-8
ISBN 13: 978-1-323-12555-7

About the Author

Rebecca J. Donatelle, Ph.D.

Oregon State University

Rebecca Donatelle has served as a faculty member in the Department of Public Health, College of Health and Human Sciences, at Oregon State University for the last two decades. In that role, she has chaired the department and been program coordinator for the Health Promotion and Health Behavior Program (bachelor's degree, master of public health, and Ph.D. degree programs), as well as served on over 50 national, state, regional, and university committees focused on improving student academic success and improving the public's health. Most importantly to her, she has also taught and mentored thousands of undergraduate and graduate students. She is proud of the many outstanding accomplishments of her students! Many of these students gained community-based intervention and research skills while working on Dr. Donatelle's funded projects, and those experiences have led to exciting career paths nationally and internationally. Others have gone on to receive advanced degrees in public health and have assumed leadership roles in a wide range of academic, community, and health care system positions. "I believe that my successes are measured in large part by the successes of the students I have worked with and their contributions to the improved health of others," says Donatelle.

Dr. Donatelle has a Ph.D. in community health/health promotion and health education, with specializations in health behaviors, aging, and chronic disease prevention, from the University of Oregon; a master of science degree in health education from the University of Wisconsin, La Crosse; and a bachelor of science degree from the University of Wisconsin, La Crosse, with majors in health/physical education and English. In recent years, Dr. Donatelle has received several professional awards for leadership, teaching, and service within the university and for her work on developing nationally ranked undergraduate and graduate programs in the health promotion/health behavior areas.

Her primary research and scholarship areas have focused on finding scientifically appropriate means of motivating behavior change among resistant populations. Specifically, her work uses incentives, social and community supports, and risk communication strategies in motivating diverse populations to change their risk behaviors. She has worked with pregnant women who smoke in an effort to motivate them to quit smoking, obese women of all ages who are at risk for cardiovascular disease and diabetes, prediabetic women at risk for progression to type 2 diabetes, and a wide range of other health issues and problems. Earlier research projects have focused on decision making and factors influencing the use of alternative and traditional health care providers for treatment of low back pain, illness and sick role behaviors, occupational stress and stress claims, and worksite health promotion.

Brief Contents

Contents

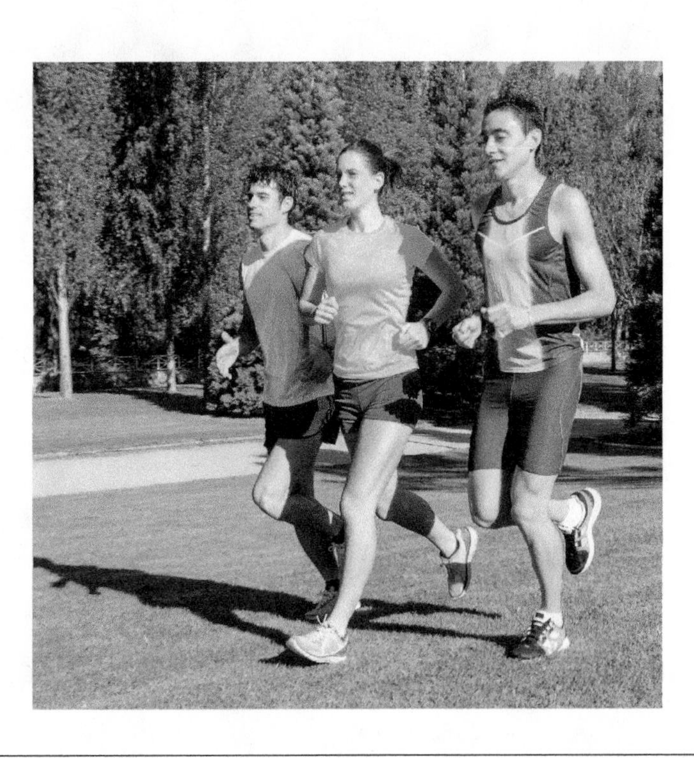

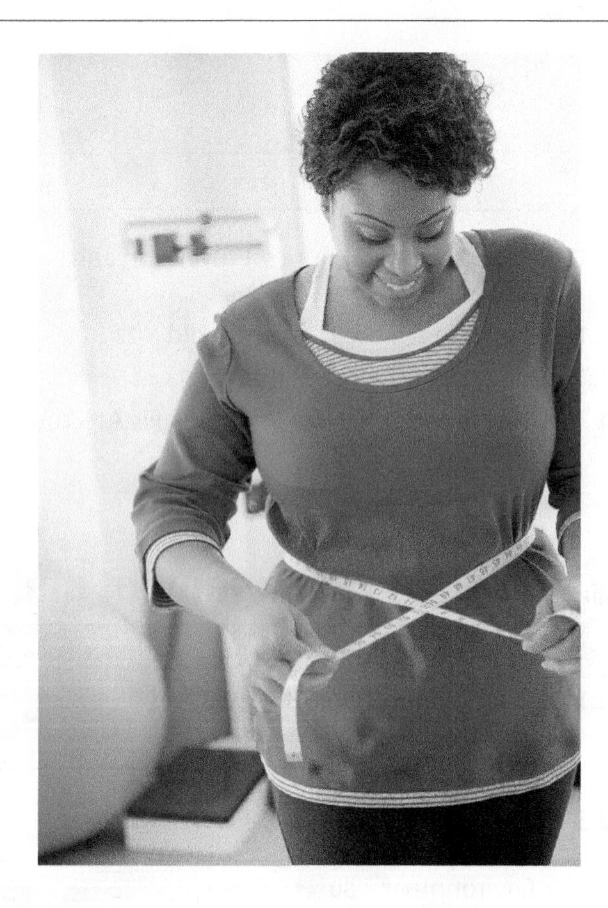

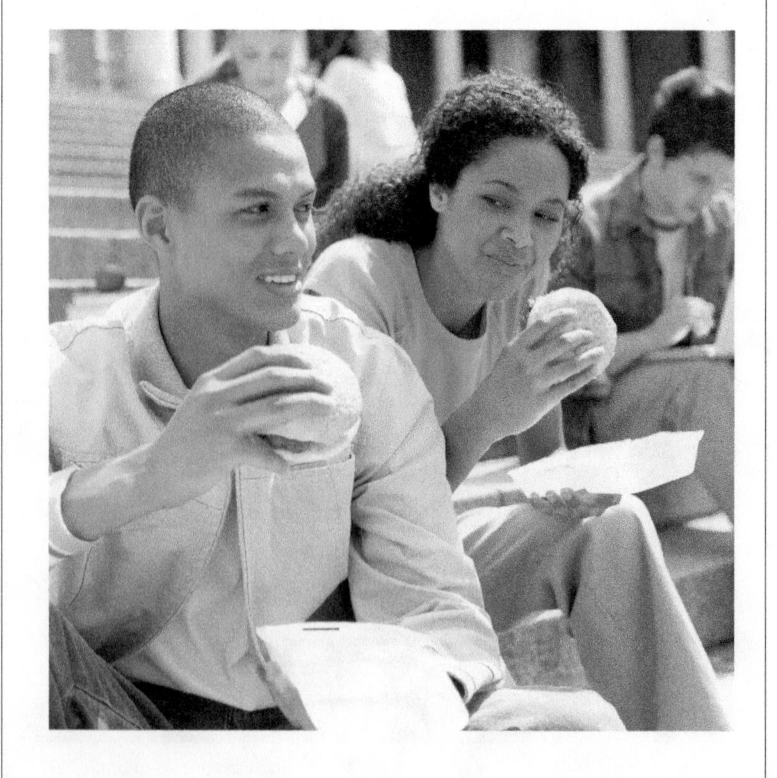

4 Stress 81

5 CVD, Cancer, and Diabetes 103

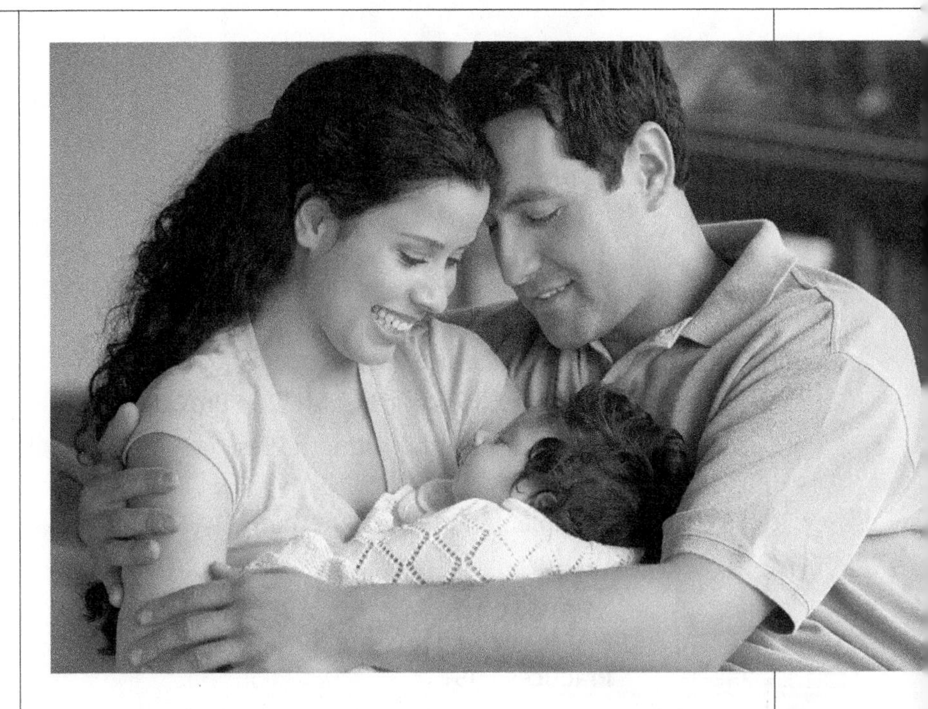

6 Consumerism and Complementary and Alternative Medicine 141

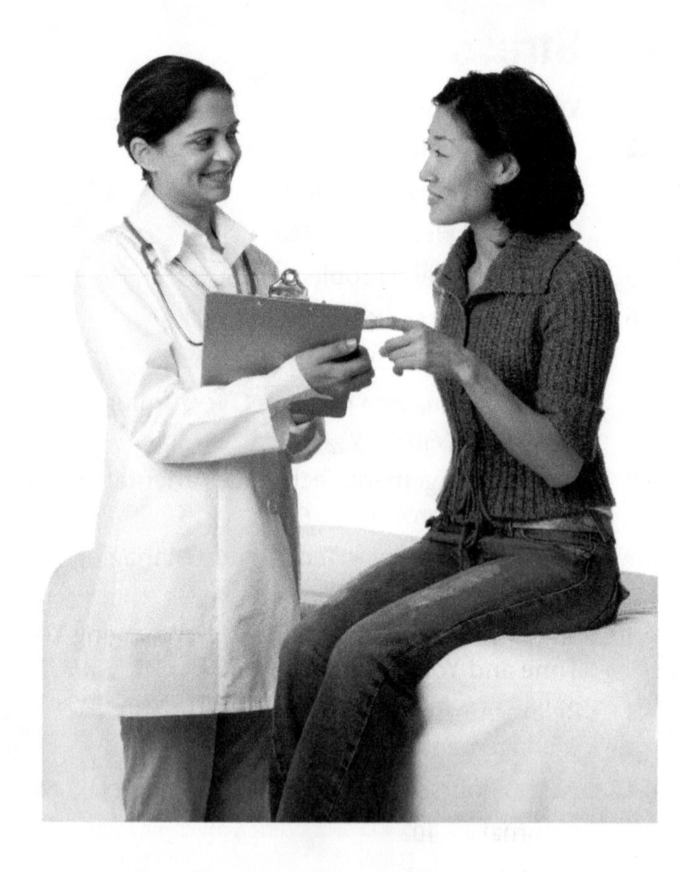

Preface

For students today, health is headline news. Whether it's the latest cases of life-threatening *E. coli* infections from eating infected produce, a deadly Ebola epidemic threatening to kill millions, a new environmental catastrophe brought on by global warming, or increasing rates of obesity and diabetes, the issues often seem overwhelming. However, although many things that influence our health are beyond our control, we are lucky that we do have control over many of the health risks we face. Health is multifaceted, and achieving it is a personal and societal responsibility.

As I have taught personal health courses over the past two decades, I have seen changes in students, especially regarding their health, their health concerns, and the way they assimilate information and make decisions about their health and the health of those around them. A new mode of instruction and a new approach to learning is required for instructors and textbook authors to present and relay scientifically valid information, create learning environments that meet diverse needs, and motivate students to engage in their own learning experiences. Students today want their information to be organized and concise. They want to know what they should be learning, see the relevance in knowing the information so that they can apply it to real world situations, and be able to test themselves to confirm that they understand the material. What's more, students and their instructors want to be able to demonstrate that they know more about their health, see things with a more critical eye, and have options for making changes to improve their health and the health of others as a result of a particular course or course sequence. When they want to delve more deeply into a given topic, they will have the skills and resources to get more information. For these reasons and more, I decided that the time had come to bring to fruition a new textbook that would change the health text marketplace. I decided to tap the creative minds of my colleagues and students and work with a great publishing company in writing *My Health: The MasteringHealth Edition*.

Key Features of This Text

My Health: The MasteringHealth Edition maintains many features that this text is known for, including the following:

- **The modular organization,** which presents information in one- and two-page spreads, helping students to pace their learning and highlighting the most essential, up-to-date information about each topic in a synthesized, easy-to-understand format.
- **Student learning outcomes,** which give instructors and students a measurable goal for each module and are matched specifically to the content in each module in the text. These take the guesswork out of the question that students inevitably ask: "What do I need to know for this exam or this performance outcome?"
- **Check Yourself questions** to help students confirm that they have mastered the content of each module.
- **Assess Yourself modules,** which provide opportunities for students to assess their current behaviors, with at least one Assess Yourself at the end of every chapter.
- **Skills for Behavior Change boxes,** which are featured in many modules and are designed to help students develop the skills necessary to use what they have learned in making practical and important improvements in their health behaviors.
- **Striking figures and photos** on every page to engage students and encourage learning.
- **A streamlined approach,** with feature-box material integrated into the text so that students can follow the narrative without interruptions, quickly navigate through the material, and apply what they have learned.

Student learning outcomes are a critical part of this book. Learning outcomes are a powerful tool to set clear expectations for students and to assess their level of mastery of a subject area. Outcomes for this text were developed based on foundational personal health content appropriate for college level learners. These outcomes were then revised and edited based on careful review and input from health instructors and other experts from representative colleges and universities throughout the country (their names are listed later in the Acknowledgments section). Each module has a specific outcome that students must try to achieve to be successful. This mastery approach helps students hone in on the relevant information and focus attention on achieving this learning outcome.

At the end of each module, students are challenged by Check Yourself questions. If students can successfully answer these questions, then they are ready to move on to the next module. If they have difficulty answering the questions, they are able to go back through the material and focus on key points until they have mastered the module content.

We know that students are often pressed for time and may only be able to read through a few pages of this book in one sitting. With the learning outcomes and the Check Yourself questions, students can learn the material in one or two modules, test themselves, and know that they have accomplished a measurable portion of their reading goal, even if they can only complete part of a reading assignment.

In addition to the modular organization, learning outcomes, and Check Yourself questions, you will notice Skills for Behavior Change boxes throughout the chapters. Using the skills learned from these boxes, students can engage in behaviors that will contribute to improved health. You will also see that these are the only feature boxes in the text. In order to keep the book streamlined and focused on essential points, the type of information that traditionally has been relegated to a feature box has been included in the text, if it is important for student understanding, or it has been omitted. I hope that you will agree that this provides students with a clear, concise presentation of the most important health information.

New to This Edition

Video Tutors

Video tutors highlight a book figure in an engaging video, covering key concepts such as how drugs act on the brain, reading food labels, and the benefits of regular exercise. Using a QR code reader, students can easily access the Video Tutors on their mobile device—just scan the code and the Video Tutor loads instantly.

Study Plan

Each module now has a numbered Learning Outcome, giving students a road map for their reading. Each chapter concludes with a Study Plan, which summarizes key points of the chapter and provides review questions to check understanding, both tied to the chapter's learning outcomes.

Chapter-by-Chapter Revisions

My Health: The MasteringHealth Edition has been thoroughly updated to reflect the most cutting-edge, scientifically valid, and relevant information available and includes additional references that will allow students to glean additional information from key sources in the area. Portions of modules have been reorganized to improve the flow of topics, while figures, tables, and photos have all been added, improved on, and updated. The following is a chapter-by-chapter listing of some of the most noteworthy changes, updates, and additions.

Chapter 1: Fitness

- Expanded coverage of SMART fitness goals and objectives
- New coverage of physical inactivity
- New coverage of alcohol and exercise

Chapter 2: Weight Management and Body Image

- New Skills for Behavior Change box on portion distortion
- New figure showing an overview of methods to measure body composition
- Expanded coverage of treatment of anorexia and bulimia
- New table on popular diet programs

Chapter 3: Nutrition

- New module on the health benefits of functional foods
- New content on the Dietary Reference Intakes (DRIs)

Chapter 4: Stress

- Increased coverage of mindfulness
- New section on happiness and flourishing
- New section named "Men and Women Respond to Stress Differently"
- New section on shift and persist

Chapter 5: CVD, Cancer, and Diabetes

- New table on the signs of a heart attack in men and women
- New Skills for Behavior Change box on recognizing the signs of a stroke
- Increased coverage on diabetes prevalence rates and risks
- New Skills for Behavior Change box on reducing your risk for diabetes
- New module on diabetes diagnosis and treatment

Chapter 6: Consumerism and Complementary and Alternative Medicine

- New table on common nonherbal supplements
- New figure on where our health care dollars are spent

Supplementary Materials

Available with *My Health: The MasteringHealth Edition* is a comprehensive set of ancillary materials designed to enhance learning and to facilitate teaching.

Instructor Supplements

- **MasteringHealth.** MasteringHealth coaches students through the toughest health topics. Instructors can assign engaging tools to help students visualize, practice, and understand crucial content, from the basics of health to the fundamentals of behavior change. **Coaching Activities** guide students through key health concepts with interactive mini-lessons, complete with hints and wrong-answer feedback. **Reading Quizzes** (20 questions per chapter) ensure students have completed the assigned reading before class. ***ABC News* Videos** stimulate classroom discussions and include multiple-choice questions with feedback for students. **NutriTools Coaching Activities** in the nutrition chapter allow students to combine and experiment with different food options and learn firsthand how to build healthier meals. **MP3s** relate to chapter content and come with multiple-choice questions that provide wrong-answer feedback. **Learning Catalytics** provides open-ended questions students can answer in real time. Through targeted assessments, Learning Catalytics helps students develop the critical-thinking skills they need for lasting behavior change.
- **Teaching Toolkit DVD.** The Teaching Toolkit DVD includes everything instructors need to prepare for their course and deliver a dynamic lecture in one convenient place. Resources include the following: *ABC News* videos, Video Tutor videos, clicker questions, Quiz Show questions, PowerPoint lecture outlines, all figures and tables from the text, PDFs and Microsoft Word files of the *Instructor Resource and Support Manual* and the Test Bank, the Computerized Test Bank, the User's Quick Guide, *Teaching with Student Learning Outcomes, Teaching with Web 2.0, Behavior Change Log Book and Wellness Journal, Eat Right!, Live Right!*, and *Take Charge of Your Health* worksheets.
- ***ABC News* Videos** and **Video Tutors.** Fifty-one new *ABC News* videos, each 5 to 10 minutes long, and 22 brand-new brief videos accessible via QR codes in the text help instructors stimulate critical discussion in the classroom. Videos are provided already linked within PowerPoint lectures and are also available separately in large-screen format with optional closed captioning on the Teaching Toolkit DVD and through MasteringHealth.

- ***Instructor Resource and Support Manual.*** This teaching tool provides chapter summaries and outlines of each chapter. It includes information on available PowerPoint lectures, integrated *ABC News* video discussion questions, tips and strategies for managing large classrooms, ideas for in-class activities, and suggestions for integrating MasteringHealth and MyDietAnalysis into your classroom activities and homework assignments.
- **Test Bank.** The Test Bank incorporates Bloom's Taxonomy, or the higher order of learning, to help instructors create exams that encourage students to think analytically and critically, rather than simply to regurgitate information. Test Bank questions are tagged to global and book-specific student learning outcomes.
- **User's Quick Guide.** Newly redesigned to be even more useful, this valuable supplement acts as your road map to the Teaching Toolkit DVD.
- ***Teaching with Student Learning Outcomes.*** This publication contains essays from 11 instructors who are teaching using student learning outcomes. They share their goals in using outcomes and the processes that they follow to develop and refine them, and they provide many useful suggestions and examples for successfully incorporating outcomes into a personal health course.
- ***Teaching with Web 2.0.*** From Facebook to Twitter to blogs, students are using and interacting with Web 2.0 technologies. This handbook provides an introduction to these popular online tools and offers ideas for incorporating them into your personal health course. Written by personal health and health education instructors, each chapter examines the basics about each technology and ways to make it work for you and your students.
- ***Behavior Change Log Book and Wellness Journal.*** This assessment tool helps students track daily exercise and nutritional intake and create a long-term nutritional and fitness prescription plan. It also includes a Behavior Change Contract and topics for journal-based activities.

Student Supplements

- **The Study Area of MasteringHealth** is organized by learning areas. *Read It* houses the Pearson eText 2.0, with which users can create notes, highlight text in different colors, create bookmarks, zoom, click hyperlinked words for definitions, and change page view. Pearson eText 2.0 also links to associated media files. *See It* includes 51 *ABC News* videos on important health topics and the key concepts of each chapter. *Hear It* contains MP3 Study Tutor files and audio case studies. *Do It* contains critical-thinking questions and Web links. *Review It* contains study quizzes for each chapter. *Live It* helps jump-start students' behavior-change projects with assessments and resources to plan change; students can fill out a Behavior Change Contract, journal and log behaviors, and prepare a reflection piece.
- ***Behavior Change Log Book and Wellness Journal.*** This assessment tool helps students track daily exercise and nutritional intake and create a long-term nutrition and fitness prescription plan. It includes Behavior Change Contracts and topics for journal-based activities.
- ***Eat Right! Healthy Eating in College and Beyond.*** This booklet provides students with practical nutrition guidelines, shopper's guides, and recipes.
- ***Live Right! Beating Stress in College and Beyond.*** This booklet gives students useful tips for coping with stressful life challenges both during college and for the rest of their lives.
- **Digital 5-Step Pedometer** Take strides to better health with this pedometer, which measures steps, distance (miles), activity time, and calories, and provides a time clock.
- **MyDietAnalysis** (www.mydietanalysis.com). Powered by ESHA Research, Inc., MyDietAnalysis features a database of nearly 20,000 foods and multiple reports. It allows students to track their diet and activity using up to three profiles and to generate and submit reports electronically.

Flexible Options

My Health: The MasteringHealth Edition is also available in alternate print and electronic versions:

- **CourseSmart eTextbooks** are an exciting new choice for students looking to save money. As an alternative to purchasing the print textbook, students can subscribe to the same content online and save 40% off the suggested list price of the print text. Access the CourseSmart eText at www.coursesmart.com.
- **Books a la Carte** offers the exact same content as *My Health: The MasteringHealth Edition* in a convenient, three-hole-punched, loose-leaf version. Books a la Carte offers a great value for your students—this format costs 35% less than a new textbook!
- Creating a customized version of the book from the **Pearson Custom Library**, with only the chapters that you select, is also possible. Contact your Pearson sales representative for more details.

A Note on the Text

From my earliest years of college instruction, I have believed that in order to motivate students to focus on their health, they needed to understand the complex health world that people live in, to appreciate how the macroenvironment and culture influence health decision making, and to understand that there is no "best" recipe for health. Helping students access the best information available and motivating them to ask the right questions and be thoughtful in their analysis of issues, as well as mindful in their approach to healthy change, has been a part of my overall approach to teaching, learning, and writing.

Today's students have been raised on a steady dose of health information, some of which sounds good, but may be highly questionable in terms of accuracy. Helping them sift through the changing sands of health information, examine their own risks, and make positive changes that affect them, their loved ones, and others in the community is key to improving health. Writing a text such as this one has helped keep me current in my teaching and tuned in to the needs of twenty-first-century students and those who teach classes such as this one. This text, focused on a more technology-based, interactive, and challenging approach to learning, cuts to the chase in delivering essential information and thought-provoking questions. Consistent with an ever-evolving and "information at your fingertips" approach, this format is designed to help students navigate the seemingly endless world of health and bring it to life in a colorful and fresh format. In keeping with the times, this text is a "work in continual progress," and it will benefit greatly from your feedback and suggestions. As an author, I'd love to hear from you!

Acknowledgments

Writing and developing a textbook is truly a team effort. Each step along the way in planning, developing, and translating critical health information to students and instructors requires a tremendous amount of work from many dedicated professionals, including contributors who are at the top of their games in their knowledge of health science and behaviors and publishing professionals who personify all that is the absolute "best" in terms of qualities an author looks for in bringing a text to fruition. I cannot help but think how fortunate I have been to work with the gifted contributors to this text and the extraordinary publishing professionals at Pearson. Through time constraints, exhaustive searches for cutting-edge background research, and the writing process, these contributors were outstanding.

From painstaking efforts in development, design, editing, and editorial decision making to highly skilled marketing and dedicated sales efforts, the Pearson group handled every detail, every obstacle with patience, professionalism, and painstaking attention to detail. From this author's perspective, these personnel personify key aspects of what it takes to be successful in the publishing world: (1) drive and motivation; (2) commitment to excellence; (3) fantastic job and performance skills; (4) a vibrant, youthful, forward-thinking and enthusiastic approach; and (5) personalities that motivate an author to continually strive to produce market-leading texts. I have been amazed at the way that this team continually works to be well ahead of the curve in terms of cutting-edge information. Asking "what do students need to know" and "what will help instructors and students thrive in today's high-pressure academic settings" was at the heart of our efforts. I am deeply indebted to everyone who has played a role in making this book come alive for students and get into the hands of instructors.

In particular, credit goes to my development editor for this edition, Erin Schnair, who worked with Susan Malloy and Jessica Picone in painstakingly merging and synthesizing content and provided additional insight and expertise in making this new edition accessible to students. Erin did an extraordinary job of streamlining and revising material to fit within the constraints of the modular outline, while retaining accuracy and readability. Without her, this book would not exist—thank you!

Further praise and thanks go to the highly skilled and hardworking executive editor Sandra Lindelof, who was responsible for the conceptualization of this text and helped spearhead its initial development in the marketplace, doing the necessary work to procure the cutting-edge technology and skilled professionals that were key to its success. Her successor, Michelle Cadden, quickly took charge of the list after Sandy's departure and worked closely with Susan and Jessica to ensure that this text provided the necessary framework to meet the needs of an increasingly demanding group of instructors and students.

Although these women were key contributors to the finished work, there were many other people who worked on *My Health: The MasteringHealth Edition*. Thanks go to Angela Urquhart and Andrea Archer at Thistle Hill Publishing Services, who reliably kept us on track with flexibility and dedication. Design director Mark Ong refreshed the visually impactful design while keeping students and instructors in mind. We could not have created this book without his creativity and dedication. Mark also created the remarkable cover, which we feel perfectly conveys the unique qualities of the text. Denise Wright of Southern Editorial gets major kudos for overseeing the supplements package. Director of Media Development Laura Tommasi put together an innovative and comprehensive set of assets for *My Health: The MasteringHealth Edition*. Additional thanks go to the rest of the team at Pearson, especially Editorial Assistant Leah Sherwood, Program Manager Team Lead Mike Early, Project Manager Team Lead Nancy Tabor, and Director of Development Barbara Yien.

The editorial and production teams are critical to a book's success, but I would be remiss without thanking another key group who ultimately help determine a book's success: the textbook sales group and Executive Marketing Manager Neena Bali. With Neena's support, the Pearson sales representatives traverse the country, promoting the book, making sure that instructors know how it compares to the competition, and providing support to customers. From directing an outstanding marketing campaign to the everyday tasks of being responsive to instructor needs, Neena does a superb job of making sure that *My Health* gets into instructors' hands and that adopters receive the service they deserve. In keeping with my overall experiences with Pearson, the marketing and sales staff is among the best of the best. I am very lucky to have them working with me on this project and want to extend a special thanks to all of them!

This book was developed in part from material from my other textbooks, *Access to Health* and *Health: The Basics*. I would like to thank the contributors to those books, particularly Dr. Patricia Ketcham (Oregon State University and immediate past president of the American College Health Association); Dr. Susan Dobie, associate professor in the School of Health, Physical Education, and Leisure Services at the University of Northern Iowa; Dr. Kathy Munoz, professor in the Department of Kinesiology and Recreation Administration at Humboldt State University; Dr. Erica Jackson, associate professor in the Department of Public and Allied Health Sciences at Delaware State University; Dr. Karen Elliot, senior instructor in the Health Promotion and Health Behavior Program at Oregon State University; and Laura Bonazzoli, who has been instrumental in writing key Focus On chapters and updating material and content for several editions of these texts. A special thanks to Niloofar Bavarian (Oregon State University), who drafted the original student learning outcomes on which the book is based.

Thanks also to the talented people who contributed to the supplements package: Denise and her team at Southern Editorial who updated the *Instructor Resource and Support Manual*; Brent

Goff, who updated the Test Bank; and Melanie Healey (University of Washington-La Crosse), who updated the PowerPoint lecture slides and PowerPoint quiz show slides.

Reviewers

This book is the result of not only my efforts, but also the invaluable contributions of the many reviewers. From the initial idea to the fine-tuning of each and every learning outcome, the thoughtful comments from reviewers shaped this book in many ways. I am extremely grateful for your feedback.

I am forever grateful to all of those who contributed in large and small ways to the success of this text. It really does take a village to make things happen, and this village was extraordinary!

Rebecca J. Donatelle, PhD

Second Edition Reviewers

Debbie Allison
Guilford Technical Community College

Nicole Clark
Indiana University of Pennsylvania

Henry Counts
University of South Carolina

Teresa Dolan
Lincoln University

Kathy Finley
Indiana University Bloomington

Ari Fisher
Louisiana State University

Chris Isenbarth
Weber State University

Ellen Larson
Northern Arizona University

Cynthia Smith
Central Piedmont Community College

MasteringHealth Faculty Advisor Board Reviewers

Kris Jankovitz
California Polytechnic State University

Stasi Kasianchuk
Oregon State University

Lynn Long
University of North Carolina at Wilmington

Ayanna Lyles
California University of Pennsylvania

Steven Namanny
Utah Valley University

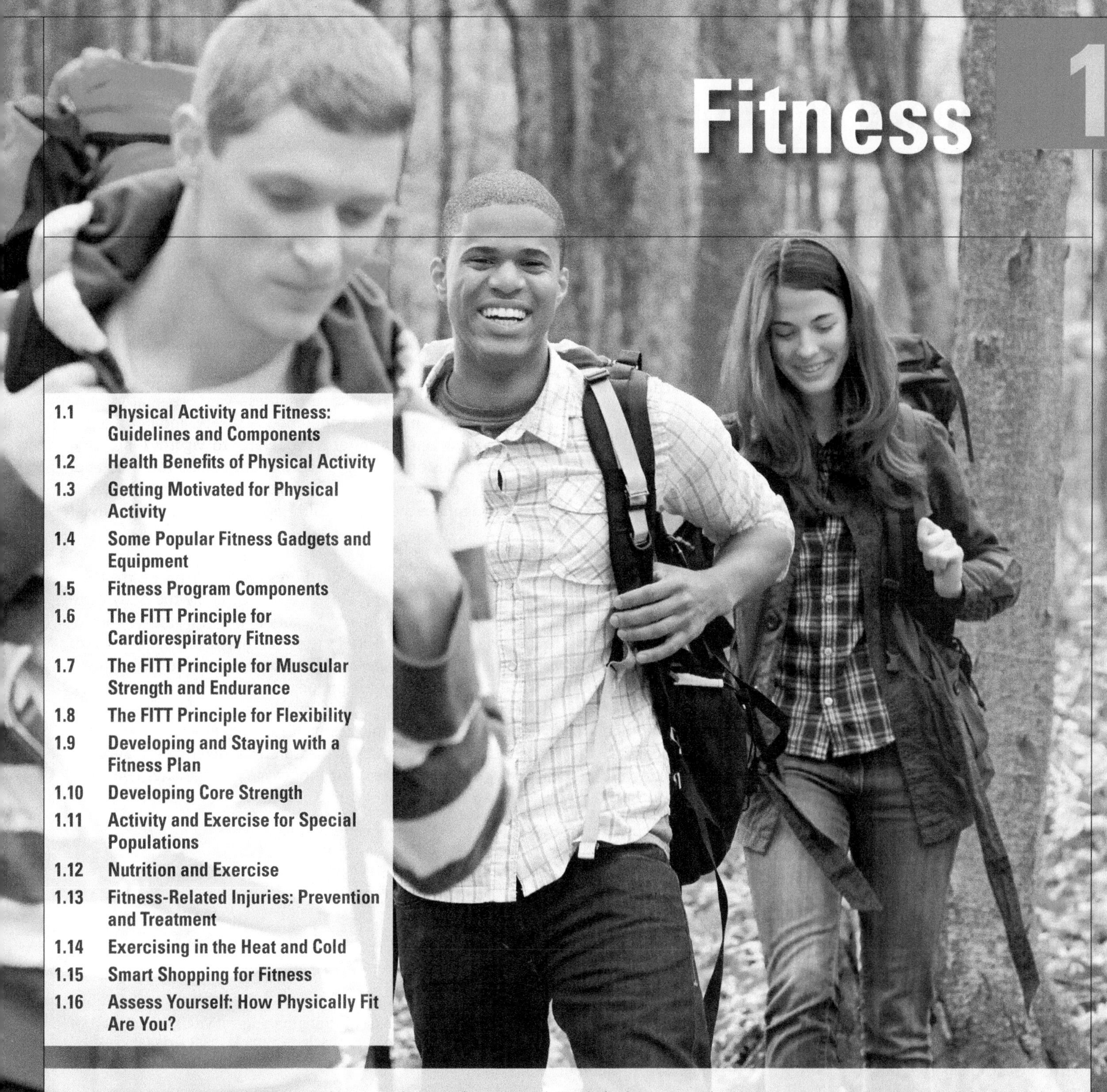

Fitness 1

Most Americans are aware of the wide range of physical, social, and mental health benefits of physical activity—and that they should be more physically active. Physiological changes resulting from regular physical activity reduce the likelihood of coronary artery disease, high blood pressure, type 2 diabetes, obesity, and other chronic diseases. Engaging in physical activity regularly also helps to control stress and increase self-esteem.

Despite these benefits, however, 23.1 percent of American adults engage in no leisure-time physical activity[1]—a situation linked to current high incidences of obesity, type 2 diabetes, and other chronic and mental health diseases.[2]

In general, college students are more physically active than are older adults, but a recent survey indicated that 56 percent of college women and 49.3 percent of college men do not meet recommended guidelines for engaging in moderate or vigorous physical activities.[3]

College is a great time to develop attitudes and behaviors that can increase the quality and quantity of your life. This chapter offers knowledge and strategies to help you get moving.

1.1

Physical Activity and Fitness: Guidelines and Components

learning outcome

1.1 Distinguish among physical activity for health, for fitness, and for performance.

Physical activity is any body movement that works your muscles, uses more energy than when resting, and enhances health.[4] Physical activities can vary by intensity. For example, walking to class on flat ground typically requires little effort, while walking to class uphill is more intense and harder to do. The three general categories of physical activity are defined by their purpose: physical activity for health, physical activity for physical fitness, and physical activity for performance.

Exercise is defined as planned, structured, and repetitive bodily movement done to improve or maintain one or more components of physical fitness, such as cardiorespiratory endurance, muscular strength or endurance, or flexibility. Although all exercise is physical activity, not all physical activity would be considered exercise. For example, walking from your car to class is physical activity, whereas going for a brisk 30-minute walk is considered exercise.

Physical Activity for Health

Researchers have found that "there is irrefutable evidence of the effectiveness of regular physical activity in the primary and secondary prevention of several chronic diseases (e.g., cardiovascular disease, diabetes, cancer, hypertension, obesity, depression, and osteoporosis)."[5] Adding more physical activity to your day can benefit your health. In fact, if the number of adults meeting the 2008 Physical Activity Guidelines (Table 1.1) increased by 25 percent, there would be 1.3 million fewer deaths per year and the life expectancy would increase. In the United States, physical inactivity is responsible for 6.7 percent of the cases of coronary heart disease, 8.3 percent cases of type 2 diabetes, 12.4 percent cases of breast cancer, and 12.0 percent cases of colon cancer, and it accounts for approximately 10.8 percent of deaths.[6]

Physical Activity for Fitness

Physical fitness refers to a set of health- and performance-related attributes. The health-related attributes—cardiorespiratory fitness, muscular strength and endurance, flexibility, and body composition—allow one to perform moderate- to vigorous-intensity physical activities on a regular basis without getting too tired and with energy left over to handle physical or mental emergencies. Figure 1.1 identifies the major health-related components of physical fitness.

Cardiorespiratory Fitness **Cardiorespiratory fitness** is the ability of the heart, lungs, and blood vessels to supply the body with oxygen efficiently. The primary category of physical activity known to improve cardiorespiratory fitness is **aerobic exercise**. The word *aerobic* means "with oxygen" and describes any exercise that requires oxygen to make energy for prolonged activity. Aerobic activities such as swimming, cycling, and jogging are among the best exercises for improving or maintaining cardiorespiratory fitness.

Cardiorespiratory fitness is measured by determining **aerobic capacity** (or **power**), the volume of oxygen the muscles consume during exercise. Maximal aerobic power (VO_{2max}) is defined as the

TABLE 1.1 **Physical Activity Guidelines for Americans**

Key Guidelines for Health*	For Additional Fitness or Weight Loss Benefits*	PLUS
150 min/week moderate intensity OR 75 min/week of vigorous intensity OR Equivalent combination of moderate and vigorous intensity (i.e., 100 min moderate intensity + 25 min vigorous intensity)	300 min/week moderate intensity OR 150 min/week of vigorous intensity OR Equivalent combination of moderate and vigorous intensity (i.e., 200 min moderate intensity + 50 min vigorous intensity) OR More than the previously described amounts	Muscle strengthening activities for *all* the major muscle groups at least 2 days/week

*Accumulate this physical activity in sessions of 10 minutes or more at one time.
Source: Office of Disease Prevention and Health Promotion, U.S. Department of Health and Human Services, *2008 Physical Activity Guidelines for Americans: Be Active, Healthy, and Happy!* ODPHP Publication no. U0036 (Washington, DC: U.S. Department of Health and Human Services, 2008), available at www.health.gov.

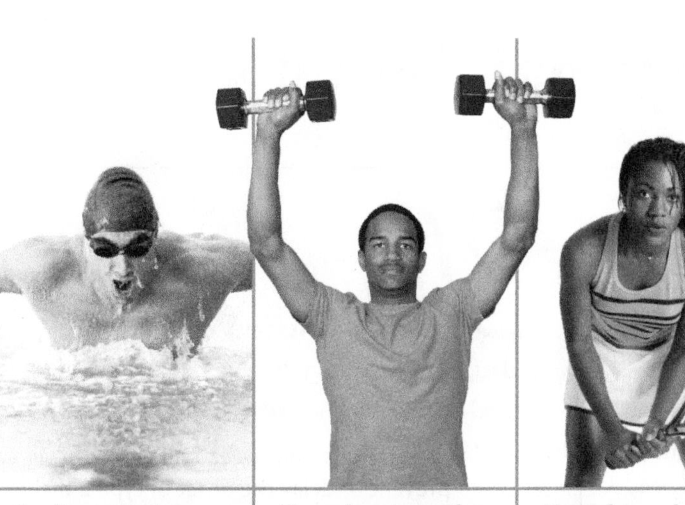
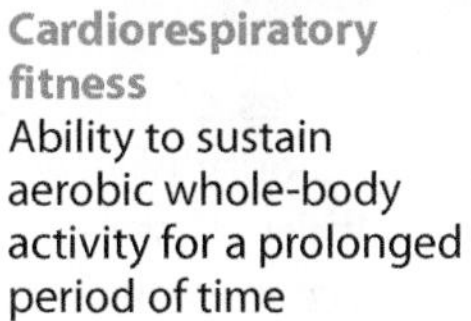
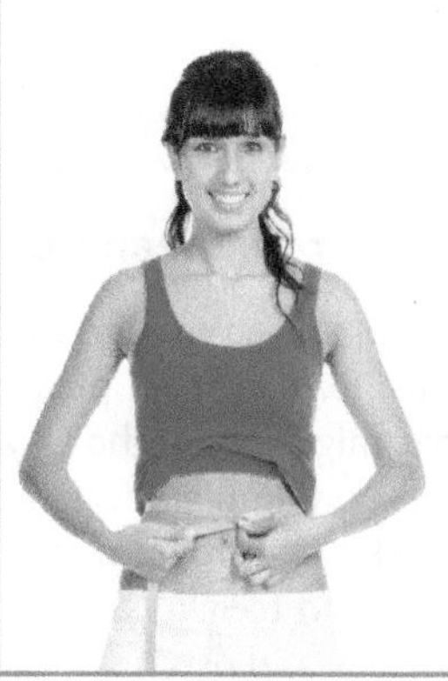

Figure 1.1 Components of Physical Fitness

maximal volume of oxygen that the muscles consume during exercise. The most common measure of maximal aerobic capacity is a walk or run test on a treadmill. For greatest accuracy, this is done in a lab and requires special equipment and technicians to measure the precise amount of oxygen entering and exiting the body during the exercise session. Submaximal tests can be used to get a more general sense of cardiorespiratory fitness; one such test, the 1-mile walk test, is described in the Assess Yourself module at the end of this chapter.

Muscular Strength **Muscular strength** refers to the amount of force a muscle or group of muscles is capable of exerting in one contraction. A common way to assess the strength of a particular muscle group is to measure the maximum amount of weight you can move one time (and no more), or your one repetition maximum (1 RM).

Muscular Endurance **Muscular endurance** is the ability of a muscle or group of muscles to exert force repeatedly without fatigue or the ability to sustain a muscular contraction. The more repetitions of an endurance activity (e.g., push-ups) you can perform successfully, or the longer you can hold a certain position (e.g., wall sit), the greater your muscular endurance. General muscular endurance is often measured using the number of curl-ups an individual can do; this test is described in the Assess Yourself module at the end of this chapter.

Flexibility **Flexibility** refers to the range of motion, or the amount of movement possible, at a particular joint or series of joints: the greater the range of motion, the greater the flexibility. One of the most common measures of general flexibility is the sit-and-reach test, described in the Assess Yourself module at the end of this chapter.

Body Composition **Body composition**, the fifth and final component of a comprehensive fitness program, describes the relative proportions and distribution of fat and lean (muscle, bone, water, organs) tissues in the body.

Physical Activity for Performance

Physical fitness for athletes involves attributes that improve their ability to perform athletic tasks. These attributes can also help general exercisers increase fitness levels and their ability to perform daily tasks. These skill-related components of physical fitness (also called sports skills) are the following: *agility, balance, coordination, power, speed,* and *reaction time*. Participating regularly in any sport or activity can improve your sport skills, as can performing drills that mimic a sport-specific skill.

check yourself

- **What are the differences between physical activity for health, for fitness, and for performance?**
- **What is the difference between exercise and physical activity?**
- **What are the core components of physical fitness?**

1.2 Health Benefits of Physical Activity

learning outcome

1.2 List the health benefits of physical activity.

The first step in starting a physical fitness program is identifying your goals for that program. You should next consider the things that might get in the way of your achieving those goals. Once you have contemplated these factors, you are ready to create an individual exercise program to meet your physical fitness goals. Before we start, and to help you get motivated, let's take a look at the many physical and psychological benefits of physical activity.

What Are the Health Benefits of Regular Physical Activity?

Regular participation in physical activity improves more than 50 different physiological, metabolic, and psychological aspects of human life. Figure 1.2 summarizes some of these major health-related benefits.

Reduced Risk of Cardiovascular Diseases Aerobic exercise is good for the heart and lungs and reduces risk for heart-related diseases. It improves blood flow and eases performance of everyday tasks. Regular exercise makes the cardiovascular and respiratory systems more efficient by strengthening the heart muscle, enabling more blood to be pumped with each stroke, and increasing the number of *capillaries* (small blood vessels that allow gas exchange between blood and surrounding tissues) in trained skeletal muscles, which supply more blood to working muscles. Exercise also improves the respiratory system by increasing the amount of oxygen inhaled and distributed to body tissues.[7]

Regular physical activity can reduce hypertension, or chronic high blood pressure—a form of cardiovascular disease and a significant risk factor for coronary heart disease and stroke.[8] Regular aerobic exercise also reduces low-density lipoproteins (LDLs, or "bad" cholesterol), total cholesterol, and triglycerides (a blood fat), thus reducing plaque buildup in the arteries while increasing high-density lipoproteins (HDLs, or "good" cholesterol), which are associated with lower risk for coronary artery disease.[9]

Reduced Risk of Metabolic Syndrome and Type 2 Diabetes Regular physical activity reduces the risk of metabolic syndrome, a combination of heart disease and diabetes risk factors that produces a synergistic increase in risk.[10] Specifically, metabolic syndrome includes high blood pressure, abdominal obesity, low levels of HDLs, high levels of triglycerides, and impaired glucose tolerance.[11] Regular participation in moderate-intensity physical activities reduces risk for these factors both individually and collectively.[12]

Research indicates that a healthy dietary intake combined with sufficient physical activity could prevent many current cases of type 2 diabetes.[13] In a major national clinical trial, researchers found that exercising 150 minutes per week and eating fewer calories and less fat could prevent or delay the onset of type 2 diabetes.[14]

30 minutes of physical activity a day—all at once or in three 10-minute sessions—provides health benefits.

Reduced Cancer Risk After decades of research, most cancer epidemiologists believe that the majority of cancers are preventable and can be avoided by healthier lifestyle and environmental choices.[15] In fact, a report recently released by the World Cancer Research Fund in conjunction with the American Institute for Cancer Research stated that one-third of cancers could be prevented by being physically active and eating well.[16]

Regular physical activity appears to lower the risk for some specific types of cancer, particularly colon and rectal cancer.[17] Regular exercise is also associated with lower risk for breast cancer. Research on exercise and breast cancer risk has found that the earlier in life a woman starts to exercise, the lower her breast cancer risk.[18]

Improved Bone Mass and Reduced Risk of Osteoporosis A common affliction for older people is *osteoporosis,* a disease characterized by low bone mass and deterioration of bone tissue, which increases fracture risk. Regular weight-bearing and strength-building physical activities are recommended to maintain bone health and prevent osteoporotic fractures. Although both men and women can be affected by osteoporosis, it is more common in women. Women (like men) have much to gain by remaining physically active as they age—bone mass levels are significantly higher among active individuals than among sedentary persons.[19] However, it appears that the full bone-related benefits of physical activity can be achieved only with sufficient hormone levels (estrogen in women; testosterone in men) and adequate calcium, vitamin D, and total caloric intakes.[20]

Improved Weight Control For many people, the desire to lose weight or maintain a healthy weight is the main reason for physical activity. Physical activity requires your body to generate energy through calorie expenditure; if calories expended exceed calories consumed over a span of time, the net result will be weight loss.

Physical activity also increases metabolic rate, keeping it elevated for several hours following vigorous physical activities. This increase in metabolic rate can lead to body composition changes that favor weight management. Increased physical activity also improves your chances of maintaining weight loss. If you are currently at a healthy body weight, regular physical activity can prevent significant weight gain.[21]

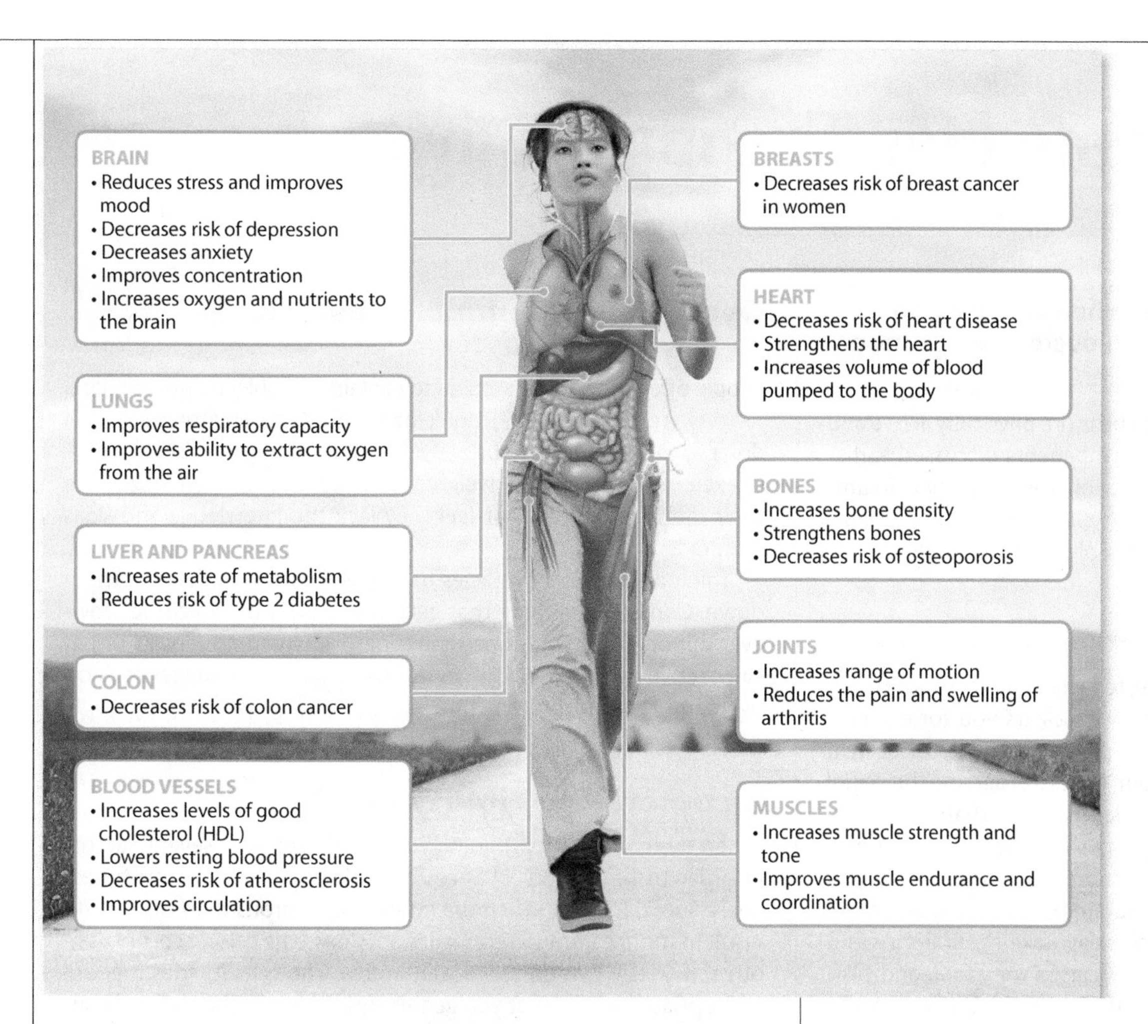

Figure 1.2 Some Health Benefits of Regular Exercise

VIDEO TUTOR
Health Benefits of Regular Exercise

Improved Immunity Research shows that regular moderate-intensity physical activity reduces individual susceptibility to disease.[22] Just how physical activity alters immunity is not well understood. We do know that moderate-intensity physical activity temporarily increases the number of white blood cells (WBCs), which are responsible for fighting infection.[23] Often the relationship of physical activity to immunity, or more specifically to disease susceptibility, is described as a J-shaped curve. In other words, susceptibility to disease decreases with moderate activity, but then increases as you move to more extreme levels of physical activity or exercise or if you continue to exercise without adequate recovery time.[24] Athletes engaging in marathon-type events or very intense physical training programs have been shown to be at greater risk for upper respiratory tract infections (colds and flu).[25]

Improved Back Strength Regular whole-body exercise, as well as exercises targeting the specific muscles of the back (and the rest of the core), create a strong platform for the entire body. A strong and healthy back helps you maintain proper posture and avoid posture-related stress in the neck, shoulders, hips, knees, and ankles. It also gives you a good foundation for a range of exercise and reduces the likelihood of injury.

Improved Mental Health and Stress Management Most people who engage in regular physical activity are likely to notice the psychological benefits, such as feeling better about oneself and an overall sense of well-being. Although these mental health benefits are difficult to quantify, they are frequently mentioned as reasons for continuing to be physically active.

Physical activity contributes to mental health in several ways. Learning new skills, developing increased ability and capacity in recreational activities, and sticking with a physical activity plan all improve self-esteem. In addition, regular physical activity can improve a person's physical appearance, further increasing self-esteem.

Regular aerobic activity can improve the way the body handles stress through its effect on neurotransmitters associated with mood enhancement. Physical activity might also help the body recover from the stress response more quickly as fitness increases.[26]

Increasing evidence suggests that regular physical activity improves cognitive function across the life span. Research has associated regular activity with improved academic and standardized test performance in school.[27] Regular aerobic activity has also been associated with improved function in adults and with the prevention and improvement of dementia in adults.[28]

Longer Life Span Experts have long debated the relationship between physical activity and longevity. Several studies indicate significant decreases in long-term health risk and increases in years lived, particularly among those who have several risk factors and who use physical activity as a means of risk reduction. Results from a study of nearly a million participants showed that the greatest benefits from physical activity occurred in sedentary individuals who added a little physical activity to their lives, with additional benefits added as physical activity levels were increased.[29]

check yourself

- **What are five health benefits of physical activity?**

1.3 Getting Motivated for Physical Activity

learning outcome

1.3 Explain factors to consider when choosing an exercise activity and ways to overcome common obstacles to physical activity.

There are many reasons for wanting to be more physically active and physically fit, including the many health benefits discussed earlier in this text. Taking some time to reflect on your personal circumstances, goals, and desires regarding physical fitness will probably make it easier for you to come up with a plan you can stick to.

What If I Have Been Inactive for a While?

If you have been physically inactive for the past few months or longer, first make sure that your physician clears you for exercise. Consider consulting a personal trainer or fitness instructor to help you get started. In this phase of your fitness program, the *initial conditioning stage*, you may begin at levels lower than those recommended for physical fitness. Starting slowly will ease you into a workout regime with a minimum of soreness. For example, you might start your cardiorespiratory program by simply moving more and reducing your sedentary time each day. Take the stairs instead of the elevator, walk farther from your car to the store, and plan for organized movement each day, such as a 10- to 15-minute walk. In addition, you can start your muscle fitness program with simple body weight exercises, emphasizing proper technique and body alignment before adding any resistance.

Overcoming Common Obstacles to Physical Activity

People offer a variety of excuses to explain why they do not exercise, ranging from personal ("I don't have time") to environmental ("I don't have a safe place to be active"). Some people may be reluctant to exercise if they are overweight, are embarrassed to work out with their more "fit" friends, or feel they lack the knowledge and skills required.

Think about your obstacles to physical activity and write them down. Consider anything that gets in your way of exercising, however minor. Once you honestly evaluate why you are not as physically active as you want to be, review Table 1.2 for suggestions on overcoming your hurdles.

Incorporating Fitness into Your Life

When designing your program, you should consider several factors in order to boost your chances of achieving your physical fitness goals. Some activities are more intense or vigorous than others and result in more calories used; Figure 1.3 shows the caloric cost of various activities when done for 30 minutes. Choose activities that are appropriate for you, that you genuinely like doing, and that are convenient. For example, you might choose jogging because you like to run and there are beautiful trails nearby, rather than swimming, since you do not really like the water and the pool is difficult to get to. Likewise, choose activities suitable for your current fitness level. If you are overweight or obese and have not exercised in months, do not sign up for the advanced aerobics classes. Start slow, plan fun activities, and progress to more challenging activities as your physical fitness improves. You may choose to simply walk more in an attempt to achieve the recommended goal of 10,000 steps per day; keep track with a pedometer

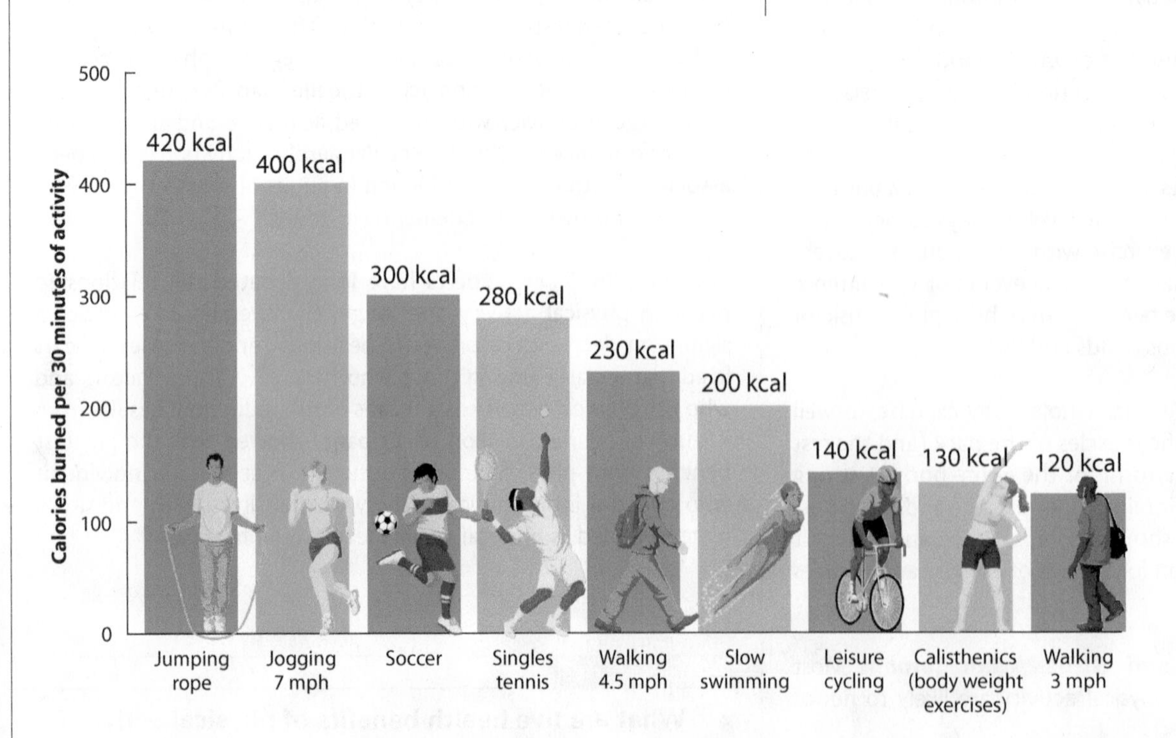

Figure 1.3 Calories Burned by Different Activities
The harder you exercise, the more energy you expend. Estimated calories burned for various moderate and vigorous activities are listed for a 30-minute bout of activity.

TABLE **1.2** **Overcoming Obstacles to Physical Activity**

Obstacle	Possible Solution
Lack of time	• Look at your schedule. Where can you find 30-minute time slots? Perhaps you need to focus on shorter times (10 minutes or more) throughout the day. • Multitask. Read while riding an exercise bike or listen to lectures or podcasts while walking. • Be physically active during your lunch and study breaks as well as between classes. Skip rope or throw a Frisbee with a friend. • Select activities that require less time, such as brisk walking or jogging. • Ride your bike to class, or park (or get off the bus) farther from your destination.
Social influence	• Invite family and friends to be active with you. • Join a class to meet new people. • Explain the importance of exercise and your commitment to physical activity to people who may not support your efforts. • Find a role model to support your efforts. • Plan for physically active dates—go dancing or bowling.
Lack of motivation, willpower, or energy	• Schedule your workout time just as you would any other important commitment. • Enlist the help of an exercise partner to make you accountable for working out. • Give yourself an incentive. • Schedule your workouts when you feel most energetic. • Remind yourself that exercise gives you more energy. • Get things ready for your workout; for example, if you choose to walk in the morning, set out your walking clothes the night before, or pack your gym bag before going to bed.
Lack of resources	• Select an activity that requires minimal equipment, such as walking, jogging, jumping rope, or calisthenics. • Identify inexpensive resources on campus or in the community. • Use active forms of transportation. • Take advantage of no-cost opportunities, such as playing catch in the park/green space on campus.

Source: Adapted from National Center for Chronic Disease Prevention and Health Promotion, "How Can I Overcome Barriers to Physical Activity?," Updated February 2011, www.cdc.gov.

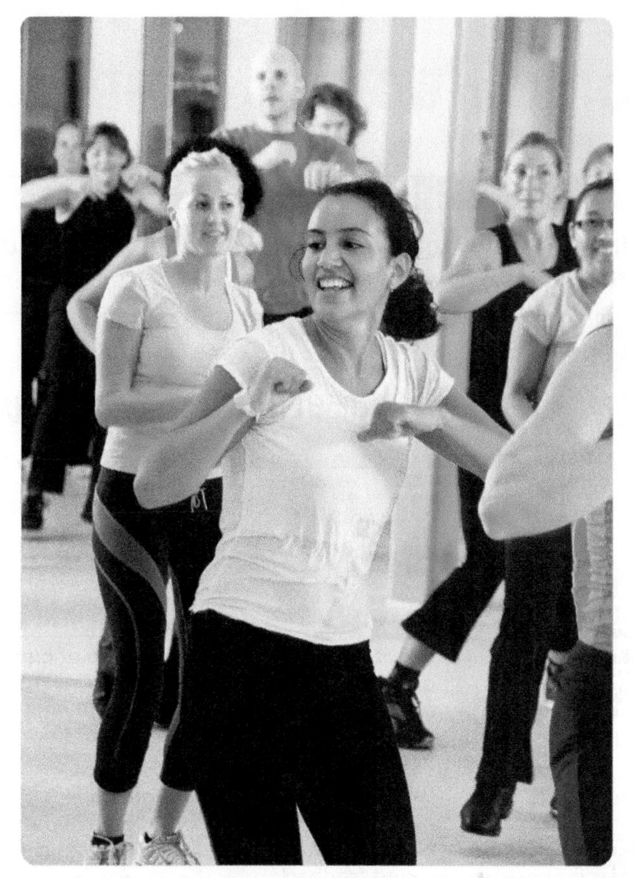

How can I motivate myself to be more physically active?

One great way to motivate yourself is to sign up for an exercise class. Find something that interests you—dance, yoga, aerobics, martial arts, acrobatics—and get yourself involved. The structure, schedule, social interaction, and challenge of learning a new skill can be terrific motivators that make exercising and being physically active exciting and fun.

(or step counter; see Table 1.3 for more on this handy gadget and other fitness equipment you may consider purchasing or using at a health club). Try to make exercise a part of your routine by incorporating it into something you already have to do—such as getting to class or work.

check yourself

- **What are some common obstacles people face when deciding to be more physically active?**
- **How can these obstacles be overcome?**
- **What factors should you consider when choosing an exercise activity?**

1.4 Some Popular Fitness Gadgets and Equipment

learning outcome

1.4 **Identify common types of fitness equipment and their uses.**

TABLE 1.3 Some Popular Fitness Gadgets and Equipment

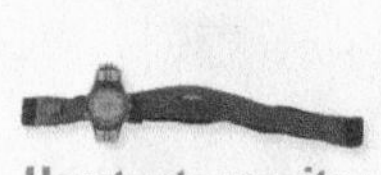 Heart rate monitor	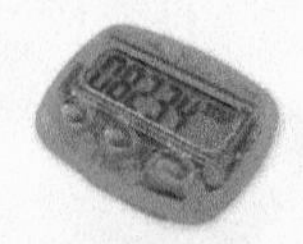 Pedometer	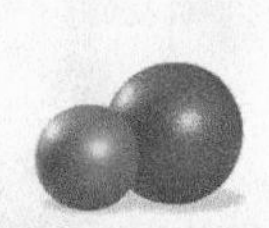 Stability ball	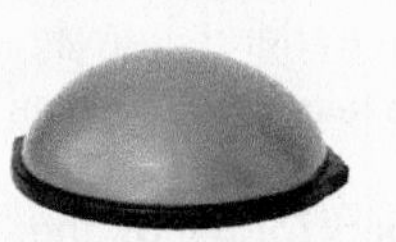 Balance Board	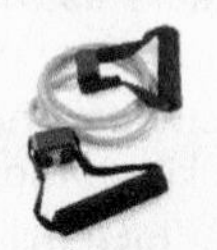 Resistance band	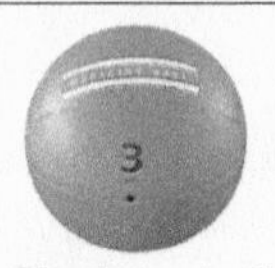 Medicine ball
Chest strap with watch device that measures heart rate during training. • Instant feedback about intensity of your workout. • Strap can be uncomfortable. Cost: $50–$200	Battery-operated device, usually worn on belt, that measures steps taken. Some models also monitor calories, distance, and speed. • Great motivation and feedback. • Must be calibrated for height, weight, and stride length. Cost: $25–$50	Ball made of burst-resistant vinyl used for strengthening core muscles or improving flexibility. • Balls must be inflated correctly to be most effective. Cost: $25–$50	Board with rounded bottom used to improve balance, core muscle strength, and flexibility. • Great for improving agility, coordination, reaction skills, and ankle strength. • Can be difficult for new users. Cost: $40–$80	Rubber or elastic material, sometimes with handles, used to build muscular strength and endurance or for flexibility. • Lightweight, durable, and portable. Cost: $5–$15	Heavy ball, about 14 inces in diameter, used in rehabilitation and strength training. Weight varies from 2–25 lb. • Can be used in plyometric training and to develop core strength. • If used incorrectly, risk of lower back injuries. Cost: $10–$150

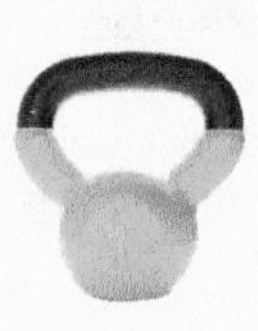 Kettlebell	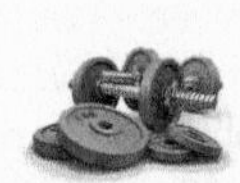 Free Weights	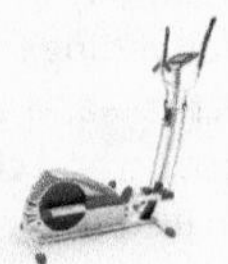 Elliptical Trainer	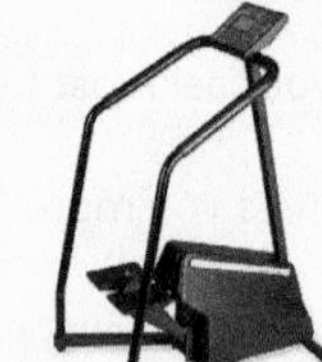 Stair Climber	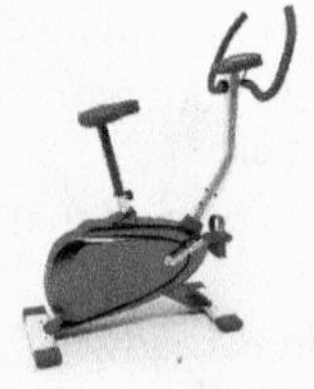 Stationary Bike	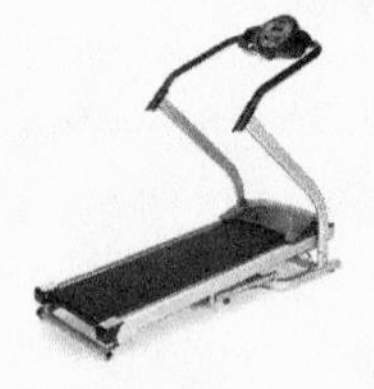 Treadmill
Heavy ball with a handle used for full body muscular strength and endurance exercises. Weight varies from 5 to 100 lb. • Movements can be complex; if used incorrectly, potential for lower back and/or wrist injuries. Cost: $10–$150	Dumbbells or barbells, often with adjustable weight. • Build muscular strength and endurance. • Potential for injury with incorrect form; concentrate on alignment and core strength. Cost: $10–$300	Stationary exercise machine that simulates walking or running without impact on bones and joints. Some include arm movements. • Nonimpact; less wear and tear on the joints and risk of shin splints. Cost: $300–$4,000	Stationary exercise machine that provides low-impact lower body workout by stair climbing. • Nonimpact; less wear and tear on the joints and risk of shin splints. • Various programs are available. Cost: $200–$3,000	Lower body exercise machine designed to simulate bike riding. • Generally easy to use; does not require balance. • Comes with varied resistance programs. • Recumbent styles offer less strain on back and knees. Cost: $200–$2,000	Exercise machine for walking or running on a moving platform. • Generally easy to use; comes with emergency shutoff. • Lower impact on joints than running on most pavements. Cost: $500–$4,000

check yourself

- **What are five types of fitness equipment? Which would you be likely to use and why?**

1.5 Fitness Program Components

learning outcome

1.5 Describe how to set SMART goals and list the parts of the FITT principle.

Set SMART Goals

Your physical fitness goals and objectives should be both achievable and in line with what you truly want. To set successful goals, try using the *SMART* system. SMART goals are **s**pecific, **m**easurable, **a**ction-oriented, **r**ealistic, and **t**ime-oriented. A vague goal would be "Improve fitness by exercising more." A SMART goal would be:

- *Specific*—"I'll participate in a resistance training program that targets all of the major muscle groups 3–5 days per week."
- *Measurable*—"I'll improve my fitness classification to average."
- *Action-oriented*—"I'll meet with a personal trainer to learn how to safely do resistance exercises and to plan a workout."
- *Realistic*—"I'll increase the weight I can lift by 20 percent."
- *Time-oriented*—"I'll try my new weight program for 8 weeks, then reassess."

Use the FITT Principle

The **FITT (frequency, intensity, time, and type)** principle shown in Figure 1.4 can be used to devise a workout plan. To achieve the desired level of fitness, consider the following elements:

- **Frequency** refers to how often you must exercise.
- **Intensity** refers to how hard your workout must be.
- **Time**, or *duration*, refers to how many minutes or repetitions of an exercise are required per session.
- **Type** refers to the kind of exercises performed.

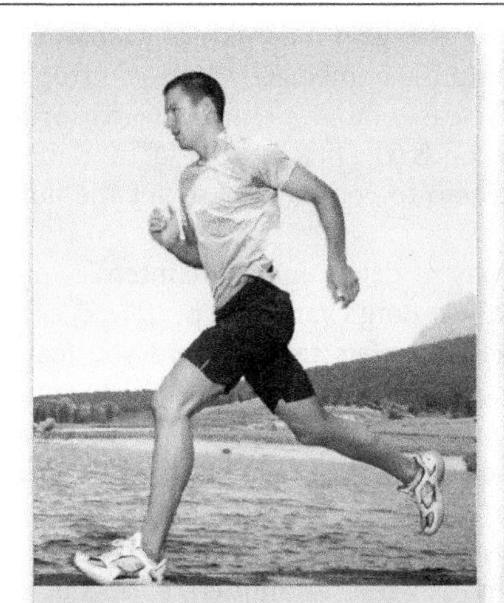

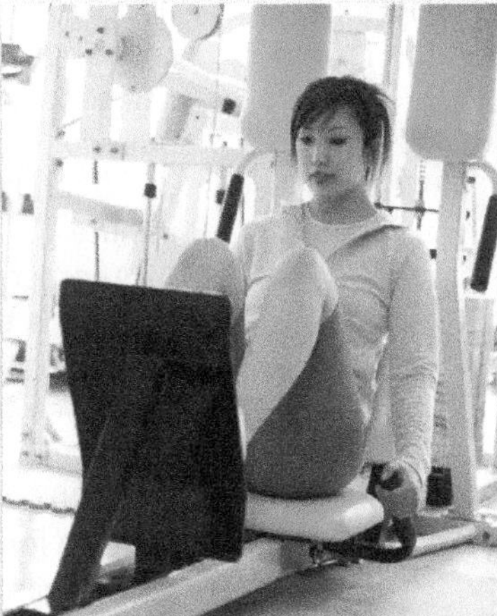

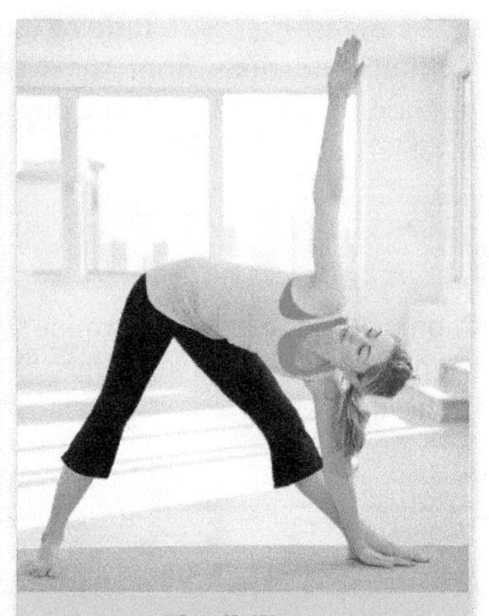

	Cardiorespiratory Endurance	Muscular Fitness	Flexibility
Frequency	3–5 days per week	2–3 days per week	Minimally 2–3 days per week
Intensity	64%–96% of maximum heart rate	60%–80% of 1 RM	To the point of mild tension
Time	20–60 minutes	8–10 exercises, 2–4 sets, 8–12 reps	10–30 seconds per stretch, 2–4 reps
Type	Any rhythmic, continuous, large muscle group activity	Resistance training (with body weight and/or external resistance) for all major muscle groups	Stretching, dance, or yoga exercises for all major muscle groups

Figure 1.4 The FITT Principle Applied to Cardiorespiratory Fitness, Muscular Strength and Endurance, and Flexibility

check yourself

- **What is an example of a SMART goal for fitness?**
- **What are the four parts of the FITT principle?**

1.6 The FITT Principle for Cardiorespiratory Fitness

learning outcome

1.6 List the FITT requirements for cardiorespiratory fitness.

The most effective aerobic exercises for building cardiorespiratory fitness are total-body activities involving the large muscle groups of your body. The FITT prescription for cardiorespiratory fitness includes 3 to 5 days per week of vigorous, rhythmic, continuous activity, at 64 to 95 percent of your estimated maximal heart rate, for 20 to 60 minutes.[30]

Frequency

To improve your cardiorespiratory fitness, you must exercise vigorously at least three times a week or moderately at least five times a week. If you are a newcomer to exercise, you can still make improvements by doing less intense exercise but doing it more days a week, following the recommendations from the Centers for Disease Control and Prevention (CDC) for moderate physical activity 5 days a week (refer to Table 1.1).

Intensity

The most common methods used to determine the intensity of cardiorespiratory endurance exercises are target heart rate, rating of perceived exertion, and the talk test. The exercise intensity required to improve cardiorespiratory endurance is a heart rate between 64 and 96 percent of your maximum heart rate. To calculate this target **heart rate**, first estimate your maximal heart rate with the formula 206.9 − (0.67 × age). Following is an example based on a 20-year-old. Substitute your age to determine your target heart rate training range, then multiply by 0.64 and 0.94 to determine the lower and upper limits of your target range. Figure 1.5 shows a range of target heart rates.

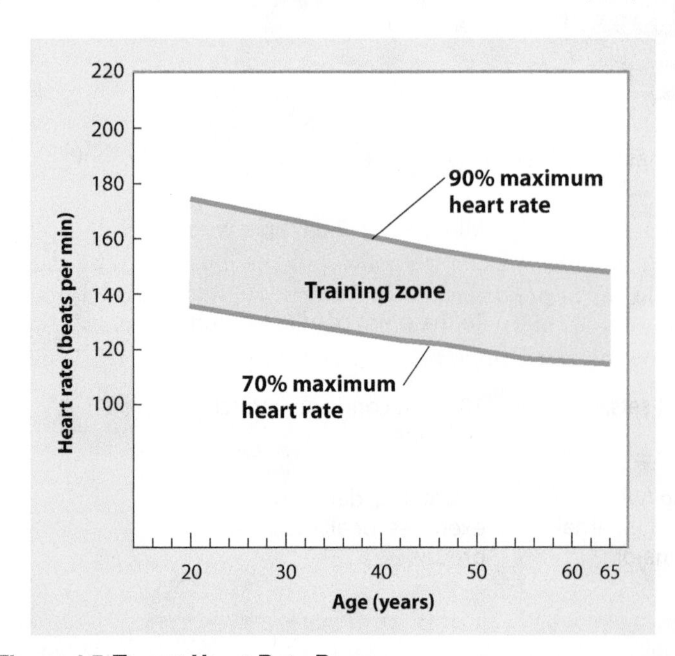

Figure 1.5 Target Heart Rate Ranges
These ranges are based on calculating the maximum heart rate as 206.9 − (0.67 × age), and the training zone as 64 percent to 96 percent of maximum heart rate. Individuals with low fitness levels should start below or at the low end of these ranges.

1. 206.9 − (0.67 × 20) = 193.5 (target heart rate for a 20-year-old)
2. 193.5 × 0.64 = 123.8 (lower target limit)
3. 193.5 × 0.94 = 181.89 (upper target limit)

Target range = 124–182 beats per minute

Take your pulse during your workout to determine how close you are to your target heart rate. Lightly place your index and middle fingers (not your thumb) over one of the major arteries in your neck, or on the artery on the inside of your wrist (Figure 1.6). Start counting your pulse immediately after you stop exercising, as your heart rate decreases rapidly. Using a watch or a clock, take your pulse for 6 seconds (the first pulse is "0") and multiply this number by 10 (add a zero to your count) to get the number of beats per minute.

Another way of determining the intensity of cardiorespiratory exercise is to use Borg's rating of perceived exertion (RPE) scale. Perceived exertion refers to how hard you feel you are working, which you might base on your heart rate, breathing rate, sweating, and level of fatigue. This scale uses a rating from 6 (no exertion at all) to 20 (maximal exertion). An RPE of 12 to 16 is generally recommended for training the cardiorespiratory system.

The easiest method of measuring cardiorespiratory exercise intensity is the "talk test." A "moderate" level of exercise (heart rate at 64 to 76 percent of maximum) is a conversational level of exercise. At this level you are able to talk with a partner while exercising.

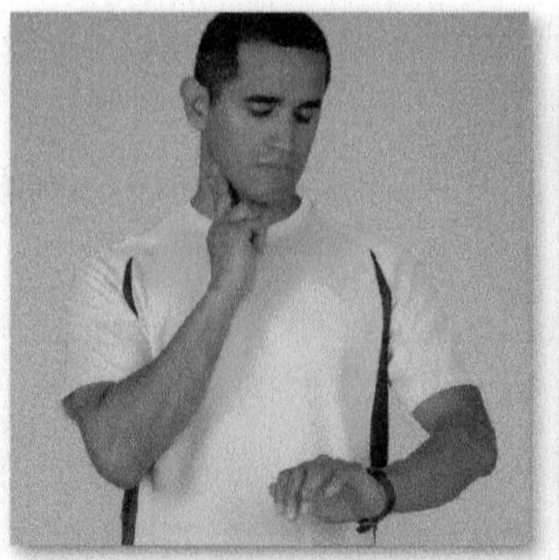

a Carotid pulse

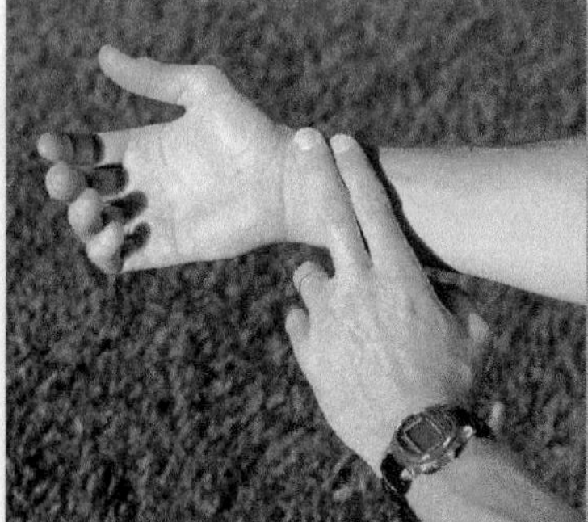

b Radial pulse

Figure 1.6 Taking a Pulse
Palpation of the carotid (neck) or radial (wrist) artery is a simple way of determining heart rate.

If you can talk but only in short fragments and not sentences, you may be at a "vigorous" level of exercise (heart rate at 76 to 96 percent of maximum). If you are breathing so hard that talking is difficult, the intensity of your exercise may be too high. Conversely, if you are able to sing or laugh heartily while exercising, the intensity of your exercise is insufficient for maintaining and/or improving cardiorespiratory fitness.

Time

For cardiorespiratory fitness benefits, the American College of Sports Medicine (ACSM) recommends that vigorous activities be performed for at least 20 minutes at a time, and moderate activities for at least 30 minutes.[31] You can also set a time goal for the entire week, as long as you keep your sessions to at least 10 minutes (150 minutes per week for moderate intensity, and 75 minutes per week for vigorous intensity).

Type

Any sort of rhythmic, continuous, and vigorous physical activity that can be done for 20 or more minutes will improve cardiorespiratory fitness. Examples include walking briskly, cycling, jogging, fitness classes, and swimming.

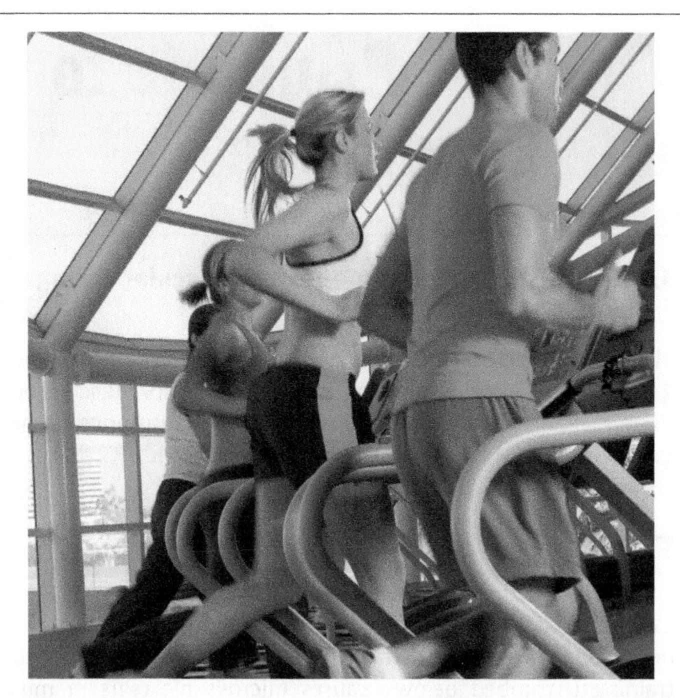

A typical 30-minute workout on a cardiorespiratory training device generates 50 watt hours of electricity—enough to operate a laptop for an hour. At least 20 colleges as well as several independent fitness clubs throughout the United States have retrofitted aerobic machines with equipment that converts the kinetic energy produced by the exercisers into renewable electric energy to help power the club.

Incorporating Cardiorespiratory Fitness into Daily Life

Before we became a car culture, much of our transportation was human powered. Bicycling and walking historically were important means of transportation and recreation in the United States. These modes not only helped keep people in good physical shape, but they also had little or no impact on the environment. Even in the first few decades after the automobile started to be popularized, people continued to get around under their own power. Since World War II, however, the development of automobile-oriented communities has led to a steady decline of bicycling and walking. Currently, only about 10 percent of trips are made by foot or bike.[32]

The more we use our cars to get around, the more congested our roads, the more polluted our air, and the more sedentary our lives become. That is why many people are now embracing a movement toward more active transportation. *Active transportation* means getting out of your car and using your own power to get from place to place—whether walking, riding a bike, skateboarding, or roller skating. Each of these activities can also be incorporated into your life as a form of exercise that contributes to cardiorespiratory fitness.

The following are just a few of the many reasons to make active transportation a bigger part of your life:[33]

- **You will be adding more exercise into your daily routine.** People who walk, bike, or use other active forms of transportation to complete errands are physically active.
- **Walking or biking can save you money.** With rising gas prices and parking fees, in addition to increasing car maintenance and insurance costs, fewer automobile trips could add up to considerable savings. During the course of a year, regular bicycle commuters who ride 5 miles to work can save about $500 on fuel and more than $1,000 on other expenses related to driving.
- **Walking or biking may save you time!** Cycling is usually the fastest mode of travel door to door for distances up to 6 miles in city centers. Walking is simpler and faster for distances of about a mile.
- **You will enjoy being outdoors.** Research is emerging on the physical and mental health benefits of nature and being outdoors. So much of what we do is inside, with recirculated air and artificial lighting, that our bodies are deficient in fresh air and sunlight.
- **You will be making a significant contribution to the reduction of air pollution.** Driving less means fewer pollutants being emitted into the air. Annually, personal transportation accounts for the consumption of approximately 136 billion gallons of gasoline, or the production of 1.2 billion tons of carbon dioxide. Leaving your car at home just 2 days a week will reduce greenhouse gas emissions by an average of 1,600 pounds per year.

check yourself

- **What are the FITT requirements for cardiorespiratory fitness?**
- **How can you incorporate cardiorespiratory fitness into your daily life?**

1.7 The FITT Principle for Muscular Strength and Endurance

learning **outcome**

1.7 List the FITT requirements for muscular strength and endurance.

The FITT prescription for muscular strength and endurance includes 2 to 3 days per week of exercises that train the major muscle groups, using enough sets and repetitions and enough resistance to maintain or improve muscular strength and endurance.[34]

Frequency

For frequency, the FITT principle recommends performing 8 to 10 exercises that train the major muscle groups 2 to 3 days a week. It is believed that overloading the muscles, a normal part of resistance training (described below), causes microscopic tears in muscle fibers. The rebuilding process that increases the muscle's size and capacity takes about 24 to 48 hours. Thus, resistance-training exercise programs should include at least 1 day of rest between workouts before the same muscles are overloaded again. But don't wait too long between workouts—one of the important principles of strength training is the idea of *reversibility.* Reversibility means that if you stop exercising, the body responds by deconditioning. Within 2 weeks, muscles begin to revert to their untrained state.[35] The saying "use it or lose it" applies here!

Intensity

To determine the intensity of exercise needed to improve muscular strength and endurance, you need to know the maximum amount of weight you can lift (or move) in one contraction. This value is called your **one repetition maximum (1 RM)** and can be individually determined or predicted from a 10 RM test. Once your 1 RM is determined, it is used as the basis for intensity recommendations for improving muscular strength and endurance. Muscular strength is improved when resistance loads are greater than 60 percent of your 1 RM, whereas muscular endurance is improved using loads of less than 60 percent of your 1 RM.

Everyone begins a resistance-training program at an initial level of strength. To become stronger, you must *overload* your muscles, that is, regularly create a degree of tension in your muscles greater than that to which you are accustomed. Overloading your muscles forces them to adapt by getting larger, stronger, and capable of producing more tension. If you "underload" your muscles, you will not increase strength. If you create too great an overload, you may experience muscle injury, muscle fatigue, and potentially a loss in strength. Once your strength goal is reached, no further overload is necessary; your challenge at that point is to maintain your level of strength by engaging in a regular (once or twice per week) total-body resistance exercise program.

Time

The time recommended for muscular strength and endurance exercises is measured not in minutes of exercise, but rather in repetitions and sets. The types of demands that you put on your body will result in the kind of adaptation that will follow.

Repetitions and Sets. To increase muscular strength, you need higher intensity and fewer repetitions and sets. Use a resistance of at least 60 percent of your 1 RM, performing 8 to 12 repetitions per set, with two to four sets performed overall. If improving muscular endurance is your goal, use less resistance and more repetitions and sets. The recommendations for improving muscular endurance are to perform one to two sets of 15 to 25 repetitions using a resistance that is less than 50 percent of your 1 RM.

Rest Periods. The amount of rest between exercises is key to an effective strength-training workout. Resting between exercises can

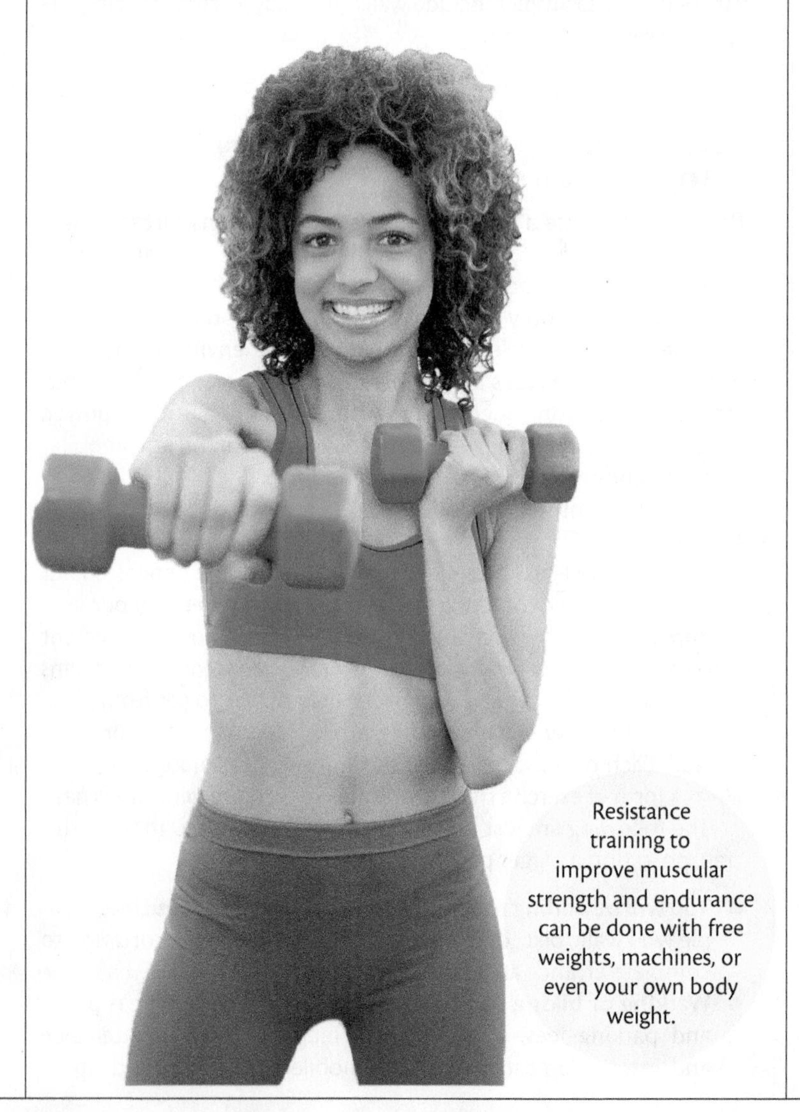

Resistance training to improve muscular strength and endurance can be done with free weights, machines, or even your own body weight.

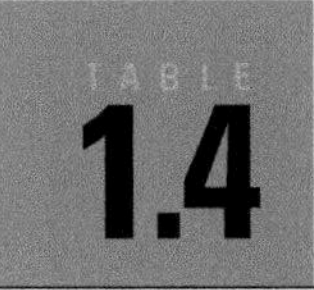

TABLE 1.4 Methods of Providing Exercise Resistance

Calisthenics (Body Weight Resistance)	Free Weights (Fixed Resistance)	Weight Machines (Variable Resistance)
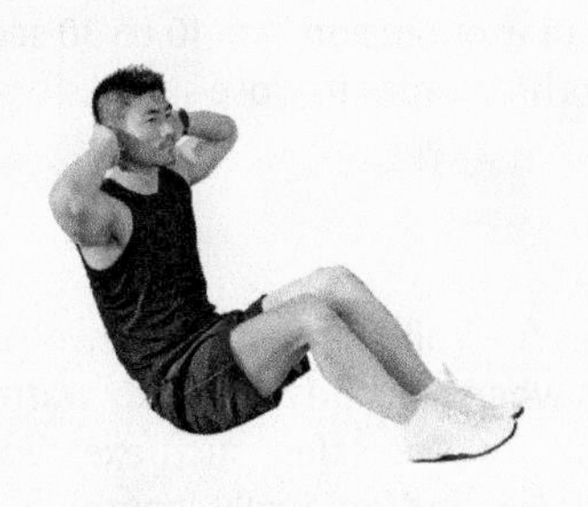	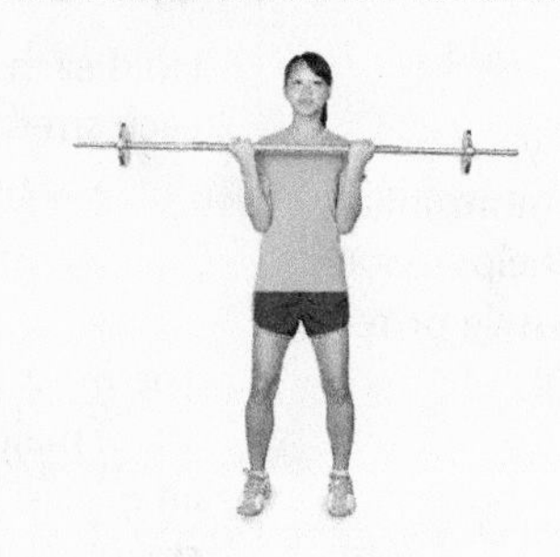	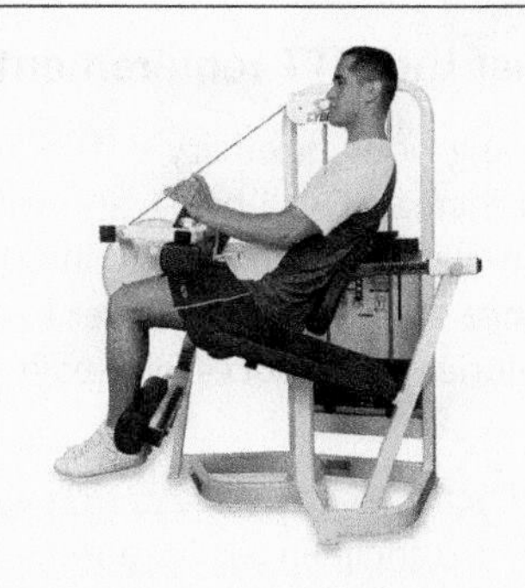
• Using your own body weight to develop muscular strength, endurance. • Improves overall muscular fitness—in particular core strength and overall muscle tone.	• Provides constant resistance throughout full range of movement. • Requires balance and coordination; promotes development of core strength.	• Resistance is altered so the muscle's effort is consistent throughout full range of motion. • Provides more controlled motion and isolates certain muscle groups.
Examples: Push-ups, pull-ups, curl-ups, dips, leg raises, chair sits. For an extra challenge, you can do these exercises on a stability ball or balance board.	**Examples:** Barbells, dumbbells, medicine balls, and kettlebells. Resistance bands can be used for resistance instead of weights.	**Examples:** Weight machines in gyms, homes (Nautilus or Bowflex), and rehabilitation centers.

reduce fatigue and help with performance and safety in subsequent sets. A rest period of 2 to 3 minutes is recommended when using the guidelines for general health benefits. However, the rest period when working to develop strength or endurance will vary. Note that the rest period refers specifically to the muscle group being exercised, and it is possible to alternate muscle groups. For example, you can alternate a set of push-ups with a set of curl-ups; the muscle groups worked in one set can rest while you are working the other muscle groups.

Type

To improve muscular strength or endurance, resistance training is most often recommended using either your own body weight or devices that provide a fixed or variable resistance (see Table 1.4). Some cardiorespiratory training activities also enhance muscular endurance: Thousands of repetitions are performed during a 20-minute (or longer) workout using relatively low resistance when jogging or when training on an exercise device such as a stationary bicycle, rowing machine, or stair-climbing machine.

When selecting the type of strength-training exercises to do, keep several important principles in mind. The first of these is *specificity.* According to the specificity principle, the effects of resistance-exercise training are specific to the muscles exercised; only the muscle or muscle group that is overloaded responds to the demands placed upon it. For example, if you regularly do curls, the muscles involved—your biceps—will become larger and stronger, but the other muscles in your body will not change. This sort of training may put opposing muscle groups—in this case the triceps—at increased risk for injury. To improve total body strength, you must include exercises for all the major muscle groups. You must also ensure that your overload is sufficient to increase strength and not only endurance.

Another important concept to consider is *exercise selection.* Exercises that work a single joint (e.g., chest presses) are effective for building specific muscle strength, whereas multiple-joint exercises (e.g., a squat coupled with an overhead press) are more effective for increasing overall muscle strength. Selecting 8 to 10 exercises targeting all major muscle groups is generally recommend and will ensure that exercises are balanced for opposing muscle groups.

Finally, for optimal training effects, it is important to pay attention to *exercise order.* When training all major muscle groups in a single workout, complete large-muscle group exercises (e.g., the bench press or leg press) before small-muscle group exercises, multiple-joint exercises before single-joint exercises (e.g., biceps curls, triceps extension), and high-intensity exercises before lower-intensity exercises.

check yourself

- **What are the FITT requirements for muscular strength and endurance?**

1.8

The FITT Principle for Flexibility

learning outcome

1.8 List the FITT requirements for flexibility.

Improving your flexibility enhances the efficiency of your movements, increases well-being, and reduces stress. Furthermore, inflexible muscles are susceptible to injury; flexibility training helps reduce incidence and severity of lower back problems and muscle or tendon injuries and reduces joint pain and deterioration.[36]

Frequency

The FITT principle calls for a minimum of 2 to 3 days per week for flexibility training; daily training is even better.

Intensity

Hold static (still) stretching positions at an individually determined "point of tension." You should feel tension or mild discomfort in the muscle(s) stretched, but not pain.[37]

Time

Hold each stretch at the "point of tension" for 10 to 30 seconds for each stretch; repeat two or three times in close succession.[38]

Type

The most effective exercises for building flexibility involve stretching of major muscle groups when the body is already warm, such as after cardiorespiratory activities. The safest such exercises involve **static stretching**, which slowly and gradually lengthens a muscle or group of muscles and their attached tendons.[39] With each repetition, your range of motion improves temporarily due to the slightly lessened sensitivity of tension receptors in the stretched muscles; when done regularly, range of motion increases.[40] Figure 1.7 shows some basic stretching exercises.

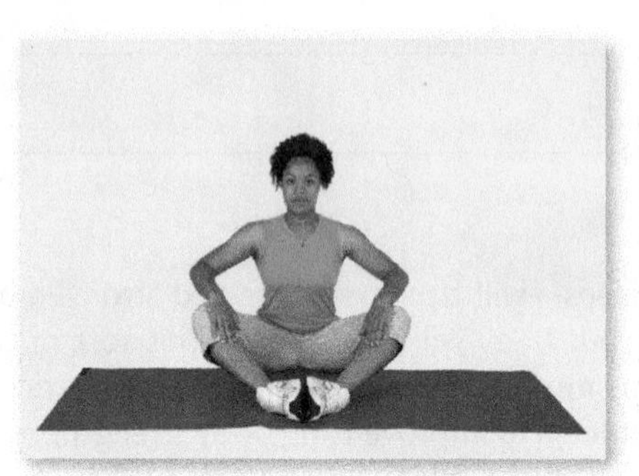

(a) Stretching the inside of the thighs

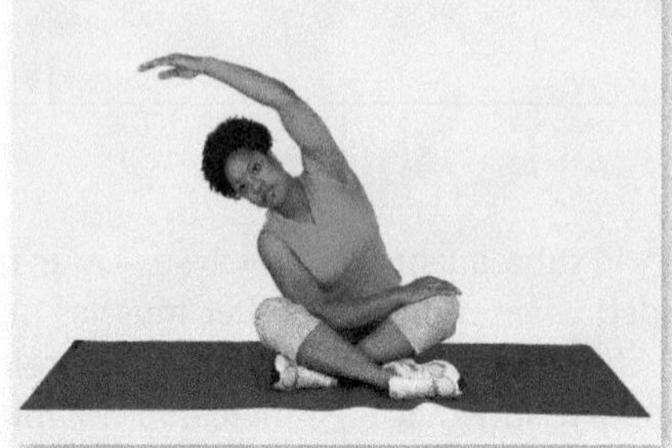

(b) Stretching the upper arm and the side of the trunk

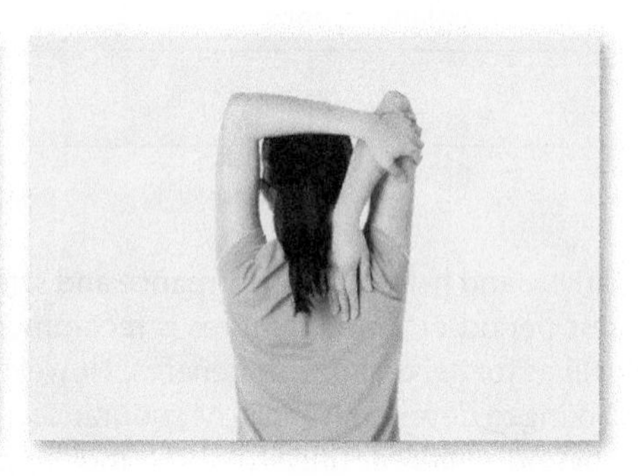

(c) Stretching the triceps

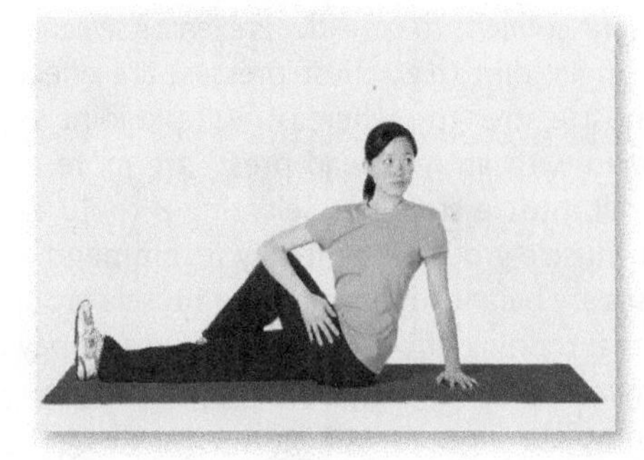

(d) Stretching the trunk and the hip

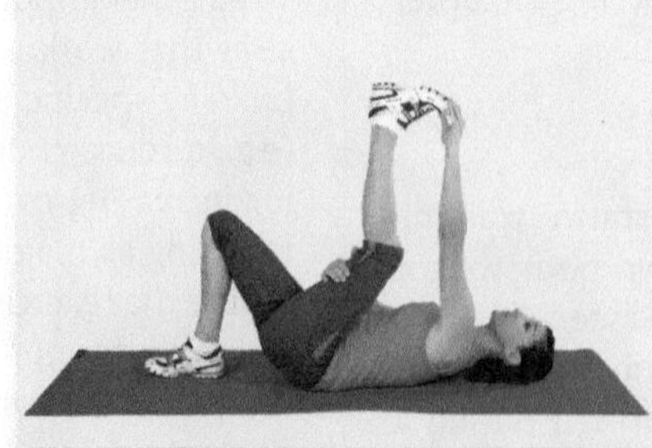

(e) Stretching the hip, back of the thigh, and the calf

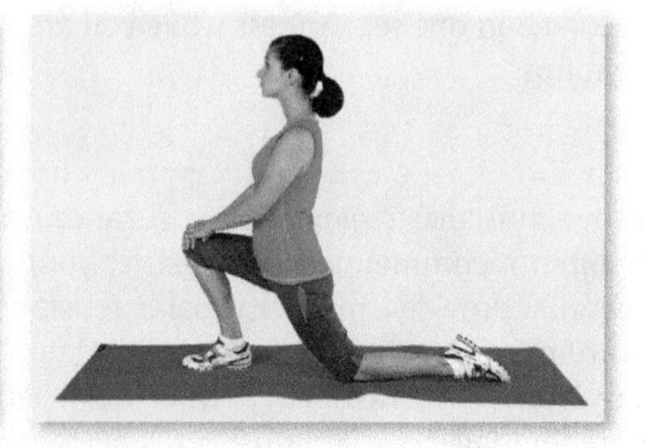

(f) Stretching the front of the thigh and the hip flexor

Figure 1.7 Stretching Exercises to Improve Flexibility and Prevent Injury

Use these stretches as part of your warm-up and cool-down. Hold each stretch for 10 to 30 seconds, and repeat two to three times for each limb.

check yourself

- **What are the FITT requirements for flexibility?**

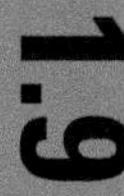

Developing and Staying with a Fitness Plan

learning outcome

1.9 Describe how to stay with and adjust your fitness program over time.

As your physical fitness improves, in order to continue to improve and/or maintain your level of fitness you will need to adjust your frequency, intensity, time, and type of exercise.

Develop a Progressive Plan

Begin an exercise regimen by picking an exercise and gradually increasing workout frequency. For example, in week 1, you might exercise 3 days for 20 minutes per day, and then move to 4 days in week 3 or 4. Then, consider increasing your duration to 30 minutes per session over the next couple of weeks. In general, an increase of 5 to 10 minutes a session every 1 to 2 weeks is tolerated by most during the first month.

Be sure to vary your type of exercise—variety is a fundamental strength training principle also relevant to cardiorespiratory fitness and flexibility training. Changes in one or more parts of your workout not only produce a higher level of physical fitness and reduce the risk of overuse injuries (because different muscle groups are used), but also keep you motivated and interested.

It's also important to reevaluate your overall goals and plans every month or so. Too often, people deciding to become more physically active (or make any other behavior change) work hard on getting started, then lose steam as they go on. To keep yourself motivated, review your progress, make changes when necessary, and continue to reevaluate regularly.

Design Your Exercise Session

A comprehensive workout includes a warm-up, cardiorespiratory and/or resistance training, and then a cool-down to finish the session.

Warm-ups involve large body movements, generally using light cardiorespiratory activities, followed by range-of-motion exercises of the muscle groups to be used during the exercise session. Usually 5 to 15 minutes long, a warm-up is shorter when you are geared up and ready to go and longer when you are struggling to get moving or your muscles are cold or tight. Warm-ups slowly increase heart rate, blood pressure, breathing rate, and body temperature; improve joint lubrication; and increase muscles' and tendons' elasticity and flexibility.

The next stage of your workout, immediately following the warm-up, may involve cardiorespiratory training, resistance training, or a little of both. If you are in a fitness center, you may choose to use one or more of the aerobic training devices for the recommended time frame. If completing aerobic and resistance exercise in the same session, it is often recommended to perform your aerobic exercise first. This order will provide additional warm-up for the resistance session, and your muscles will not be fatigued for the aerobic workout.

Cool-down includes 5 to 10 minutes of low-intensity activity and 5 to 10 minutes of stretching. Because of the body's increased temperature, the cool-down is an excellent time to stretch to improve flexibility. The cool-down gradually reduces heart rate, blood pressure, and body temperature; reduces the risk of blood pooling in the extremities; and helps speed recovery between exercise sessions.

Skills for Behavior Change

PLAN IT, START IT, STICK WITH IT!

The most successful physical activity program is one that is realistic and appropriate for your skill level and needs.

- **Make it enjoyable.** Pick activities you like to do so you will make the effort and find the time to do it.
- **Start slowly.** If you have been physically inactive for a while or are a first-time exerciser, any type and amount of physical activity is a step in the right direction. Keep in mind that it is an achievement to get to the fitness center or to put your sneakers on for a walk! Make sure you start slowly and let your body adapt so that your new physical activity or exercise does not cause excess pain the next day (a real reaction to using muscles you have not used much or as intensely before). Do not be discouraged; you will be able to increase your activity each week, and soon you will be on your way to meeting the physical activity recommendations and your personal goals.
- **Make only one lifestyle change at a time.** It is not realistic to change everything at once. Plus, success with one behavioral change will increase your belief in yourself and encourage you to make other positive changes.
- **Set reasonable expectations for yourself and your physical fitness program.** You will not become "fit" overnight. It takes several months to really feel the benefits of your physical activity. Be patient.
- **Choose a time to exercise and stick with it.** Set priorities and keep to a schedule. Try exercising at different times of the day to learn what works best for you. Yet be flexible, so if something comes up that you cannot work around, you will find time later that day or evening to do some physical activity. Be careful of an all-or-none attitude.
- **Keep a record of your progress.** Include the intensity, time, type of physical activities, and your emotions and personal achievements.
- **Take lapses in stride.** Sometimes life gets in the way. Start again and do not despair; your commitment to physical fitness has ebbs and flows like everything else in life.

check yourself

- **What are strategies for staying with and adjusting your fitness program over time?**

1.10 Developing Core Strength

learning outcome

1.10 Explain the benefits of a strong core.

Yoga, tai chi, and Pilates have become increasingly popular in the United States. All three forms of exercise have the potential to improve **core strength**, flexibility, balance, coordination, and agility. They also develop the mind–body connection through concentration on breathing and body position.

Core Strength Training

The body's core muscles, including deep back and abdominal muscles that attach to the spine and pelvis, are the foundation for all movement.[41] Contraction of these muscles provides the basis of support for movements of the upper and lower body and powerful movements of the extremities. A weak core generally results in poor posture, low back pain, and muscle injuries. A strong core provides a stable center of gravity and so a more stable platform for movements, thus reducing the chance of injury.

You can develop core strength using exercises such as calisthenics, yoga, and Pilates. Core strength does not happen from one single exercise, but rather from a structured regime of postures and exercises.[42] Holding yourself in a front or reverse plank ("up" and reverse of a push-up position) and holding or doing abdominal curl-ups are examples of exercises that increase core strength. The use of instability devices (stability ball, wobble boards, etc.) and exercises to train the core have also become popular.[43]

Yoga

Yoga, based on ancient Indian practices, blends the mental and physical aspects of exercise—a union of mind and body that participants often find relaxing and satisfying. If done regularly, yoga improves flexibility, vitality, posture, agility, balance, coordination, and muscular strength and endurance. Many people report an improved sense of general well-being, too.

The practice of yoga focuses attention on controlled breathing as well as physical exercise and incorporates a complex array of static stretching exercises expressed as postures (*asanas*). During a session, participants move to different asanas and hold them for 30 seconds or longer.

Some forms of yoga are more meditative in their practice, whereas others are more athletic. *Ashtanga yoga,* also called "power yoga," focuses on a series of poses done in a continuous, repeated flow, with controlled breathing. *Bikram yoga,* also known as *hot yoga,* is unique in that classes are held in rooms heated to 105°F, which practitioners claim helps the potential for increasing flexibility.

See It! Videos

Yoga is a great way to exercise your body and your mind. Watch **Beginner's Guide to Yoga** in the Study Area of MasteringHealth.

Tai Chi

Tai chi is an ancient Chinese form of exercise that combines stretching, balance, muscular endurance, coordination, and meditation. It increases range of motion and flexibility while reducing muscular tension. Tai chi involves a series of positions called *forms* that are performed continuously. Tai chi is often described as "meditation in motion" because it promotes serenity through gentle movements, connecting the mind and body.

Pilates

Pilates was developed by Joseph Pilates in 1926 as an exercise style that combines stretching with movement against resistance, frequently aided by devices such as tension springs or heavy rubber bands. It teaches body awareness, good posture, and easy, graceful body movements while improving flexibility, coordination, core strength, muscle tone, and economy of motion.

Pilates differs from yoga and tai chi in that it includes sequences of movements specifically designed to increase strength. Some Pilates exercises are carried out on specially designed equipment, whereas others can be performed on mats.

Strengthening core body muscles can also enhance flexibility and help lower stress levels.

check yourself

- **What are some benefits of having a strong core?**
- **What types of exercise increase core strength?**

1.11 Activity and Exercise for Special Populations

learning outcome

1.11 Explain challenges and considerations related to physical activity for older people and those with common health conditions.

All individuals can benefit from a physically active lifestyle. People with the considerations mentioned here should consult a physician before beginning an exercise program.

Asthma

For individuals with asthma, regular physical activity strengthens respiratory muscles, improves immune system functioning, and helps in weight maintenance.

Before engaging in exercise, ensure that your asthma is under control. Ask about adjusting medications (for example, your doctor may recommend you use your inhaler 15 minutes prior to exercise). When exercising, keep your inhaler nearby. Warm up and cool down properly; it is particularly important that you allow your lungs and breathing rate to adjust slowly. Protect yourself from asthma triggers when exercising. Finally, if you have symptoms while exercising, stop and use your inhaler; if an asthma attack persists, call 9-1-1.[44]

Obesity

Limitations such as heat intolerance, shortness of breath during physical activity, lack of flexibility, frequent musculoskeletal injuries, and difficulty with balance in weight-bearing activities need to be addressed. Programs for individuals who are obese should emphasize physical activities that can be sustained for 30 minutes or more, such as walking, swimming, or bicycling, with caution recommended in heat or humidity. Start slow (5 to 10 minutes of activity at 55% to 65% of maximal heart rate), then work up to at least 30 to 60 minutes of exercise per day—150 to 300 minutes per week. Obese individuals can improve health with cardiorespiratory and resistance-training activities.[45]

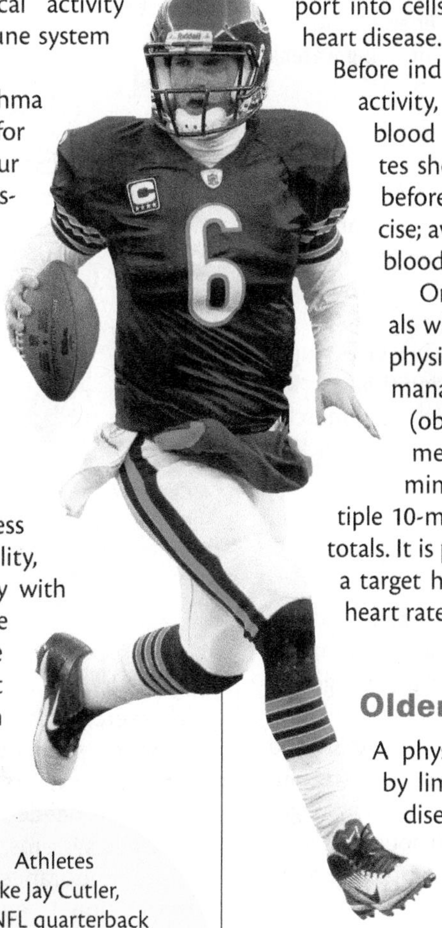

Coronary Heart Disease and Hypertension

Although regular physical activity reduces risk of coronary heart disease, vigorous activity acutely increases risk of sudden cardiac death and heart attack. Individuals with coronary heart disease must consult their physicians and might need to participate in a supervised exercise program for individuals with heart disease.[46]

Physical activity is an integral component for the prevention and treatment of hypertension. Using the FITT prescription, individuals who are hypertensive should engage in physical activity on most, if not all, days at moderate intensity for 30 minutes or more.[47]

Athletes like Jay Cutler, an NFL quarterback and a type 1 diabetic, are living proof that chronic conditions needn't prevent you from achieving your physical activity goals.

Diabetes

Physical activity benefits individuals with diabetes by controlling blood glucose (for type 2 diabetics) by improving insulin transport into cells, controlling body weight, and reducing risk of heart disease.

Before individuals with type 1 diabetes engage in physical activity, they must learn how to manage their resting blood glucose levels. Individuals with type 1 diabetes should have an exercise partner; eat 1 to 3 hours before exercise; eat complex carbohydrates after exercise; avoid late-evening physical activities; and monitor blood glucose before, during, and after exercise.

One of the most important factors for individuals with type 2 diabetes is the time or length of their physical activity. Because a critical objective of the management of type 2 diabetes is to reduce body fat (obesity), the longer exercise periods are recommended—at least 30 minutes, working up to 60 minutes per session or 300 minutes per week. Multiple 10-minute sessions can be used to accumulate these totals. It is prudent to reduce the intensity of the activity to a target heart rate range of 40 to 60 percent of maximal heart rate.

Older Adults

A physically active lifestyle increases life expectancy by limiting development and progression of chronic diseases and disabling conditions; the general recommendation for older adults is to engage in regular physical activity. For individuals with arthritis, osteoarthritis, and other musculoskeletal problems, non-weight-bearing activities, such as cycling and swimming or other water exercises, are recommended.[48]

check yourself

- **What should older people and those with health conditions be aware of when choosing a program of physical exercise?**
- **Have you had to make any accommodations in your fitness program due to an existing health condition?**

1.12 Nutrition and Exercise

learning outcome

1.12 Explain nutritional habits that support healthy exercise.

To make the most of your workouts, follow the recommendations from the MyPlate plan and make sure that you eat sufficient carbohydrates, the body's main source of fuel. Your body stores carbohydrates as glycogen primarily in the muscles and liver and then uses this stored glycogen for energy when you are physically active. Fats are also an important source of energy, packing more than double the energy per gram of carbohydrates. Protein plays a role in muscle repair and growth, but is not normally a source of energy. Another important nutrient to consider is water (or fluids containing water).

Timing Your Food Intake

When you eat is almost as important as what you eat. Eating a large meal before exercising can cause upset stomach, cramping, and diarrhea, because your muscles have to compete with your digestive system for energy. After a large meal, wait 3 to 4 hours before you begin exercising. Smaller meals (snacks) can be eaten about an hour before activity. Not eating at all before a workout can cause low blood sugar levels that, in turn, cause weakness and slower reaction times.

It is also important to refuel after your workout. Help your muscles recover and prepare for the next bout of activity by eating a snack or meal that contains plenty of carbohydrates plus a bit of protein.

Staying Hydrated

In addition to eating well, staying hydrated is crucial for active individuals wanting to maintain a healthy, fully functional body. How much fluid do you need to stay well hydrated? Keep in mind that the goal of fluid replacement is to prevent excessive dehydration (greater than 2% loss of body weight). The ACSM and the National Athletic Trainers Association recommend consuming 5 to 7 mL per kg of body weight (approximately 0.7 to 1.07 oz per 10 pounds of body weight), 4 hours prior to exercise.[49] Drinking fluids during exercise is also important, though it is difficult to provide guidelines for how much or when because intake should be based on time, intensity, and type of activity performed. A good way to monitor how much fluid you need to replace is to weigh yourself before and after your workout. The difference in weight is how much you should drink. So, for example, if you lost 2 pounds during a training session, you should drink 32 ounces of fluid.[50]

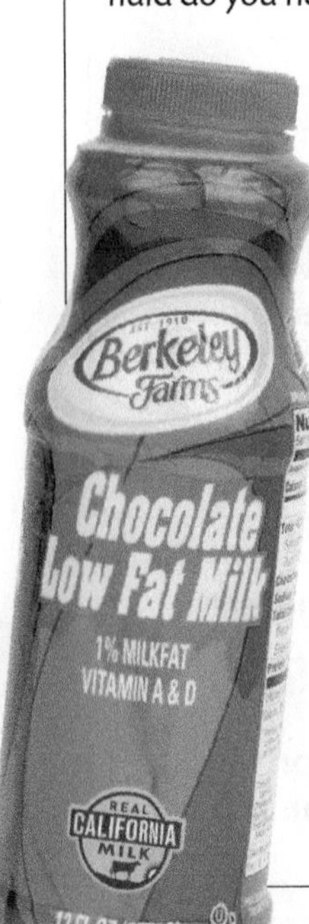

For hydration, electrolytes, carbohydrates, and protein, low-fat chocolate milk may be the ideal post-workout drink.

How much do I need to drink before, during, and after physical activity?

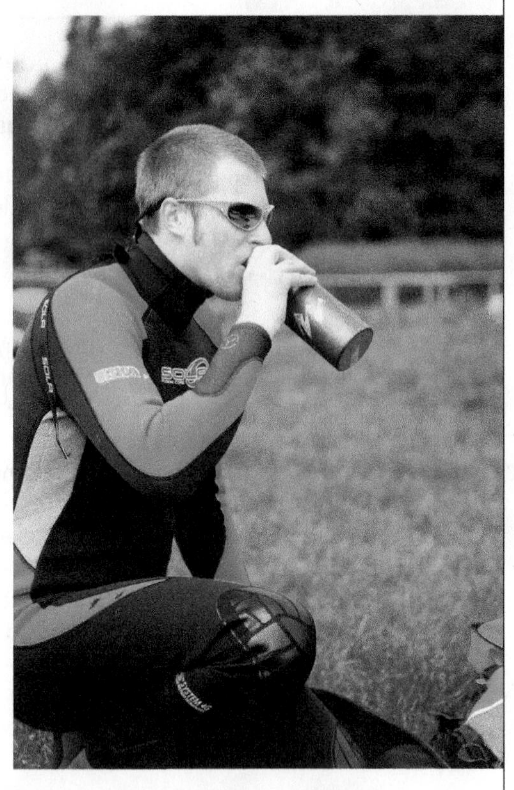

The American College of Sports Medicine and the National Athletic Trainers' Association recommend consuming 14 to 22 ounces of fluid several hours prior to exercise and about 6 to 12 ounces per 15 to 20 minutes during—assuming you are sweating.

What are the best fluids to drink? For exercise sessions lasting less than 1 hour, plain water is sufficient for rehydration. If your exercise session exceeds 1 hour—and you sweat profusely—consider a sports drink containing electrolytes. The electrolytes in these products are minerals and ions such as sodium and potassium needed for proper functioning of your nervous and muscular systems. Replacing electrolytes is particularly important for endurance athletes engaging in long bouts of exercise or competition. In endurance events lasting more than 4 hours, an athlete's overconsumption of plain water can dilute the sodium concentration in the blood with potentially fatal results, an effect called **hyponatremia** or **water intoxication**.

What about mixing alcohol and exercise? Drinking alcohol can contribute to weight gain, derailing efforts to stay fit. Additionally, a hangover from drinking the night before leads to dehydration and other negative symptoms that can inhibit exercise performance. Consuming

See It! Videos

Will that fancy sports drink help you exercise better? Watch **Sports Drinks Science: Is It Hype?** in the Study Area of MasteringHealth.

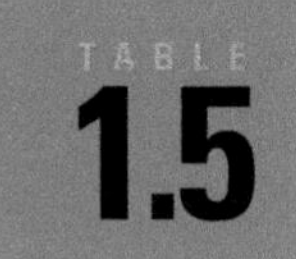

TABLE 1.5 Performance-Enhancing Dietary Supplements and Drugs—Their Uses and Effects

Substance	Primary Uses	Side Effects
Creatine Naturally occurring compound that helps supply energy to muscle	• Improve post-workout recovery • Increase muscle mass • Increase strength • Increase power	• Weight gain, nausea, muscle cramps • Large doses have a negative effect on the kidneys
Ephedra and ephedrine Stimulant that constricts blood vessels and increases blood pressure and heart rate Illegal; banned by FDA in 2006; banned by sports organizations	• Lose weight • Increase performance	• Nausea, vomiting • Anxiety and mood changes • Hyperactivity • In rare cases, seizures, heart attack, stroke, psychotic episodes
Anabolic steroids Synthetic versions of the hormone testosterone Nonmedical use is illegal; banned by major sports organizations	• Improve strength, power, and speed • Increase muscle mass	• In adolescents, stops bone growth; therefore reduces adult height • Masculinization of females; feminization of males • Mood swings • Severe acne, particularly on the back • Sexual dysfunction • Aggressive behavior • Potential heart and liver damage
Steroid precursors Substances that the body converts into anabolic steroids, e.g., androstenedione (andro), dehydroepiandrosterone (DHEA) Nonmedical use is illegal; banned by major sports organizations	• Converted in the body to anabolic steroids to increase muscle mass	• In addition to side effects noted with anabolic steroids: body hair growth, increased risk of pancreatic cancer
Human growth hormone Naturally occurring hormone secreted by the pituitary gland that is essential for body growth Nonmedical use is illegal; banned by major sports organizations	• Antiaging agent • Improve performance • Increase muscle mass	• Structural changes to the face • Increased risk of high blood pressure • Potential for congestive heart failure

Sources: Mayo Clinic Staff, "Performance-Enhancing Drugs and Your Teen Athlete," MayoClinic.com, August 2013, www.mayoclinic.com; Office of Diversion Control, Drug and Chemical Evaluation Section, "Drugs and Chemicals of Concern: Human Growth Hormone," August 2013, www.deadiversion.usdoj.gov; Office of Dietary Supplements, National Institutes of Health, "Ephedra and Ephedrine Alkaloids for Weight Loss and Athletic Performance," Reviewed July 2004, http://ods.od.nih.gov.

alcohol immediately before or during exercise also impairs judgment and motor coordination. After the workout, it's important to rehydrate with water (or other recovery fluids) and refuel first before drinking any alcohol.

Dietary Supplements

Today there is a burgeoning market for dietary supplements that claim to deliver the nutrients needed for muscle recovery, as well as some that include additional "performance-enhancing" ingredients. Supplements do not require FDA approval, and ingredients may cause side effects and interact with prescription medicines. See Table 1.5 for a list of some of the most popular performance-enhancing drugs and supplements, their purported benefits, and associated risks.

check yourself

- **What are some of the most important nutritional aspects of fitness?**
- **How does hydration affect exercise?**

1.13

Fitness-Related Injuries: Prevention and Treatment

learning outcome

1.13 Distinguish between traumatic injuries and overuse injuries, and discuss how to prevent common fitness-related injuries.

The two basic types of fitness-related injuries are traumatic and overuse injuries. **Traumatic injuries** occur suddenly and violently, typically by accident. Typical traumatic injuries are broken bones, torn ligaments and muscles, contusions, and lacerations.

Many traumatic injuries are unavoidable—for example, spraining your ankle by landing on another person's foot after jumping up for a rebound in basketball. Others are preventable through proper training, appropriate equipment and clothing, and common sense. If your traumatic injury causes a noticeable loss of function and immediate pain or pain that does not go away after 30 minutes, consult a physician.

Overtraining is the most frequent cause of injuries related to physical fitness training. Doing too much intense exercise, too much exercise without variation, or not allowing for sufficient rest and recovery time can increase the likelihood of **overuse injuries**. Overuse injuries occur because of the cumulative, day-after-day stresses placed on tendons, muscles, and joints.

Common Overuse Injuries

Common sites of overuse injuries are the hip, knee, shoulder, and elbow joints. Three of the most common overuse injuries are plantar fasciitis, shin splints, and runner's knee.

Plantar Fasciitis *Plantar fasciitis* is an inflammation of the plantar fascia, a broad band of dense, inelastic tissue (fascia) that runs from the heel to the toes on the bottom of your foot. The main function of the plantar fascia is to protect the nerves, blood vessels, and muscles of the foot from injury. In repetitive weight-bearing physical activities such as walking and running, the plantar fascia may become inflamed. Common symptoms are pain and tenderness under the ball of the foot, at the heel, or at both locations.[51] The pain of plantar fasciitis is particularly noticeable during your first steps in the morning. If not treated properly, this injury may progress to the point that weight-bearing activities are too painful to endure.

Shin Splints *Shin splints*, a general term for any pain that occurs on the front part of the lower legs, is used to describe more than 20 different medical conditions. The most common type of shin splints occurs along the inner side of the tibia and is usually a combination of muscle irritation and irritation of the tissues attaching the muscles to the bone. Specific pain on the tibia or on the fibula (the adjacent smaller bone) should be examined for a possible stress fracture.

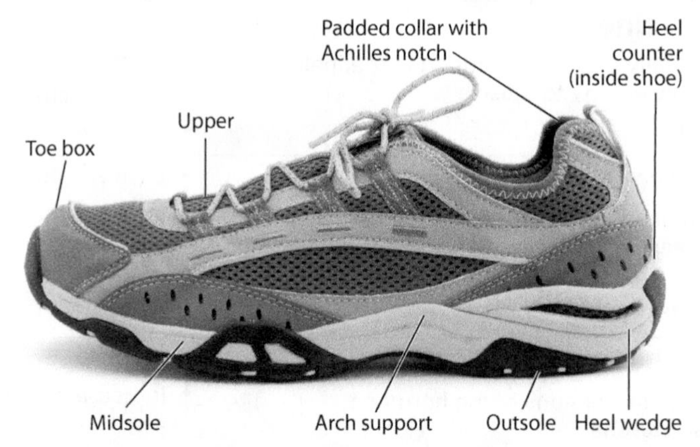

Figure 1.8 Anatomy of a Running Shoe
A good running shoe should fit comfortably; allow room for your toes to move; have a firm, but flexible, midsole; and have a firm grip on your heel to prevent slipping.

Sedentary people who start a new weight-bearing physical activity program are at the greatest risk for shin splints, although well-conditioned aerobic exercisers who rapidly increase their distance or pace may also be at risk.[52] Running and exercise classes are the most frequent cause of shin splints, but those who do a great deal of walking (such as postal carriers and restaurant workers) may also develop them.

Runner's Knee *Runner's knee* describes a series of problems involving the muscles, tendons, and ligaments of the knee. The most common cause is abnormal movements of the patella (kneecap). Women are more commonly affected because their wider pelvis results in a lateral pull on the patella by the muscles that act on the knee. In women (and some men), this causes irritation to cartilage on the back of the patella and to nearby tendons and ligaments. The main symptom is pain experienced when downward pressure is applied to the kneecap after the knee is straightened fully. Additional symptoms include pain, swelling, redness, and tenderness around the patella, and a dull aching pain in the center of the knee.[53]

Treatment of Fitness-Training Related Injuries

First-aid treatment for virtually all fitness-training related injuries involves **RICE**: rest, ice, compression, and elevation. *Rest* is required to avoid further irritation of the injured body part. *Ice* is applied to relieve pain and constrict the blood vessels to reduce internal or external bleeding. To prevent frostbite, wrap the ice or cold pack in a layer of wet toweling or

Applying ice to an injury such as a sprain can help relieve pain and reduce swelling, but never apply the ice directly to the skin, as that could lead to frostbite.

elastic bandage before applying to your skin. A new injury should be iced for approximately 20 minutes every hour for the first 24 to 72 hours. *Compression* of the injured body part can be accomplished with a 4- or 6-inch-wide elastic bandage; this applies indirect pressure to damaged blood vessels to help stop bleeding. Be careful, though, that the compression wrap does not interfere with normal blood flow. Throbbing or pain indicates that a compression wrap should be loosened. *Elevation* of an injured extremity above heart level also helps control internal or external bleeding by forcing the blood to flow upward to reach the injured area.

Preventing Injuries

Using common sense and identifying and using proper gear and equipment can help you avoid an injury. Varying your physical activities and setting appropriate and realistic short- and long-term goals will also help. It is important to listen to your body when working out. Warning signs include muscle stiffness and soreness, bone and joint pains, and whole-body fatigue that simply does not go away.

Appropriate Footwear Proper footwear decreases the likelihood of foot, knee, and back injuries. Biomechanics research has revealed that running is a collision sport—with each stride, a runner's foot collides with the ground with a force three to five times the runner's body weight.[54] Force not absorbed by a shoe is transmitted upward into the foot, leg, thigh, and back. Although our bodies can absorb forces such as these, they may be injured by the cumulative effect of repetitive impact. A shoe's ability to absorb shock is therefore critical—not just for runners, but for anyone engaged in weight-bearing activities.

In addition to providing shock absorption, an athletic shoe should provide a good fit for maximum comfort and performance (see Figure 1.8). To get the best fit, shop at a sports or fitness specialty store where there is a large selection to choose from and there are salespeople available who are trained in properly fitting athletic shoes. Because different activities place different stresses on your feet and joints, you should choose shoes specifically designed for your sport or activity. Shoes of any type should be replaced once they lose their cushioning.

Protective Equipment It is essential to use well-fitted, appropriate protective equipment for your physical activities. For some activities, that means choosing what is best for you and your body. For example, using the correct racquet with the proper tension helps prevent the general inflammatory condition known as tennis elbow. Likewise, eye injuries can occur in virtually all physical activities, although some activities (such as baseball, basketball, and racquet sports) are more risky than others.[55] As many as 90 percent of eye injuries could be prevented by wearing appropriate eye protection, such as goggles with polycarbonate lenses.[56]

Wearing a helmet while bicycle riding is an important safety precaution. An estimated 66 to 88 percent of head injuries among cyclists can be prevented by wearing a helmet.[57] Of the college students who rode a bike in the past 12 months, 39.2 percent reported never wearing a helmet, and 24 percent said they wore one only sometimes or rarely.[58] The direct medical costs from cyclists' failure to wear helmets is an estimated $81 million a year.[59] Cyclists aren't the only ones who should be wearing helmets—so should people who skateboard, use kick-scooters, ski, in-line skate, play contact sports, and snowboard. Look for helmets that meet standards established by the American National Standards Institute or the Snell Memorial Foundation.

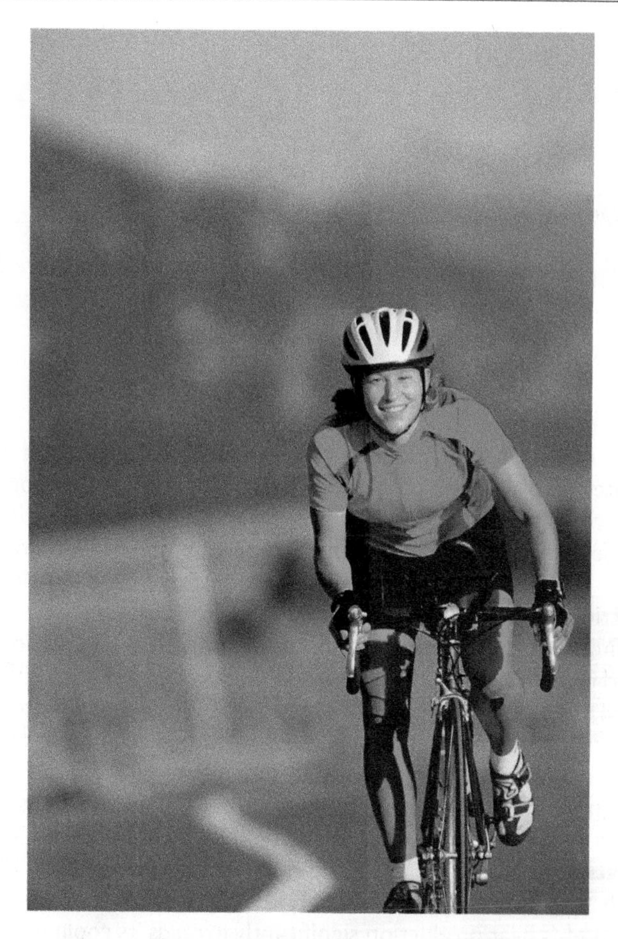

What can I do to avoid injury when I am physically active?

Reducing risk for exercise-related injuries requires common sense and some preventative measures. Wear protective gear, such as helmets, knee pads, elbow pads, eyewear, and supportive footwear, that is appropriate for your activity. Vary your activities to avoid overuse injuries. Dress for the weather, try to avoid exercising in extreme conditions, and always stay properly hydrated. Finally, respect your personal physical limitations, listen to your body, and respond effectively to it.

check yourself

- **What is the difference between traumatic injuries and overuse injuries?**
- **How can you prevent and treat fitness-related injuries?**

1.14 Exercising in the Heat and Cold

learning outcome

1.14 Describe signs and prevention of heat-related injuries and hypothermia.

Exercising in the Heat

Exercising in hot or humid weather increases the risk of a heat-related injury, in which the body's rate of heat production can exceed its ability to cool. The three heat stress illnesses, by increasing severity, are heat cramps, heat exhaustion, and heatstroke.

Heat cramps, heat-related involuntary and forcible muscle contractions that cannot be relaxed, can usually be prevented by intake of fluid and electrolytes lost during sweating. **Heat exhaustion** is a mild form of shock, in which blood pools in the arms and legs away from the brain and major organs, caused by excessive water loss because of intense or prolonged exercise or work in a hot and/or humid environment. Symptoms include nausea, headache, fatigue, dizziness and faintness, and, paradoxically, "goose bumps" and chills. In sufferers from heat exhaustion, the skin is cool and moist. **Heatstroke**, or *sunstroke*, is a life-threatening emergency condition with a high morbidity and mortality rate.[60] Heatstroke occurs when the body's heat production significantly exceeds its cooling capacities. Core body temperature can rise from normal (98.6°F) to 105°F to 110°F; this rapid increase can cause brain damage, permanent disability, or death. Common signs of heatstroke are dry, hot, and usually red skin; very high body temperature; and rapid heart rate. If you experience any of these symptoms, stop exercising immediately.

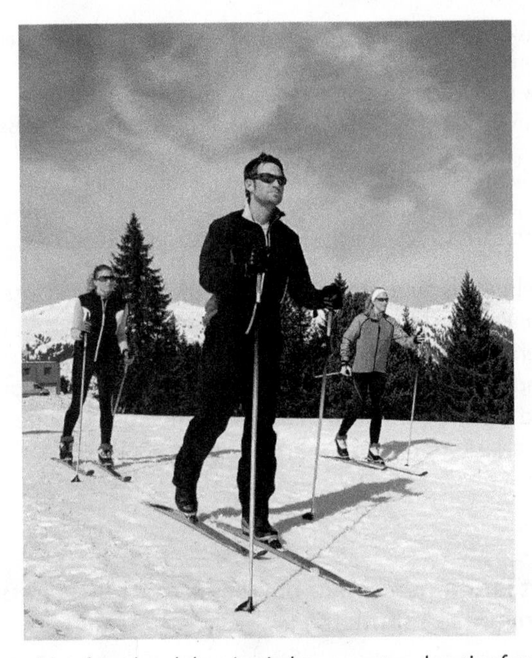

Staying with a friend and dressing in layers are two key tips for making cold weather exercise both safe and fun.

Move to the shade or a cool spot to rest, and drink plenty of cool fluids. If heatstroke is suspected, seek medical attention immediately.

Heat stress illnesses may also occur when the danger is not so obvious. Serious or fatal heat stroke may result from prolonged immersion in a sauna, hot tub, or steam bath or from exercising in a "sauna suit." Similarly, exercising in the heat with heavy clothing and equipment, such as a football uniform, puts one at risk.[61]

To prevent heat stress, follow certain precautions. If possible, acclimatize yourself to hot or humid climates through 10 to 14 days of gradually increased activity in the hot environment. Replace fluids before, during, and after exercise. Wear light, breathable clothing appropriate for the activity and environment. Use common sense—for example, when the temperature is 85°F and the humidity 80 percent, postpone a lunchtime run until evening when it is cooler.

Pay particular attention to your pets if you take them running or walking with you. Pets can quickly succumb to heatstroke and rely on you for hydration. They can also quickly burn their pads on hot pavement. Be responsible and take care of yourself and your pets.

Exercising in the Cold

When you exercise in cool weather, especially in windy conditions, your body's rate of heat loss is frequently greater than its rate of heat production. This may lead to **hypothermia**—a condition in which the body's core temperature drops below 95°F.[62] Hypothermia doesn't require frigid temperatures; it can result from prolonged, vigorous exercise in 40°F to 50°F temperatures, particularly if there is rain, snow, or strong wind.

As body core temperature drops from the normal 98.6°F to about 93.2°F, shivering begins, which increases body temperature using the heat given off by muscle activity. You may also experience cold hands and feet, poor judgment, apathy, and amnesia. Shivering ceases as core temperatures drop to between 87°F and 90°F, a sign the body has lost its ability to generate heat. Death usually occurs at body core temperatures between 75°F and 80°F.[63]

To prevent hypothermia, analyze weather conditions, including wind and humidity, before engaging in outdoor activity. Have a friend join you for cold-weather outdoor activities and wear layers of appropriate clothing to prevent excessive heat loss and frostbite. Keep your head, hands, and feet warm. Do not allow yourself to become dehydrated.

check yourself

- **What are the signs and treatment of heat cramps, heat exhaustion, and heatstroke?**
- **How can you prevent hypothermia?**

Smart Shopping for Fitness

learning outcome

1.15 List important factors to keep in mind when choosing fitness equipment, facilities, and clothing.

You can achieve your personal physical fitness goals without becoming a member of a fitness or wellness center, without buying equipment, and without spending lots of money on the latest fitness fashions. All you need is a good pair of shoes, comfortable clothing to suit the environment you will be physically active in, your own body to use as resistance, and a safe place for activity. However, you may enjoy the outing or experience created by going to a fitness or wellness center or prefer to have some exercise equipment in your home. The following will help guide your selections.

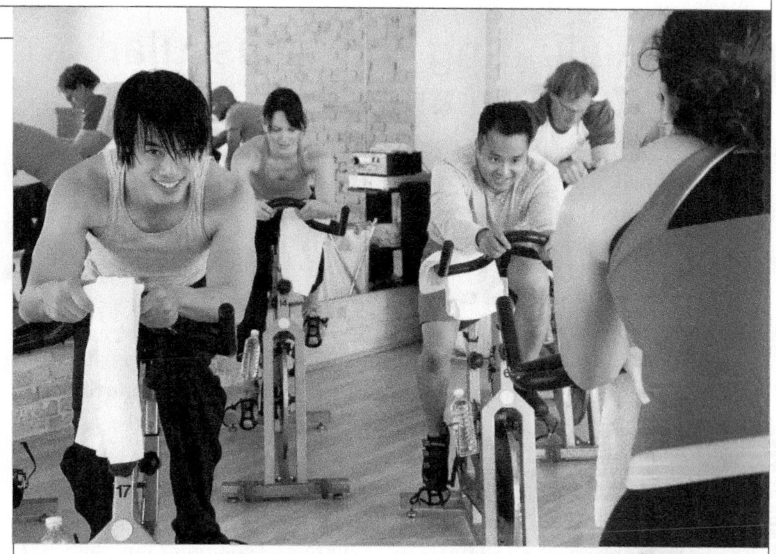

Before you sign on the dotted line, check out the classes, equipment, and personnel a fitness center offers.

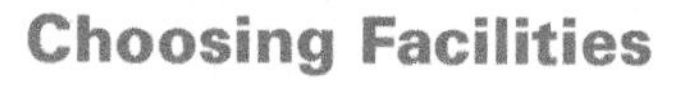

Choosing Facilities

- Visit several facilities before making a decision—and if possible during the time when you intend to use them (so you can see how busy or crowded they are at that time).
- Determine the hours of operation. Are they convenient for you?
- Consider the exercise classes offered. What is the schedule? Can you try one for free? Are classes included in the price of membership or do they cost extra?
- Consider the equipment. Is it sufficient to cover your training needs (e.g., aerobic exercise machines; resistance-training equipment, including both free weights and machines; mats; and other items to assist with stretching)? Is it kept clean and in good condition? Do they offer instruction in how to use the equipment?
- Consider the locker room. Is it kept clean? Are there lockers free for your use if you need them?
- Consider the location. How convenient is it (e.g., on your way to or from work or school, close to your home)?
- Consider the personnel (including their training in first aid and CPR), options for working with a personal trainer, and how friendly and approachable staff members are.
- Consider the financial implications. What membership benefits, student rates, or other discounts are available? Will they hold your membership for the summer, so you do not have to continue paying if you are not attending school in the area? Steer clear of clubs that pressure you for a long-term commitment and do not offer trial memberships or grace periods that allow you to get a refund.

Buying Equipment

- Ignore claims that an exercise device provides lasting "no-sweat" results in a short time.
- Question claims that an exercise device can target or burn fat or lead to miracle cures for "cellulite."
- Be skeptical of testimonials and before-and-after pictures of satisfied customers.
- Calculate the cost including shipping and handling fees, sales tax, delivery and setup charges, or long-term commitments.
- Obtain details on warranties, guarantees, and return policies.
- Consider how this piece of equipment will fit in your home. Where will you store it? Will you be able to get to it easily?
- Check out consumer reports or online resources for the best product ratings and reviews.

Buying Exercise Clothing

- Choose your exercise clothing based on comfort, not looks. It should be neither too loose nor too tight.
- Invest in a good pair of sneakers.
- Consider the environment (temperature, humidity, ventilation) when making your selection.
- Choose clothing that helps you to feel good about yourself and the activity you are undertaking.

check yourself

- **What should you keep in mind when choosing fitness equipment, facilities, and clothing?**
- **Which of these factors are most important to you?**

Assessyourself

1.16

How Physically Fit Are You?

An interactive version of this assessment is available online in MasteringHealth.

1 Evaluating Your Muscular Strength and Endurance (the 1-Minute Curl-Up Test)

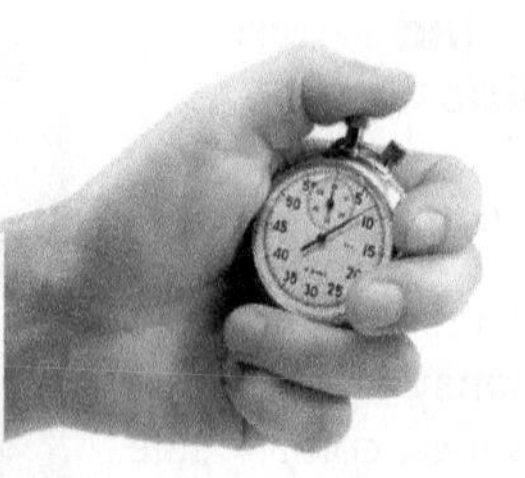

Your abdominal muscles are important for core stability and back support; this test will assess their muscular endurance.

Description/Procedure:

Lie on a mat with your arms by your sides, palms flat on the mat, elbows straight, and fingers extended. Bend your knees at a 90-degree angle. Your instructor or partner will mark your starting finger position with a piece of masking tape aligned with the tip of each middle finger. He or she will also mark with tape your ending position, 10 cm or 3 inches away from the first piece of tape, with one ending position tape for each hand.

Set a metronome to 50 beats per minute and curl up at this slow, controlled pace: one curl-up every two beats (25 curl-ups per minute). Curl your head and upper back upward, lifting your shoulder blades off the mat (your trunk should make a 30-degree angle with the mat) and reaching your arms forward along the mat to touch the ending tape. Then curl back down so that your upper back and shoulders touch the floor. During the entire curl-up, your fingers, feet, and buttocks should stay on the mat. Your partner will count the number of correct repetitions you complete. Perform as many curl-ups as you can in 1 minute without pausing, to a maximum of 25.

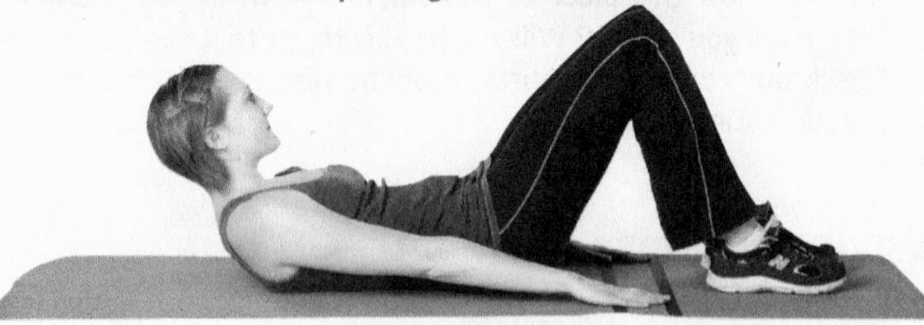

Healthy Musculoskeletal Fitness: Norms and Health Benefit Zones: Curl-Ups

Men	Excellent	Very Good	Good	Fair	Needs Improvement
Ages 20–29	25	21–24	16–20	11–15	≤ 10
Ages 30–39	25	18–24	15–17	11–14	≤ 10
Ages 40–49	25	18–24	13–17	6–12	≤ 5
Ages 50–59	25	17–24	11–16	8–10	≤ 7
Ages 60–69	25	16–24	11–15	6–10	≤ 5
Women	**Excellent**	**Very Good**	**Good**	**Fair**	**Needs Improvement**
Ages 20–29	25	18–24	14–17	5–13	≤ 4
Ages 30–39	25	19–24	10–18	6–9	≤ 5
Ages 40–49	25	19–24	11–18	4–10	≤ 3
Ages 50–59	25	19–24	10–18	6–9	≤ 5
Ages 60–69	25	17–24	8–16	3–7	≤ 2

Source: Adapted from *Canadian Physical Activity, Fitness & Lifestyle Approach: CSEP-Health & Fitness Program's Appraisal and Counselling Strategy*, 3rd edition, © 2003. Reprinted with permission from the Canadian Society for Exercise Physiology.

2 Evaluating Your Flexibility (the Sit-and-Reach Test)

This test measures the general flexibility of your lower back, hips, and hamstring muscles.

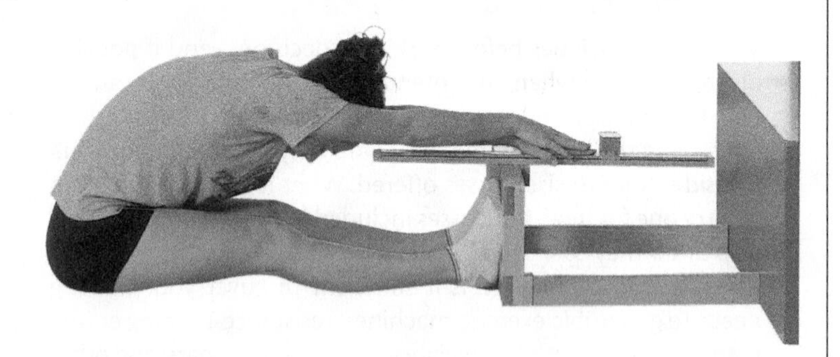

Description/Procedure:

Warm up with some light activity that involves the total body and range-of-motion exercises and stretches for the lower back and hamstrings. For the test, start by sitting upright, straight-legged on a mat with your shoes removed and soles of the feet flat against the flexometer (sit-and-reach box) at the 26-cm mark. Inner edges of the soles are placed within 2 cm of the measuring scale.

Have a partner on hand to record your measurements. Stretch your arms out in front of you and, keeping the hands parallel to each other, slowly reach forward with both hands as far as possible, holding the position for approximately 2 seconds. Your fingertips should be in contact with the measuring portion (meter stick) of the sit-and-reach box. To facilitate a longer reach, exhale and drop your head between your arms while reaching forward. Keep your knees extended the whole time and breathe normally.

Your score is the most distant point (in centimeters) reached with the fingertips; have your partner make note of this number for you. Perform the test twice, record your best score, and compare it with the norms presented in the tables.

Healthy Musculoskeletal Fitness: Norms and Health Benefit Zones: Sit-and-Reach Test

Men	Excellent	Very Good	Good	Fair	Needs Improvement	Women	Excellent	Very Good	Good	Fair	Needs Improvement
Ages 20–29	≥ 40 cm	34–39 cm	30–33 cm	25–29 cm	≤ 24 cm	Ages 20–29	≥ 41 cm	37–40 cm	33–36 cm	28–32 cm	≤ 27 cm
Ages 30–39	≥ 38 cm	33–37 cm	28–32 cm	23–27 cm	≤ 22 cm	Ages 30–39	≥ 41 cm	36–40 cm	32–35 cm	27–31 cm	≤ 26 cm
Ages 40–49	≥ 35 cm	29–34 cm	24–28 cm	18–23 cm	≤ 17 cm	Ages 40–49	≥ 38 cm	34–37 cm	30–33 cm	25–29 cm	≤ 24 cm
Ages 50–59	≥ 35 cm	28–34 cm	24–27 cm	16–23 cm	≤ 15 cm	Ages 50–59	≥ 39 cm	33–38 cm	30–32 cm	25–29 cm	≤ 24 cm
Ages 60–69	≥ 33 cm	25–32 cm	20–24 cm	15–19 cm	≤ 14 cm	Ages 60–69	≥ 35 cm	31–34 cm	27–30 cm	23–26 cm	≤ 22 cm

Note: These norms are based on a sit-and-reach box in which the zero point is set at 26 cm. When using a box in which the zero point is set at 23 cm, subtract 3 cm from each value in this table.

Source: Adapted from *Canadian Physical Activity, Fitness & Lifestyle Approach: CSEP-Health & Fitness Program's Appraisal and Counselling Strategy*, 3rd edition, © 2003. Reprinted with permission from the Canadian Society for Exercise Physiology.

3 Evaluating Your Cardiorespiratory Fitness (the 1-Mile Walk Test)

The 1-mile walk test assesses your cardiorespiratory fitness level.

Description/Procedure:

The objective of this test is to walk 1 mile as quickly as possible. This walk can be completed on an oval track or any properly measured course using a stopwatch to measure the time used. Do not eat a heavy meal for at least 2 to 3 hours prior to the test. Be sure to warm-up for 5 to 10 minutes before the test. It is best to pace yourself on this test and choose a pace/speed you think you can continue for the entire test. If you become extremely fatigued during the test, slow your pace—do not overstress yourself! If you feel faint or nauseated or experience any unusual pains in your upper body, stop and notify your instructor. Upon completion of the test, cool down and record your time and fitness category from the table below.

Cardiorespiratory Fitness Categories: 1-Mile Run Test (min)

	Fitness Category						Fitness Category				
Men	Very Poor	Poor	Average	Good	Excellent	Women	Very Poor	Poor	Average	Good	Excellent
Ages 13–19	>17:30	16:01–17:30	14:01–16:00	12:30–14:00	<12:30	Ages 13–19	>18:01	16:31–18:00	14:31–16:30	13:31–14:30	< 13:30
Ages 20–29	>18:01	16:31–18:00	14:31–16:30	13:00–14:30	< 13:00	Ages 20–29	>18:31	17:01–18:30	15:01–17:00	13:31–15:00	< 13:30
Ages 30–39	>19:00	17:31–19:00	15:31–17:30	13:30–15:30	< 13:30	Ages 30–39	>19:31	18:01–19:30	16:01–18:00	14:01–16:00	< 14:00
Ages 40+	>21:30	18:31–21:30	16:01–18:30	14:00–16:00	< 14:00	Ages 40+	>20:01	19:31–20:00	18:01–19:30	14:31–18:00	< 14:30

Source: Adapted from *Rockport Walking Fitness Test*. Copyright © 1993 by The Rockport Company, LLC. Reprinted with permission.

Your Plan for Change

The Assess Yourself activity helped you determine your current level of physical fitness. Based on your results, you may decide to improve one or more components of your physical fitness.

Today, you can:

- ◯ Visit your campus fitness facility and familiarize yourself with the equipment and resources.
- ◯ Walk between your classes; make an extra effort to take the long way to get from building to building. Use the stairs instead of the elevator.
- ◯ Take a stretch break. Spend 5 to 10 minutes between homework projects doing some stretches to release tension.

Within the next 2 weeks, you can:

- ◯ Shop for comfortable workout clothes and appropriate athletic footwear.
- ◯ Ask a friend to join you in your workout once a week. Agree on a date and time in advance so you'll both be committed to following through.
- ◯ Plan for a physically active outing with a friend or date; go dancing or bowling. Use active transportation (e.g., walk or cycle) to get to a movie.

By the end of the semester, you can:

- ◯ Establish a regular routine of engaging in physical activity or exercise at least three times a week. Mark your exercise times on your calendar and keep a log to track your progress.
- ◯ Take your workouts to the next level. If you are walking, perhaps try intermittent jogging or sign up for a fitness event such as a charity 5K.

Summary

To hear an MP3 Tutor session, scan here or visit the Study Area in **MasteringHealth**.

LO 1.1 Physical fitness involves achieving minimal levels in the health-related components of fitness: cardiorespiratory, muscular strength, muscular endurance, flexibility, and body composition. Skill-related components of fitness, such as agility, balance, reaction time, speed, coordination, and power, are essential for elite and recreational athletes to increase performance and enjoyment in sport.

LO 1.2 Benefits of regular physical activity include reduced risk of heart attack, some cancers, hypertension, and type 2 diabetes and improved blood profile, bone mass, weight control, immunity, mental health and stress management, and physical fitness. Regular physical activity can also increase life span.

LO 1.3 Commit to your lifestyle of physical activity and increased fitness levels by incorporating fitness activities into your life. If you are new to exercise, start slowly, keep your fitness program simple, and consider consulting your physician and/or a fitness instructor for recommendations. Overcome your barriers or obstacles to exercise by identifying them and then planning specific strategies to address them.

LO 1.4 Fitness gadgets and equipment can encourage you to stay motivated and provide opportunities to try different types of exercises and movements.

LO 1.5 Planning to improve fitness involves setting SMART goals and designing a program to achieve them. The FITT principle can be used to develop a progressive program of physical fitness.

LO 1.6 For general health benefits, every adult should participate in moderate-intensity activities for 30 minutes at least 5 days a week. To improve cardiorespiratory fitness, engage in vigorous, continuous, and rhythmic activities 3 to 5 days per week.

LO 1.7 Three key principles for developing muscular strength and endurance are overload, specificity of training, and variation. Muscular strength and muscular endurance are improved via resistance-training exercises multiple times per week.

LO 1.8 Flexibility is improved by engaging in two to three repetitions of static stretching exercises at least 2 to 3 days a week.

LO 1.9 A regular comprehensive workout should include a warm-up with light stretching, strength-development exercises, aerobic activities, and a cool-down period with a heavier emphasis on stretching. A fitness program should be appropriate and realistic to the individual's skill level.

LO 1.10 Core strength training is important for maintaining full mobility and stability and for preventing back injury.

LO 1.11 Individuals with special conditions, such as asthma, heart disease, and diabetes, should consult with a physician before beginning an exercise program. Obese individuals need to take precautions to avoid excessive heat and musculoskeletal injuries. Non-weight-bearing activities are recommended for older adults.

LO 1.12 Fueling properly for exercise involves eating a balance of healthy foods 3 to 4 hours before exercise. Hydrating properly for exercise is important for performance and injury prevention.

LO 1.13–1.15 Fitness training injuries are generally caused by overuse or trauma. Proper footwear and equipment can help prevent injuries. Exercise in the heat or cold requires special precautions.

Pop Quiz

Visit MasteringHealth to personalize your study plan with Chapter Review Quizzes and Dynamic Study Modules.

LO 1.1 1. The maximum volume of oxygen consumed by the muscles during exercise defines
a. target heart rate.
b. muscular strength.
c. aerobic capacity.
d. muscular endurance.

LO 1.1 2. Flexibility is the range of motion around
a. specific bones.
b. a joint or series of joints.
c. the tendons.
d. the muscles.

LO 1.3 3. Theresa wants to lower her ratio of fat to her total body weight. She wants to work on her
a. flexibility.
b. muscular endurance.
c. muscular strength.
d. body composition.

LO 1.1 4. Miguel is a runner able to sustain moderate-intensity, whole-body activity for an extended time. This ability relates to what component of physical fitness?
a. Flexibility
b. Body composition
c. Cardiorespiratory fitness
d. Muscular strength and endurance

LO 1.6 5. The "talk test" measures
a. exercise intensity.
b. exercise time.
c. exercise frequency.
d. exercise duration.

LO 1.6 6. An example of aerobic exercise is
a. brisk walking.
b. bench-pressing weights.
c. stretching exercises.
d. holding yoga poses.

LO 1.7 7. Isabella has been lifting 95 pounds while doing leg curls. To become stronger, she began lifting 105 pounds while doing leg curls. What principle of strength development does this represent?
a. Reversibility
b. Overload
c. Strain increase
d. Specificity of training

LO 1.10 8. Which of the following includes sequences of movements specifically designed to increase strength?
a. Pilates
b. Ashtanga yoga
c. Tai chi
d. Bikram yoga

LO 1.11 9. People with type 2 diabetes
a. should not engage in physical activity.
b. should avoid weight-bearing activities.
c. should limit physical activity to 30 minutes a day or less.
d. can improve blood glucose levels through physical activity.

LO 1.13 10. Overuse injuries can be prevented by
a. monitoring quantity and quality of workouts.
b. engaging in only one type of aerobic training.
c. working out daily.
d. working out with a friend.

Answers to these questions can be found on page A-1. If you answered a question incorrectly, review the module identified by the Learning Outcome. For even more study tools, visit MasteringHealth.

Weight Management and Body Image

2

The keys to weight management sound simple enough: Eat too many calories without exercising and you will gain weight; reduce calories and increase exercise, and the pounds will slide right off. But if all it took were eating less and exercising more, Americans would merely reevaluate their diets, cut calories, and exercise. Unfortunately, it's not that easy. And the problem goes beyond body weight to increasingly common issues of self-perception and disordered eating, among both men and women.

What factors predispose us to problems with weight? Although diet and exercise are clearly major contributors, genetics and physiology are also important. Learned behaviors in the home and influences at school, in social environments, in the media, and in the environments where we live, work, and play are all important to our weight profiles.[1] Experts realize that a complex web of interactive factors influences what we eat, how much we eat, and when we eat, as well as how we expend energy. Figuring out what these factors are and developing key strategies to reduce risk are key.[2]

2.1 Obesity in the United States and Worldwide

learning outcome

2.1 Examine obesity trends in the United States.

The United States currently has the dubious distinction of being among the fattest nations on Earth. Young and old, rich and poor, rural and urban, educated and uneducated Americans share one thing in common—they are fatter than virtually all previous generations.[3]

The word **obesogenic**, meaning characterized by environments that promote increased food intake, nonhealthful foods, and physical inactivity, has increasingly become an apt descriptor of our society. The maps in Figure 2.1 illustrate the rapidly increasing levels of obesity in the United States over the last two decades. Indeed, the prevalence of obesity has tripled among children and doubled among adults in recent decades.[4] While previous research has shown some stabilization in overweight and obesity rates between 2003–2004 and 2011–2012, current rates are still extremely high. More than 68 percent of U.S. adults overall (over 170 million people) are *overweight* (have a body mass index [BMI] of 25.0–29.9) or obese (have a BMI of 30.0 or higher).[5] Rates of obesity are 34.4 percent among men and 36.1 among women, with rates of extreme obesity on the rise.[6] This has staggering implications for increased risks from heart disease, diabetes, and other health complications associated with obesity.

A bright spot in the obesity profile appears to be among the very youngest populations. Rates for 2- to 5-year-olds have dropped significantly, from a high of nearly 14 percent in 2003–2004 to just over 8 percent in 2011–2012.[7] Possible reasons for this include greater public awareness; more options for healthy foods in child care centers, restaurants, and grocery stores; improved labeling; improvements in physical activity programs; and decreases in sugar consumption.

Research points to higher obesity rates and risks among some ethnic groups. Mexican American men (81 percent) and non-Hispanic whites (73 percent) are more likely to be overweight/obese than non-Hispanic blacks (69 percent). Non-Hispanic black women (80 percent) and Mexican-American women (78 percent) are more likely to be overweight or obese than are non-Hispanic white women (60 percent). In sharp contrast, nearly 58 percent of Asian populations are at a healthy weight.[8] Of youth aged 2 to 19, over 39 percent of Hispanics, Mexican Americans, and non-Hispanic blacks, as well as nearly 28 percent of non-Hispanic whites, are overweight/obese. Low parental education, low-income, and higher unemployment are related to increased risk of overweight/obesity in youth.[9]

The United States is not alone in the obesity epidemic. In fact, overweight and obesity have become the fifth leading risks for global death, and nearly 1.5 billion adults aged 20 and over and 40 million children under the age of 5 are overweight/obese.[10] While obesity was once predominantly a problem in high-income countries, today, increasing numbers of low- and middle-income countries have overweight/obesity problems.[11] The global epidemic of high rates of overweight and obesity in multiple regions of the world has come to be known as **globesity**.

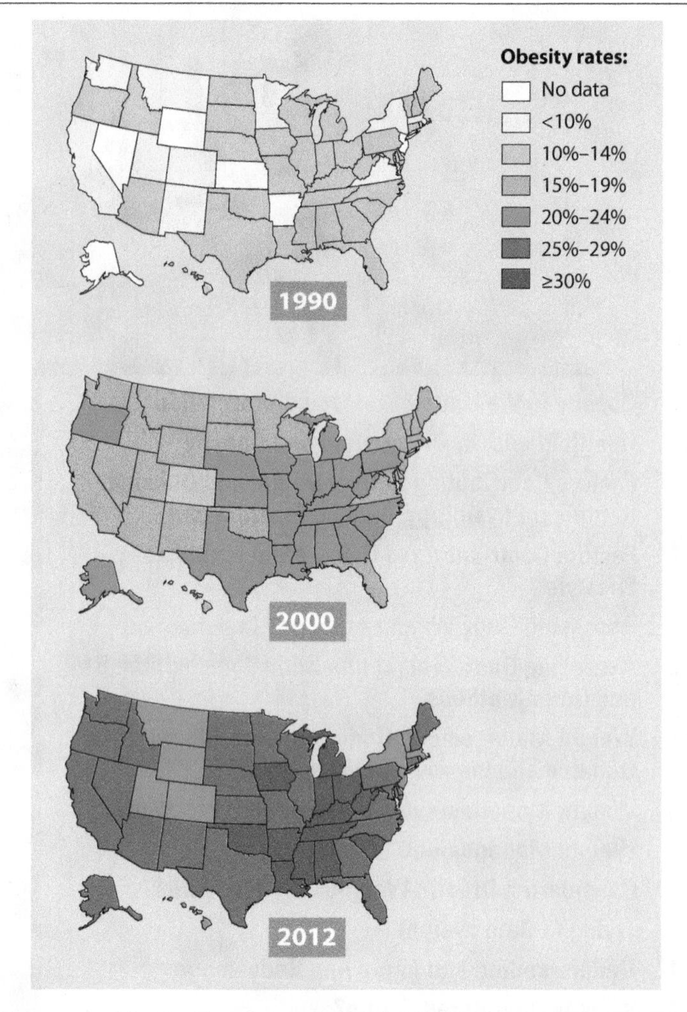

Figure 2.1 Obesity Trends among U.S. Adults, 1990, 2000, and 2012

Sources: Centers for Disease Control and Prevention (CDC), "U.S. Obesity Trends: 1999–2010," 2012, www.cdc.gov; CDC, "Prevalence of Self-Reported Obesity among U.S. Adults," 2013, www.cdc.gov.

Note: Historical maps are provided for reference only, as differences in the analysis of prevalence rates for 2012 make direct comparisons to previous years incompatible.

check yourself

- **How have levels of obesity changed in the United States over the last two decades?**
- **Why do you think disparities in obesity levels exist among certain populations in the United States?**

2.2

Health Effects of Overweight and Obesity

learning outcome

2.2 List health effects associated with overweight and obesity.

Although smoking is still the leading cause of preventable death in the United States, obesity is rapidly gaining ground on this killer as associated health problems soar. Cardiovascular disease (CVD), stroke, cancer, hypertension, diabetes, depression, digestive problems, gallstones, sleep apnea, osteoarthritis, and other ailments lead the list of life-threatening, weight-related problems. Diabetes, strongly associated with overweight and obesity, is another major concern. Nearly 26 million Americans have diabetes and another 79 million adults have prediabetes.[12] Figure 2.2 summarizes these and other potential health consequences of obesity.

Short- and long-term health consequences of obesity are not our only concern: According to new estimates, obesity accounts for nearly 21 percent of U.S. health care costs, more than double previous estimates. Morbidly obese individuals may cost between $6,500 and $15,000 more per year in additional health care costs when factors such as longer hospital stays, recovery, and increased medications are included.[13] Of course, it is impossible to place a dollar value on a life lost prematurely due to diabetes, stroke, or heart attack or to assess the cost of the social isolation of and discrimination against overweight individuals. Of growing importance is the recognition that obese individuals suffer significant disability during their lives, in terms of both mobility and activities of daily living.[14]

Other effects of overweight and obesity can be more subtle. Consequences can include depression, anxiety, low self-esteem, poor body image, and suicidal acts and thoughts; binge eating and unhealthy weight-control practices; lack of adequate health care due to doctors spending less time with and doing fewer interventions on overweight patients and doctor reluctance to perform preventive health screenings; and reluctance to visit the doctor and get necessary preventive health care services.

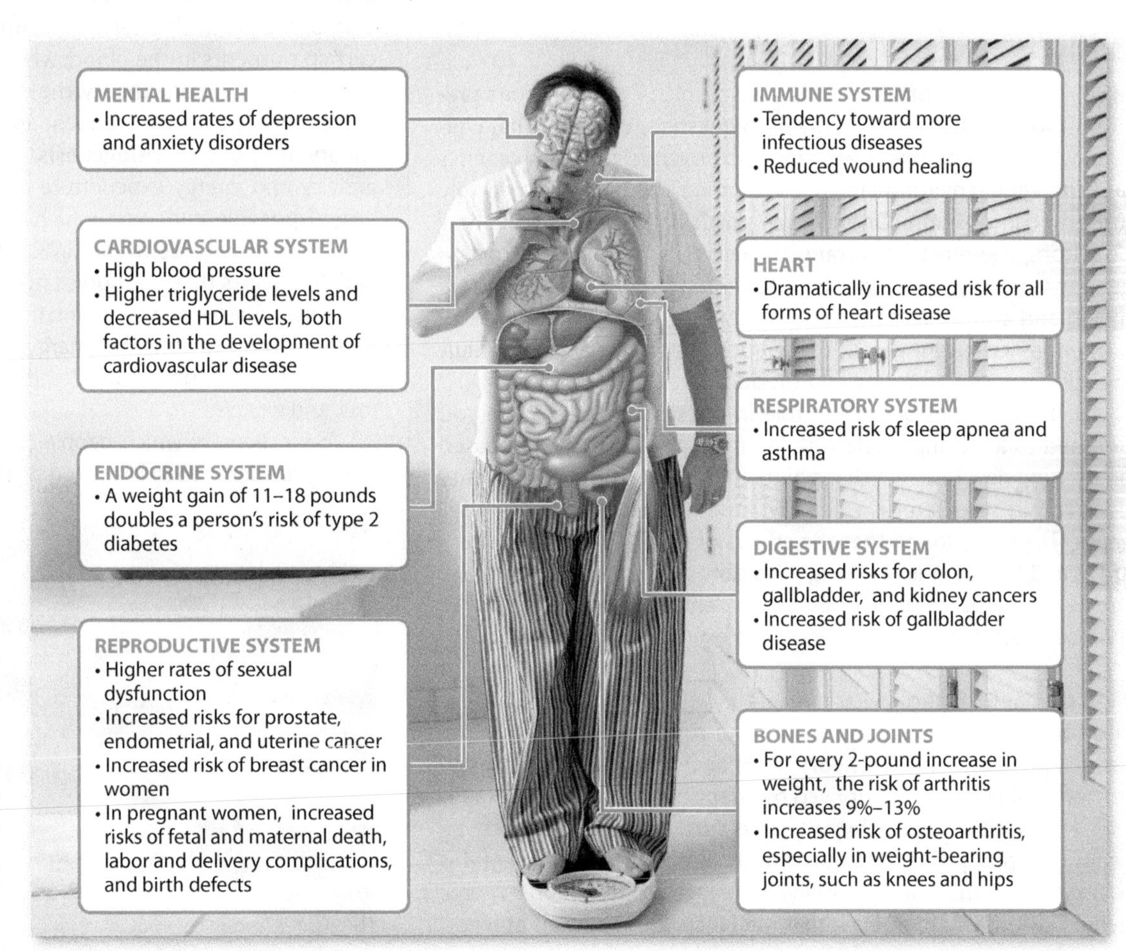

Figure 2.2 Potential Negative Health Effects of Overweight and Obesity

VIDEO TUTOR
Obesity Health Effects

check yourself

- **What are some potential effects on the body of overweight and obesity?**
- **Do you consider the most significant consequences of overweight and obesity to be physical, financial, emotional, or other?**

2.3 Factors Contributing to Overweight and Obesity: Genetics, Physiology, and the Environment

learning outcome

2.3 Explain the impact of genetics, physiology, and environment on body weight.

Several factors appear to influence why one person becomes obese and another remains thin.

Body Type and Genes

In spite of decades of research, the exact role of genes in one's predisposition toward obesity remains in question. We know that children whose parents are obese tend to be overweight. Both genetics and the gene–environment interaction are thought to play a role in body composition. One gene in particular, the *FTO gene,* may be among the most important.[15] Specifically, people with certain genetic variations may tend to graze for food more often, eat more meals, and consume more calories every day. Also, different genes may influence weight gain at certain periods of life, particularly during adolescence and young adulthood.[16]

So, if your genes play a key role in obesity tendencies, are you doomed to a lifelong battle with your weight? Probably not, based on exciting new research that points to the fact that even if obesity does run in your family, a healthy lifestyle can override "obesity" genes. The study found that the effects of the *FTO* gene on obesity are over 30 percent less among physically active adults. Those who seemed to be beating their obesity tendencies exercised at least 90 minutes a day compared to those who exercised 30 minutes.[17]

Thrifty Gene Theory Researchers have noted higher body fat and obesity levels in certain Indian and African tribes than in the general population.[18] The theory: Their ancestors struggled through centuries of famine and survived by adapting with slowed metabolism. If this "thrifty gene" hypothesis is true, certain people may be genetically programmed to burn fewer calories. Today, critics of this theory believe that there are many other factors, such as obesogenic behaviors and environments, that influence obesity development.

Physiological Factors

Metabolic Rates Although number of calories consumed is important, metabolism also helps determine weight. The **basal metabolic rate (BMR)** is the minimum rate at which the body uses energy when working to maintain basic vital functions. BMR for the average healthy adult is 1,200 to 1,800 calories per day.

The **resting metabolic rate (RMR)** includes the BMR plus any energy expended through daily sedentary activities such as food digestion, sitting, studying, or standing. The **exercise metabolic rate (EMR)** accounts for all remaining daily calorie expenditures. For most of us, these calories come from activities such as walking, climbing stairs, and mowing the lawn.

In general, the younger you are, the higher your BMR. Growth consumes a good deal of energy, and BMR is highest during infancy, puberty, and pregnancy. After age 30, a person's BMR slows down by 1 to 2 percent a year. Less activity, shifting priorities from fitness to family and career, and loss in muscle mass also contribute to weight gain in many middle-aged people.

Theories abound concerning mechanisms regulating metabolism and food intake. Some sources indicate that the hypothalamus (the part of the brain that regulates appetite) closely monitors levels of certain nutrients in the blood; when they fall, the brain signals us to eat. According to one theory, the monitoring system in obese people makes cues to eat more frequent and intense than in others. Another theory, **adaptive thermogenesis**, suggests the brain slows metabolic activity and energy expenditure as a form of defensive protection against possible starvation, which makes weight loss difficult.[19]

On the other side of the BMR equation is the **set point theory**, which suggests that our bodies fight to maintain our weight around a narrow range or at a set point. If we go on a drastic diet, our bodies slow our BMR to conserve energy. The good news is that set points can be changed, slowly and steadily, via healthy diet, steady weight loss, and exercise.

Yo-yo diets, in which people repeatedly gain weight then lose it quickly, are doomed to fail. When such dieters resume eating, their BMR

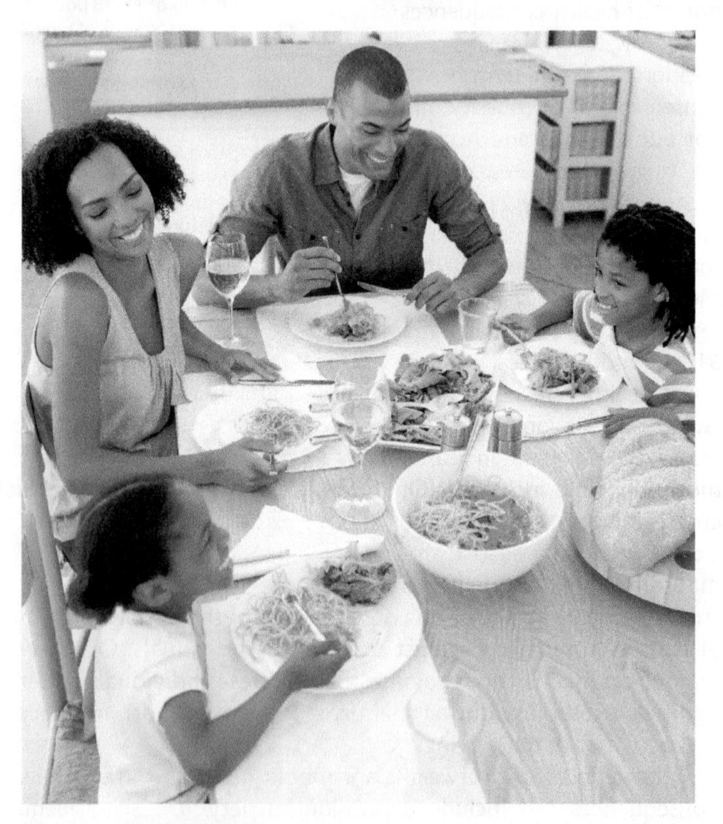

Do my genes affect my weight?
Many factors help determine weight and body type, including heredity and genetic makeup, environment, and learned eating patterns, which are often connected to family habits.

is set lower, making them almost certain to regain lost pounds. After repeated gains and losses, such people find it increasingly hard to lose weight and easy to regain it.

Hormonal Influences: Ghrelin and Leptin Obese people may be more likely than thin people to eat for reasons other than nutrition.[20] Many people have attributed obesity to problems with the thyroid gland and resultant hormone imbalances that impede the ability to burn calories. Although less than 2 percent of the obese population have a thyroid problem and can trace their weight problems to a metabolic or hormone imbalance,[21] hormones may still affect one's weight.

Problems with overconsumption may be related to **satiety**—the feeling of fullness when nutritional needs are satisfied and the stomach signals "no more." Researchers suspect that *ghrelin*, sometimes referred to as "the hunger hormone," influences satiety.[22] Ghrelin helps regulate appetite, food intake control, gastrointestinal motility, gastric acid secretion, endocrine and exocrine pancreatic secretions, glucose and lipid metabolism, and cardiovascular and immunological processes.[23] Another hormone, *leptin*, is produced by fat cells; its levels in the blood increase as fat tissue increases. Scientists believe leptin signals when you are getting full, slows food intake, and promotes energy expenditure.[24] When levels of leptin in the blood rise, appetite levels drop. Although obese people have adequate leptin and leptin receptors, the receptors do not seem to work properly—though why remains a mystery. It may be simply that environmental cues are stronger than our hunger pangs.

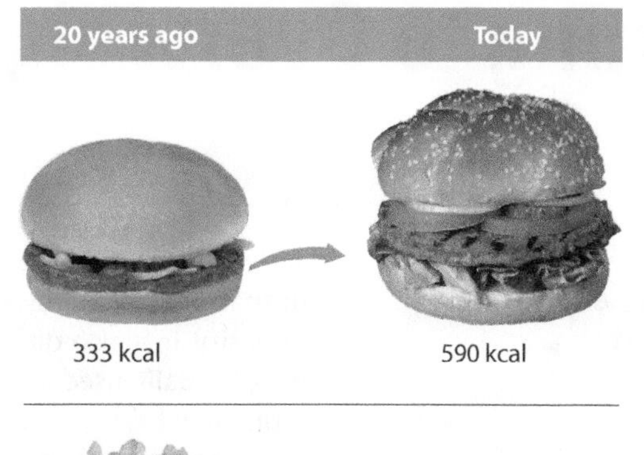

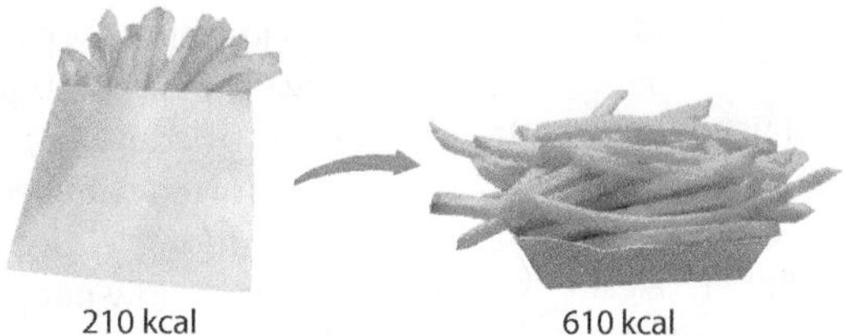

Figure 2.3 Today's Bloated Portions
The increase in average portion sizes has made it tougher than ever to manage your weight.
Source: Data are from the National Institutes of Health/National Heart, Lung, and Blood Institute (NHLBI), "Portion Distortion!," Updated February 2013, www.nhlbi.nih.gov.

Fat Cells and Predisposition to Fatness Some obese people may have excessive numbers of fat cells. An average-weight adult has approximately 25 to 35 billion fat cells, a moderately obese adult 60 to 100 billion, and an extremely obese adult as many as 200 billion.[25] This type of obesity, **hyperplasia**, usually appears in early childhood and perhaps, due to the mother's dietary habits, even prior to birth. Critical periods for development of hyperplasia are the last 2 to 3 months of fetal development, the first year of life, and from ages 9 to 13. Central to this theory is the belief that the number of fat cells in a body does not increase appreciably during adulthood. However, the ability of each cell to swell (**hypertrophy**) and shrink does carry over into adulthood. Weight gain may be tied to both the number of fat cells and the capacity of individual cells to enlarge.

Environmental Factors

Automobiles, remote controls, desk jobs, and computer use all lead us to sit more and move less; our culture also urges us to eat more. Combined, these environmental influences are a clear recipe for weight gain.

- We are bombarded with advertising for high-calorie foods at a low price and marketing of super-sized portions. Standard portions have increased dramatically in the past 20 years (Figure 2.3).
- Access to prepackaged, high-fat meals; fast food; and sugar-laden soft drinks are increasingly widespread, as are high-calorie coffee drinks and energy drinks.
- As society eats out more, higher-calorie, high-fat foods become the norm.
- Bottle-feeding infants may increase energy intake relative to breast-feeding.
- Misleading food labels confuse consumers about portion and serving sizes.

A Youthful Start on Obesity Children have always loved junk food. However, today's youth have easy access to a vast array of high-fat, high-calorie foods, have fewer physical education requirements in schools, and are more obese than ever before. Maternal nutrition, diabetes, and obesity may predispose children to overweight or obesity prior to puberty and early onset puberty.[26] Race and ethnicity also seem to be intricately interwoven with environmental factors in increasing risks to young people.[27]

Skills for Behavior Change

BEWARE OF PORTION DISTORTION

To make sure you're not overeating when you dine out, follow these strategies:

- **Order the smallest size available. Focus on taste, not quantity.**
- **Take your time, and let your fullness indicator have a chance to kick in while there is still time to quit.**
- **Dip your food in dressings, gravies, and sauces on the side rather than pour extra calories over the top.**
- **Order a healthy appetizer as your main meal along with a small side salad or veggie side.**
- **Split an entrée with a friend. Alternately, put half of your meal in a take-out box immediately, and finish the rest at the restaurant.**
- **Avoid buffets and all-you-can-eat establishments. If you go to them, use small plates and fill them with salads, veggies, and other high-protein, low-calorie, low-fat options.**

check yourself

- **What are the influences of genetics, physiology, and environment on body weight? Which do you consider most important?**
- **How does the importance of genetics and physiology affect strategies for weight management?**

2.4 Factors Contributing to Overweight and Obesity: Lifestyle

learning outcome

2.4 Explain the impact of psychosocial, economic, and lifestyle factors on body weight.

Psychosocial and Economic Factors

The relationship of weight problems to emotional needs and wants remains uncertain. Food often is used as a reward for good behavior in childhood. For adults facing economic and interpersonal stress, the bright spot in the day is often "what's for dinner." Again, the research here is controversial. What is certain is that eating is a social ritual associated with companionship, celebration, and enjoyment.

Socioeconomic factors can also affect weight control. When economic times are tough, people tend to eat more inexpensive, high-calorie processed foods. People living in poverty may have less access to fresh, nutrient-dense foods and have less time to cook nutritious meals due to shiftwork, longer commutes, or multiple jobs.[28] Unsafe neighborhoods and lack of recreational areas may make it difficult for less affluent people to exercise.[29]

Lifestyle Factors

Of all the factors affecting obesity, perhaps the most critical is the relationship between activity level and calorie intake. Determining activity levels using surveys, however, is difficult. One big problem in that people surveyed overestimate their daily exercise level and intensity. It is also difficult to determine which measures of fitness were actually used and how indicative of overall health these may ultimately be. Defining yourself as "active" can mean very different things for different people. According to data from the 2012 Health Interview Survey, 30 percent of adults reported being inactive, 20 percent of adults reported being insufficiently active, and 50 percent reported sufficient levels of activity—mostly through physical activity during leisure time.[30]

Do you know people who seemingly can eat whatever they want without gaining weight? With few exceptions, if you were to monitor the level and intensity of their activity, you would discover why. Even if their schedule does not include intense exercise, it probably includes a high level of activity.

Rather than focusing only on how much formal exercise we get in each day, health and fitness experts have begun to focus on how much time we spend sitting. If the body isn't moving, it's not burning many calories. Research indicates a dose-response association between sitting time and mortality from all causes and from cardiovascular disease, independent of leisure-time activity; that is, the more time you spend sitting, the worse your health is likely to be, regardless of whether you exercise or not. Because muscle activity burns energy, passive sitting is one of the worst things you can do if you are trying to burn calories. If you stood up while reading this chapter, the large and small muscle groups in your legs would be constantly working to keep you from falling over—and burning more calories. These little extra bouts of movement may make a big difference in daily calories burned, weight management, and overall health.

U.S. adults get **11.3** percent of total daily calories from fast foods.

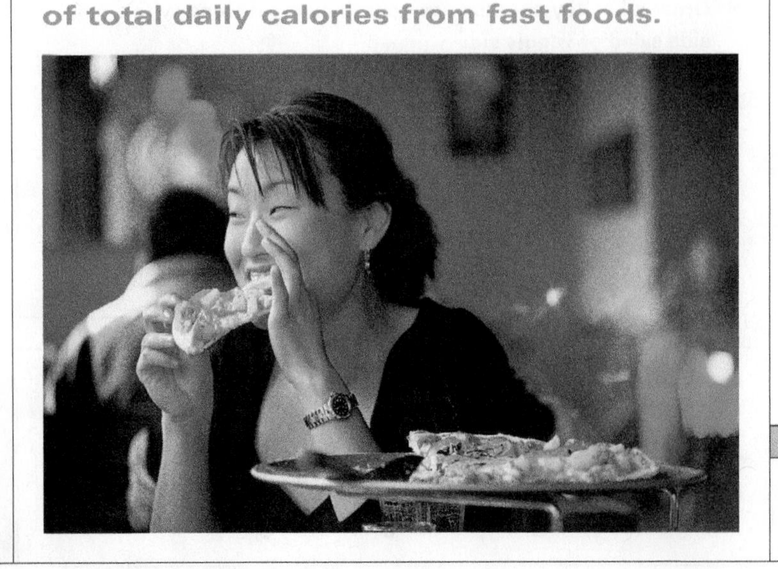

Skills for Behavior Change

FINDING THE FUN IN HEALTHY EATING AND EXERCISE

With a little creativity, you can make weight management a fun, positive part of your life. Try these tips:

- Cook and eat with friends. Share the responsibility for making the meal while you spend time with people you like.
- Experiment with new foods to add variety to your meals.
- Vary your exercise routine. Change the exercise or your location, join a team for the social aspects in addition to exercise, decide to run a race for the challenge, or learn how to skateboard for fun.

check yourself

- **What are some lifestyles changes that can contribute to weight management?**

2.5 Assessing Body Weight and Body Composition

learning outcome

2.5 Distinguish among overweight, obesity, and underweight.

Everyone has his or her own ideal weight, based on individual variables such as body structure, height, and fat distribution. Traditionally, experts used measurement techniques such as height-weight charts to determine whether an individual fell into the ideal weight, overweight, or obese category. However, these charts can be misleading because they don't take body composition (a person's ratio of fat to lean muscle) or fat distribution into account.

In fact, weight can be a deceptive indicator. Many a muscular athlete or a middle-aged adult who brags about weighing the same as in high school may be shocked to find out that he or she has relatively high fat levels based on BMI. More accurate measures of evaluating healthy weight and disease risk focus on a person's percentage of body fat and how that fat is distributed in his or her body.

Many people worry about becoming fat, but some fat is essential for healthy body functioning. Fat regulates body temperature, cushions and insulates organs and tissues, and is the body's main source of stored energy. Body fat is composed of two types of fat: essential and storage. *Essential fat* is the fat necessary for maintenance of life and reproductive functions. *Storage fat,* the nonessential fat that many of us try to shed, makes up the remainder of our fat reserves.

Overweight and Obesity

In general, **overweight** is increased body weight due to excess fat that exceeds healthy recommendations, whereas **obesity** refers to body weight that greatly exceeds health recommendations. Traditionally, *overweight* was defined as being 1 to 19 percent above one's ideal weight, based on a standard height-weight chart, and *obesity* was defined as being 20 percent or more above one's ideal weight. **Morbidly obese** people are 100 percent or more above their ideal weight. Experts now usually define *overweight* and *obesity* in terms of BMI, a measure discussed later, or percentage of body fat, as determined by some of the methods we'll discuss shortly. Although opinion varies somewhat, most experts agree that men's bodies should contain between 8 and 20 percent total body fat, and women should be within the range of 20 to 30 percent. At various ages and stages of life, these ranges also vary, but generally, men who exceed 22 percent body fat and women who exceed 35 percent are considered overweight (see Table 2.1).

Underweight

Men with only 3 to 7 percent body fat and women with approximately 8 to 15 percent are considered **underweight**, which can seriously compromise health. Extremely low body fat can cause hair loss, visual disturbances, skin problems, a tendency to fracture bones easily, digestive system disturbances, heart irregularities, gastrointestinal problems, difficulties in maintaining body temperature, and amenorrhea (in women). Rates of underweight individuals have declined in recent decades as overweight and obesity percentages have increased. Today, fewer than 4 percent of children and adolescents aged 2–19 and 2 percent of adults aged 20–74 are underweight.[31]

TABLE 2.1 **Body Fat Percentage Norms for Men and Women***

Men Age	Very Lean	Excellent	Good	Fair	Poor	Very Poor
20–29	<7%	7%–10%	11%–15%	16%–19%	20%–23%	>23%
30–39	<11%	11%–14%	15%–18%	19%–21%	22%–25%	>25%
40–49	<14%	14%–17%	18%–20%	21%–23%	24%–27%	>27%
50–59	<15%	15%–19%	20%–22%	23%–24%	25%–28%	>28%
60–69	<16%	16%–20%	21%–22%	23%–25%	26%–28%	>28%
70–79	<16%	16%–20%	21%–23%	24%–25%	26%–28%	>28%
Women Age	**Very Lean**	**Excellent**	**Good**	**Fair**	**Poor**	**Very Poor**
20–29	<14%	14%–16%	17%–19%	20%–23%	24%–27%	>27%
30–39	<15%	15%–17%	18%–21%	22%–25%	26%–29%	>29%
40–49	<17%	17%–20%	21%–24%	25%–28%	29%–32%	>32%
50–59	<18%	18%–22%	23%–27%	28%–30%	31%–34%	>34%
60–69	<18%	18%–23%	24%–28%	29%–31%	32%–35%	>35%
70–79	<18%	18%–24%	25%–29%	30%–32%	33%–36%	>36%

*Assumes nonathletes. For athletes, recommended body fat is 5 to 15 percent for men and 12 to 22 percent for women. Please note that there are no agreed-upon national standards for recommended body fat percentage.

Source: Based on data from The Cooper Institute, Dallas Texas, www.cooperinstitute.org.

check yourself

- **What are the differences between overweight and obesity?**

Assessing Body Weight and Body Composition: BMI and Other Methods

learning outcome

2.6 Compare and contrast different methods of body composition assessment.

Although people have a general sense that BMI is an indicator of how "fat" a person is, most do not really know what it assesses. **Body mass index (BMI)** is a description of body weight relative to height, numbers highly correlated with total body fat. Find your BMI in inches and pounds in Figure 2.4, or you can calculate your BMI by dividing your weight in kilograms by height in meters squared:

$$\text{BMI} = \text{weight(kg)/height squared (m}^2\text{)}$$

A BMI calculator is also available at www.nhlbi.nih.gov.

Desirable BMI levels may vary with age and by sex; however, most BMI tables for adults do not account for such variables. **Healthy weight** is defined as having a BMI of 18.5 to 24.9, the range of lowest statistical health risk.[32] A BMI of 25 to 29.9 indicates overweight and potentially significant health risks. A BMI of 30 or above is classified as obese. A BMI of 40 to 49.9 is morbidly obese, and a new category of BMI of 50 or higher has been labeled as super obese.[33] Nearly 3 percent of obese men and almost 7 percent of obese women are morbidly obese.[34]

Although useful, BMI levels don't include water, muscle, and bone mass or account for the fact that muscle weighs more than fat. BMI levels can be inaccurate for people who are under 5 feet tall, are highly muscled, or who are older and have little muscle mass. More precise methods of determining body fat, described below, should be used for these individuals.

Youth and BMI The labels *obese* and *morbidly obese* have been used for years for adults, though there is growing concern about the consequences of pinning these potentially stigmatizing labels on children.[35] BMI ranges above normal weight for children and teens are often labeled as "at risk of overweight" and "overweight." BMI ranges for children and teens take into account normal differences in body fat between boys and girls and the differences in body fat that occur at various ages. Specific guidelines for calculating youth BMI are available at the Centers for Disease Control and Prevention website, www.cdc.gov.

Key:
- Underweight
- Normal weight
- Overweight
- Obese

Height (feet and inches) \ Weight (pounds)	100		120		140		160		180		200		220		240		260
4'6"	24	27	29	31	34	36	39	41	43	46	48	51	53	55	58	60	63
4'8"	22	25	27	29	31	34	36	38	40	43	45	47	49	52	54	56	58
4'10"	21	23	25	27	29	31	33	36	38	40	42	44	46	48	50	52	54
5'0"	20	22	23	25	27	29	31	33	35	37	39	41	43	45	47	49	51
5'2"	18	20	22	24	26	27	29	31	33	35	37	38	40	42	44	46	48
5'4"	17	19	21	22	24	26	28	29	31	33	34	36	38	40	41	43	45
5'6"	16	18	19	21	23	24	26	27	29	31	32	34	36	37	39	40	42
5'8"	15	17	18	20	21	23	24	26	27	29	30	32	33	35	37	38	40
5'10"	14	16	17	19	20	22	23	24	26	27	29	30	32	33	34	36	37
6'0"	14	15	16	18	19	20	22	23	24	26	27	29	30	31	33	34	35
6'2"	13	14	15	17	18	19	21	22	23	24	26	27	28	30	31	32	33
6'4"	12	13	15	16	17	18	20	21	22	23	24	26	27	28	29	30	32
6'6"	12	13	14	15	16	17	19	20	21	22	23	24	25	27	28	29	30
6'8"	11	12	13	14	15	17	18	19	20	21	22	23	24	25	26	28	29
6'10"	11	12	13	14	15	16	17	18	19	20	21	22	23	24	25	26	27
7'0"	10	11	12	13	14	15	16	17	18	19	20	21	22	23	24	25	26

Figure 2.4 Body Mass Index
Locate the intersection of your weight and height to determine BMI. Note that BMI values have been rounded off to the nearest whole number.

Waist Circumference and Ratio Measurements

Knowing where you carry your fat may be more important than knowing how much you carry. Men and postmenopausal women tend to store fat in the abdominal area. Premenopausal women usually store fat in the hips, buttocks, and thighs. Waist circumference measurement is increasingly recognized as

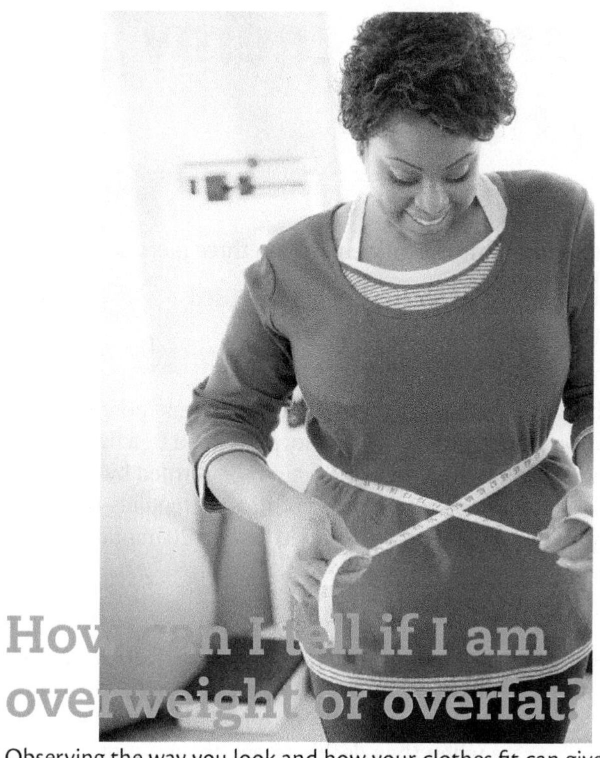

How can I tell if I am overweight or overfat?

Observing the way you look and how your clothes fit can give you a general idea of whether you weigh more or less than in the past. But for evaluating your weight and body fat levels in terms of potential health risks, it's best to use more scientific measures, such as BMI, waist circumference, waist-to-hip ratio, or a technician-administered body composition test.

a useful tool in assessing abdominal fat, which is considered more threatening to health than fat in other regions. In particular, as waist circumference increases, the risk for diabetes, cardiovascular disease, and stroke increases.[36] A waistline greater than 40 inches (102 centimeters) in men and 35 inches (88 centimeters) in women may be particularly indicative of greater health risk.[37] If a person is less than 5 feet tall or has a BMI of 35 or above, waist circumference standards used for the general population might not apply.

The **waist-to-hip ratio** measures regional fat distribution. A waist-to-hip ratio greater than 1 in men and 0.8 in women indicates increased health risks.[38] Measuring the waist-to-hip ratio is relatively inexpensive and accurate; however, it is less practical to use in clinical settings, and many believe that for most people, waist circumference and BMI are sufficient.[39]

Measures of Body Fat

There are many other ways to assess body fat levels. One low-tech way is simply to look in the mirror or consider how your clothes fit now compared with how they fit in the past. For those who wish to take a more precise measurement of their percentage of body fat, more accurate techniques are available, including caliper measurement, underwater weighing, and various body scans (Figure 2.5). These methods usually involve the help of a skilled professional and typically must be done in a lab or clinical setting. Before undergoing any procedure, make sure you understand the expense, potential for accuracy, risks, and training of the tester. Also, consider why you are seeking this assessment and what you plan to do with the results.

Underwater (hydrostatic) weighing:
Measures the amount of water a person displaces when completely submerged. Fat tissue is less dense than muscle or bone, so body fat can be computed within a 2%–3% margin of error by comparing weight underwater and out of water.

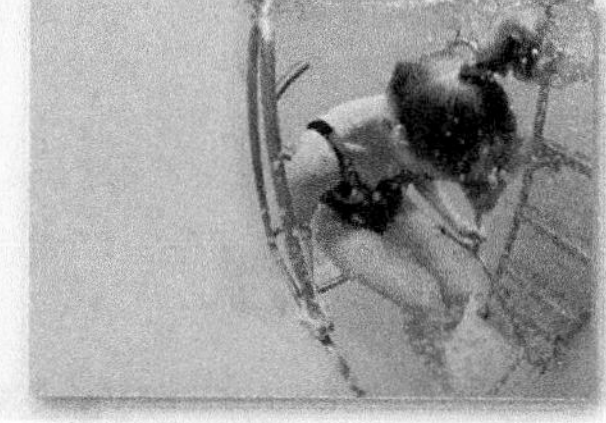

Skinfolds:
Involves "pinching" a person's fold of skin (with its underlying layer of fat) at various locations of the body. The fold is measured using a specially designed caliper. When performed by a skilled technician, it can estimate body fat with an error of 3%–4%.

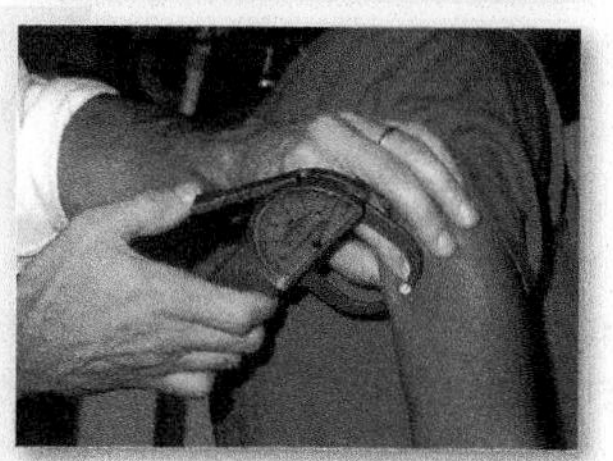

Bioelectrical impedance analysis (BIA):
Involves sending a very low level of electrical current through a person's body. As lean body mass is made up of mostly water, the rate at which the electricity is conducted gives an indication of a person's lean body mass and body fat. Under the best circumstances, BIA can estimate body fat with an error of 3%–4%.

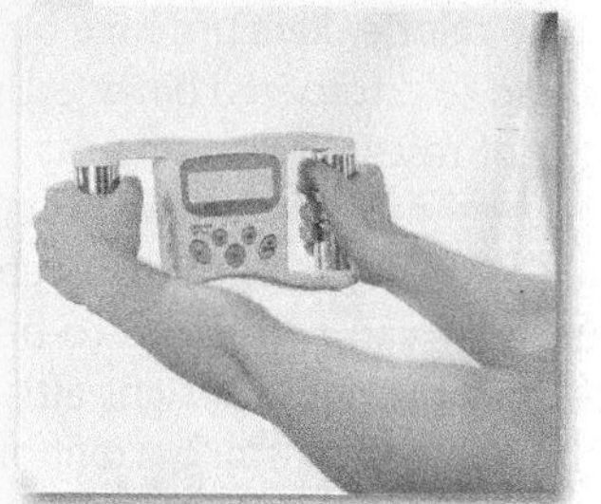

Dual-energy X-ray absorptiometry (DXA):
The technology is based on using very-low-level X-ray to differentiate between bone tissue, soft (or lean) tissue, and fat (or adipose) tissue. The margin of error for predicting body fat is 2%–4%.

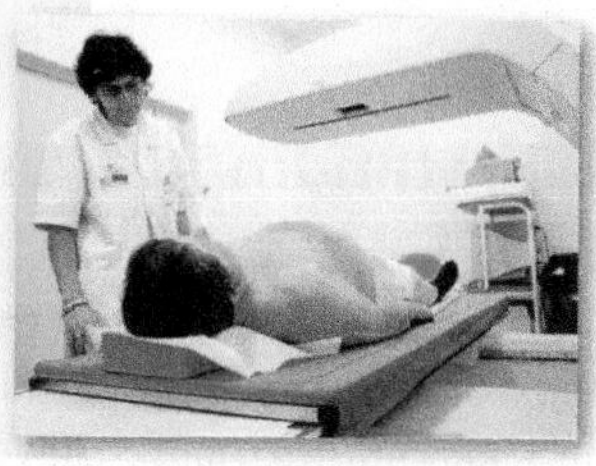

Bod Pod:
Uses air displacement to measure body composition. This machine is a large, egg-shaped chamber made from fiberglass. The person being measured sits in the machine wearing a swimsuit. The door is closed and the machine measures how much air is displaced. That value is used to calculate body fat, with a 2%–3% margin of error.

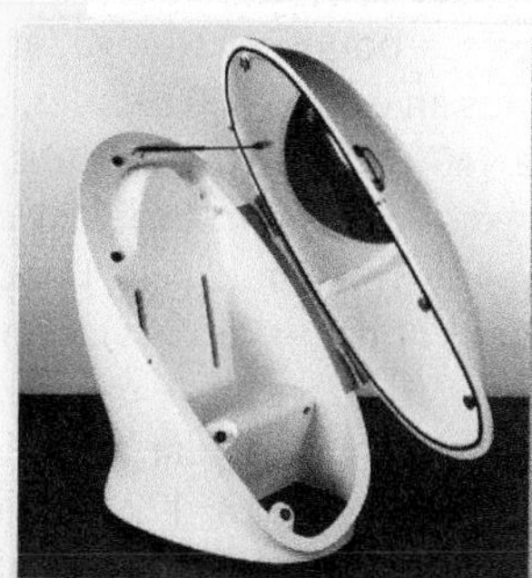

Figure 2.5 Overview of Various Body Composition Methods

Source: Adapted from J. Thompson and M. Manore, *Nutrition: An Applied Approach My Plate Edition*, 3rd ed., © 2012. Printed and electronically reproduced by permission of Pearson Education, Inc., Upper Saddle River, New Jersey.

check yourself

- **Which of the various assessment methods do you consider the most accurate? Which is the most accessible to the average person?**

2.7 Weight Management: Understanding Energy Balance and Improving Eating Habits

learning outcome

2.7 Explain how energy expenditure and energy intake affect weight management and ways to successfully manage your weight.

At some point in our lives, almost all of us will decide to lose weight or modify our diet. Many will have mixed success. Failure is often related to thinking about losing weight in terms of short-term "dieting" rather than adjusting long-term eating behaviors (such as developing the habit of healthy snacking).

Low-calorie diets produce only temporary losses and may actually lead to disordered binge eating or related problems.[40] Repeated bouts of restrictive dieting may be physiologically harmful; moreover, the sense of failure we experience each time we don't meet our goal can exact far-reaching psychological costs. Drugs and intensive counseling can contribute to positive weight loss, but, even then, many people regain weight after treatment. Maintaining a healthful body takes constant attention and nurturing over the course of your lifetime.

Understanding Calories and Energy Balance

A *calorie* is a unit of measure that indicates the amount of energy gained from food or expended through activity. Each time you consume 3,500 calories more than your body needs to maintain weight, you gain a pound of storage fat. Conversely, each time your body expends an extra 3,500 calories, you lose a pound of fat. If you consume 140 calories (the amount in one can of regular soda) more than you need every single day and make no other changes in diet or activity, you would gain 1 pound in 25 days (3,500 calories ÷ 140 calories ÷ 1 day = 25 days). Conversely, if you walk for 30 minutes each day at a pace of 15 minutes per mile (172 calories burned) in addition to your regular activities, you would lose 1 pound in 20 days (3,500 calories ÷ 172 calories ÷ 1 day = 20.3 days) due to the negative caloric balance. This is an example of the concept of energy balance described in Figure 2.6.

The Importance of Exercise

Any increase in the intensity, frequency, and duration of daily exercise can have a significant impact on total calorie expenditure because lean (muscle) tissue is more metabolically active than fat tissue. Exact estimates vary, but experts currently think that 2–50 more calories per day are burned per pound of muscle than for each pound of fat tissue. Thus, the base level of calories needed to maintain a healthy weight varies greatly from person to person.

The number of calories spent depends on three factors:

1. The number and proportion of muscles used
2. The amount of weight moved
3. The length of time the activity takes

An activity involving both the arms and legs burns more calories than one involving only the legs. An activity performed by a heavy person burns more calories than the same activity performed by a lighter person. And an activity performed for 40 minutes requires twice as much energy as the same activity performed for only 20 minutes.

Improving Your Eating Habits

Before you can change a behavior, such as unhealthy eating habits, you must first determine what causes or triggers it. Many people find it helpful to keep a chart of their eating patterns: when they feel like eating, where they are when they decide to eat, the amount of time they spend eating, other activities they engage in during the meal (watching television or reading), whether they eat alone or with others, what and how much they consume, and how they felt before they took their first bite. If you keep a detailed daily log of eating triggers for at least a week, you will discover useful clues about what in your environment or your emotional makeup causes you to want food. Typically, these

See It! Videos

A new strategy to keep off the weight? Watch **Keeping It Off** in the Study Area of MasteringHealth.

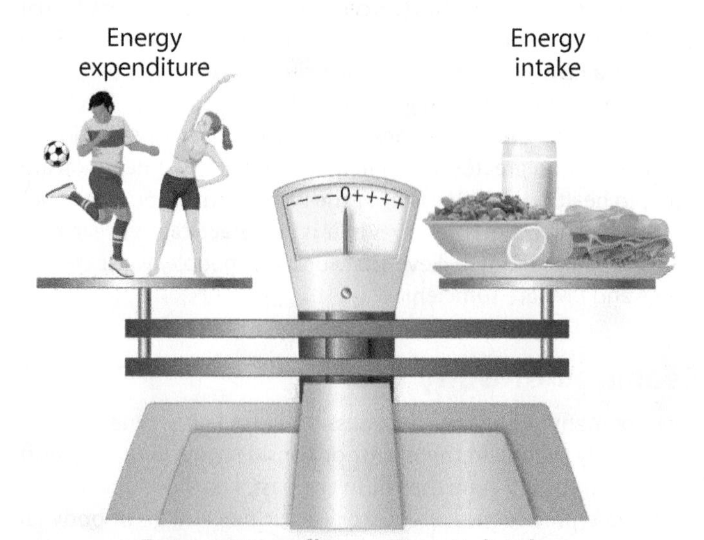

Figure 2.6 The Concept of Energy Balance
If you consume more calories than you burn, you will gain weight. If you burn more than you consume, you will lose weight. If both are equal, your weight will not change, according to this concept.

dietary triggers center on patterns and problems in everyday living rather than on real hunger pangs. Many people eat compulsively when stressed; however, for other people, the same circumstances diminish their appetite, causing them to lose weight.

Once you've evaluated your behaviors and determined your triggers, you can begin to devise a plan for improved eating. If you are unsure of where to start, seek assistance from reputable sources such as MyPlate (www.choosemyplate.gov). Registered dietitians, some physicians (not all doctors have a strong background in nutrition), health educators and exercise physiologists with nutritional training, and other health professionals can provide reliable information. Be wary of people who call themselves nutritionists; there is no such official designation. Avoid weight-loss programs that promise quick "miracle" results or those run by "trainees," often people with short courses on nutrition and exercise that are designed to sell products or services.

Before engaging in any weight-loss program, ask about the credentials of the adviser; assess the nutrient value of the prescribed diet; verify that dietary guidelines are consistent with reliable nutrition research; and analyze the suitability of the diet to your tastes, budget, and lifestyle. Any diet that requires radical behavior changes or sets up artificial dietary programs through prepackaged products that don't teach you how to eat healthfully is likely to fail. Supplements and fad diets that claim fast weight loss will invariably mean fast weight regain. The most successful plans allow you to make food choices in real-world settings and do not ask you to sacrifice everything you enjoy.

You will also need to address some of the triggers that you may have for eating that are unrelated to hunger. For example, if you tend to eat in stressful situations, try to acknowledge the feelings of stress and anxiety and develop stress management techniques to practice daily. If you find yourself eating when you are bored or tired, identify the times when you feel low energy, and fill them with activities other than eating, such as exercise breaks, or cultivate a new interest or hobby that keeps your mind and hands busy. If your trigger is feeling angry or upset, analyze your emotions and look for a noneating activity to deal with them, such as taking a quick walk or calling a friend. If it is the sight and smell of food, stop buying high-calorie foods that tempt you, or store them in an inconvenient place, out of sight. Avoid walking past or sitting or standing near the table of tempting treats at a meeting, party, or other gathering.

Some people drink diet soda to help maintain or control their weight. In fact, 11 percent of healthy weight, 19 percent of overweight, and 22 percent of obese adults drink diet sodas for weight control. They may not realize it, but in drinking diet sodas they could actually be sabotaging their weight loss plans. According to new research, overweight/obese individuals who opt for diet beverages actually consume more calories from food at meals and from snacks than people who choose sugared beverages.[41] Why is this the case? While the exact mechanism remains in question, researchers speculate that artificial sweeteners may change the way we perceive fullness and may increase appetite. Others suggest a form of "cognitive distortion" whereby we justify a few more snacks or dessert since our drinks have fewer calories.

Skills for Behavior Change

TIPS FOR SENSIBLE SNACKING

- **Keep healthy munchies around.** Buy 100 percent whole-wheat breads. If you need to spice up your snack, use low-fat or soy cheese, low-fat cream cheese, peanut butter, hummus, or other healthy favorites. Some baked or popped crackers are low in fat and calories and high in fiber. Look for these on your grocery shelves.
- **Keep "crunchies" on hand.** Apples, pears, red or green pepper sticks, carrots, and celery all are good choices. Wash the fruits and vegetables and cut them up to carry with you; eat them when a snack attack comes on.
- **Quench your thirst with hot drinks.** Hot tea, heated milk, plain or decaffeinated coffee, hot chocolate made with nonfat milk or water, or soup broths will help keep you satisfied.
- **Choose natural beverages.** Drink plain water, 100 percent juice in small quantities, or other low-sugar choices to satisfy your thirst. Avoid certain juices, energy drinks, and soft drinks that have added sugars, low fiber, and no protein. Usually, they are high in calories and low in longer-term satisfaction.
- **Eat nuts instead of candy.** Although nuts are relatively high in calories, they are also loaded with healthy fats and make a healthy snack when consumed in moderation.
- **If you must have a piece of chocolate, keep it small.** Note that dark chocolate is better than milk chocolate or white chocolate because of its antioxidant content.
- **Avoid high-calorie energy bars.** Eat these only if you are exercising hard and don't have an opportunity to eat a regular meal. If you buy energy bars, look for ones with a good mixture of fiber and protein and that are low in fat and calories.

check yourself

- **What are three potential triggers for overeating, and how can they be overcome?**
- **What steps should you take before engaging in any weight-loss program?**

2.8 Weight Management: Assessing Diet Programs

learning outcome

2.8 Identify strengths and weaknesses of popular diet programs.

People looking to lose weight and improve eating habits often turn to diet programs for advice and guidance. Table 2.2 analyzes several popular diets marketed today. For information on other plans, check out the regularly updated list of reviews on the website of the Academy of Nutrition and Dietetics at www.eatright.org.

See It! Videos

What makes one diet plan work better than another? Watch **Best Diet Plan Apparently Works** in the Study Area of MasteringHealth.

TABLE 2.2 **Analyzing Popular Diet Programs**

Diet Name	Basic Principles	Good for Diabetes and Heart Health?	Weight Loss Effectiveness	Pros, Cons, and Other Things to Consider
DASH (Dietary Approaches to Stop Hypertension)	A plan developed to fight high blood pressure. Eat fruits, veggies, whole grains, lean protein, and low-fat dairy. Avoid sweets, fats, red meat, and sodium.	Yes	Not specifically designed for weight loss.	A safe and healthy diet that can be complicated to learn. Although not designed for weight reduction, it is regarded as effective in improving cholesterol levels long term.
Mediterranean	A plan that emphasizes fruits, vegetables, fish, whole grains, beans, nuts, legumes, olive oil, and herbs and spices. Poultry, eggs, cheese, yogurt, and red wine are enjoyed in moderation; sweets and red meat are for special occasions.	Yes	Effective	Widely considered to be one of the more healthy, safe, and balanced diets. Weight loss may not be as dramatic, but long-term health benefits have been demonstrated.
Weight Watchers	The program assigns every food a point value based on its nutritional values and how hard your body has to work to burn it off. Total points allowed depend on activity level and personal weight goals.	Yes (depending on individual choices)	Effective	Experts consider Weight Watchers effective and easy to follow for both short- and long-term weight loss. Other pluses include an emphasis on group support and room for occasional indulgences. But while not as expensive as some plans, there are membership fees.
Jenny Craig	Prepackaged meals do the work of restricting calorie intake. Members get personalized meal and exercise plans, plus weekly counseling sessions.	Yes	Effective short term, long-term results dependent on adopting healthful eating later	Support and premade meals make weight loss easier; however, it may be difficult to maintain for the long run. Cons include cost—hundreds of dollars per month for food alone plus membership fees. No lactose- and gluten-free foods are available.
Atkins	Carbs (sugars and simple starches) are avoided in this plan, and protein and fat from chicken, meat, and eggs are embraced.	Not likely with so much fat eaten	Effective in short term, mixed long-term results	Atkins is extremely effective at short-term weight loss, but many experts worry that fat intake is up to three times higher than standard daily recommendations.
Paleo	Based on the theory that digestive systems have not evolved to deal with many modern foods such as diary, legumes, grains and sugar, this plan emphasizes meats, fish, poultry, fruits, and vegetables.	Unknown (too few studies)	Unknown (too few studies)	Gets low marks by health and nutrition experts due to avoidance of grains, legumes, and dairy and higher fat than the government recommends. Other cons include that it is missing essential nutrients, costly to maintain, hard to follow long term, and has had only a few very small studies done to document effectiveness.
Fast Diet (also known as the 5:2 diet or intermittent fasting diet)	Based on the theory that by drastically reducing calories on two days (500 cal/day) each week and eating normally the other five, you will lose weight	Not likely as it doesn't follow guidelines for carbohydrates	Effective but weight loss is slow unless calorie intake is monitored on non-fast days and exercise is part of regimen	Exceeds dietary guidelines for fat and protein and falls short on carbohydrate recommendation. Does encourage fruits and veggies, but feast and famine regimen is hard to sustain.

Sources: Opinions on diet pros and cons are based on *U.S. News & World Report*, "Best Diet Rankings," 2012, http://health.usnews.com; Dietary reviews available online from registered dieticians at the Academy of Nutrition and Dietetics, 2013, www.eatright.org.

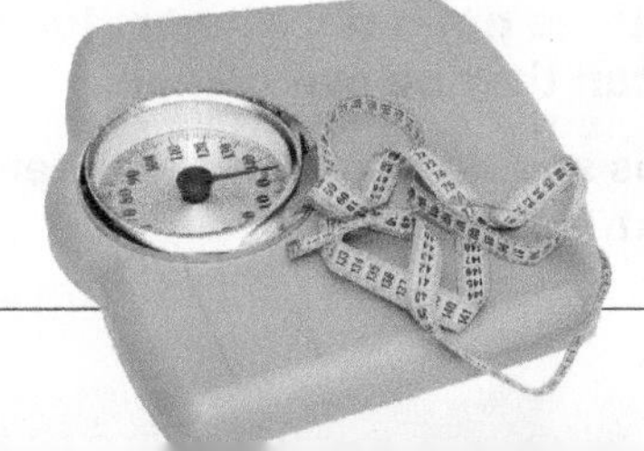

check yourself

- **What are important factors to consider when evaluating current diet programs?**

2.9 Weight Management: In Perspective

learning **outcome**

2.9 List steps to successful weight management.

Supportive friends, relatives, community resources, and policies that support healthy food choices and exercise options all increase the likelihood of successful weight loss. People of the same age, sex, height, and weight can have resting metabolic rates that differ by as much as 1,000 calories a day. This may explain why one person's extra food intake and weight gain may lead to weight loss and hunger in another person. Depression, stress, cultural influences, and the availability of high-fat, high-calorie foods can also make weight loss harder.

To reach and maintain the weight at which you will be healthy and feel your best, develop a program of exercise and healthy eating that you can maintain. It is unrealistic and potentially dangerous to try to lose weight in a short period of time. Instead, try to lose a healthy 1 to 2 pounds during the first week, and stay with this slow-and-easy regimen. Adding exercise and cutting back on calories to expend about 500 calories more than you consume each day will help you lose weight at a rate of 1 pound per week.

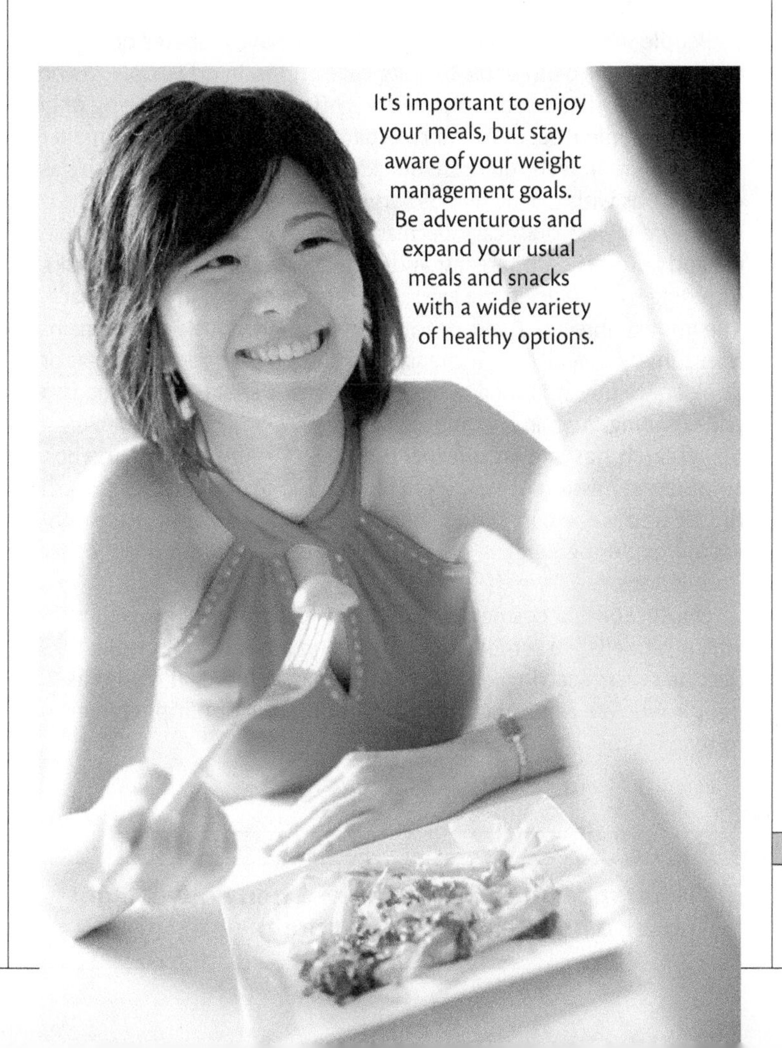

It's important to enjoy your meals, but stay aware of your weight management goals. Be adventurous and expand your usual meals and snacks with a wide variety of healthy options.

Skills for Behavior Change

KEYS TO SUCCESSFUL WEIGHT MANAGEMENT

The key to successful weight management is finding a sustainable way to control what you eat and to make exercise a priority.

- To get started, ask yourself some key questions. Why do you want to make this change right now? What are your ultimate goals?
- Write down the things you find positive about your diet and exercise behaviors. Then write down things that need to be changed. For each change you need to make, list three or four small things you could change right now.
- What resources on campus or in your community could help? Out of your friends and family members, who will help you?
- Keep a food and exercise log for 2 or 3 days. Note the good things you are doing, the things that need improvement, and the triggers you need to address.

Make a Plan

- Set realistic short- and long-term goals.
- Establish a plan. What diet and exercise changes can you make this week? Once you do 1 week, plot a course for 2 weeks, and so on.
- Look for balance. Remember that it is calories taken in and burned over time that make the difference.

Change Your Habits

- Notice whether you're hungry before starting a meal. Eat slowly, noting when you start to feel full. Stop before you are full.
- Eat breakfast. This will prevent you from being too hungry and overeating at lunch.
- Keep healthful snacks on hand for when you get hungry.
- Don't constantly deprive yourself or set unrealistic guidelines.

Incorporate Exercise

- Be active; slowly increase your time, speed, distance, or resistance levels.
- Vary your physical activity. Find activities you love; try things you haven't tried before.
- Find an exercise partner to help you stay motivated.
- Make exercise a fun break. Go for a walk in a place that interests you.

check yourself

- **What are the key components of a successful weight management plan?**

2.10 Considering Drastic Weight-Loss Measures

learning outcome

2.10 Explain measures that may be taken when body weight poses an extreme threat to health.

In certain limited instances, extreme measures may be considered to reduce weight.

In severe cases of obesity, patients may be given powdered formulas with daily values of 400 to 700 calories plus vitamin and mineral supplements. Such **very-low-calorie diets (VLCDs)** should never be undertaken without strict medical supervision.

One dangerous potential complication of VLCDs or starvation diets is *ketoacidosis*, in which a patient's blood becomes more acidic, causing severe damage to body tissues. Risk is greatest for those with untreated type 1 diabetes, anorexia nervosa, or bulimia nervosa. If fasting continues, the body turns to its last resort—protein—for energy, breaking down essential muscle and organ tissue to stay alive. Within about 10 days after the typical adult begins a complete fast, the body will have depleted its energy stores, and death may occur.

Dieters often turn to commercially marketed weight-loss supplements. U.S. Food and Drug Administration (FDA) approval is not required for over-the-counter "diet aids" or supplements, whose effectiveness is largely untested and unproven. Virtually all persons who use diet pills eventually regain their weight.[42]

In 2007, the FDA approved the first over-the-counter weight loss pill—a half-strength version of the drug orlistat (Xenical), marketed as Alli. This drug inhibits the action of lipase, an enzyme that helps the body digest fats, causing about 30 percent of fats consumed to pass through the digestive system. Side effects include gas with watery fecal discharge; frequent, often unexpected, bowel movements; and possible deficiencies of fat-soluble vitamins.

The FDA approved the drugs Belvig and Qsymia in 2012. Belvig affects serotonin levels, helping patients feel full, and Qsymia is an appetite suppressant and anti-seizure drug that reduces the desire for food.

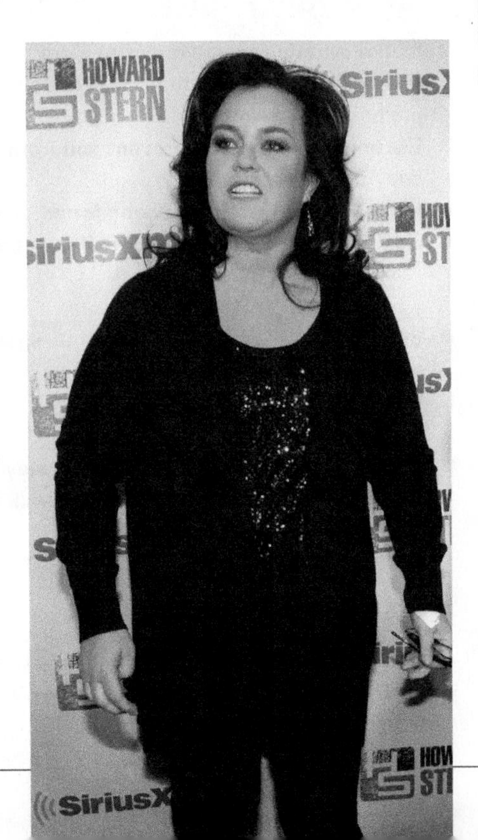

Comedian and talk show host Rosie O'Donnell underwent weight loss surgery in 2013, following a heart attack the previous year.

Several once-approved diet drugs have since been recalled due to a variety of problems like heart attacks, heart valve problems, stroke, and liver damage. View all diet drugs and supplements with caution, including these:

- **Human chorionic gonadotropin (HCG).** In prescription form, this is an approved treatment for some female fertility problems; it has recently become known as a crash-diet miracle drug. Results consistently show that hCG is no more effective for weight loss than cutting calories.[43]
- **Sibutramine (Meridia).** This prescription medication suppresses appetite by inhibiting serotonin uptake in the brain. Side effects include dry mouth, headache, and high blood pressure. The FDA has issued warnings about Meridia for people with hypertension or heart disease.[44]
- ***Hoodia gordonii.*** This plant native to Africa is a purported appetite suppressant. To date, it is not FDA approved and has not been tested in clinical trials.[45]
- **Herbal weight-loss aids.** Products containing *Ephedra* can cause rapid heart rate, seizures, insomnia, and raised blood pressure, all without significant effects on weight. *St. John's wort* and other herbs reported to suppress appetite have not been shown effective.

People who are severely overweight and have diabetes or hypertension may be candidates for surgical options. In *adjustable gastric banding*, an inflatable band partitions off the stomach, leaving only a small opening between its two parts so the stomach is smaller and the person feels full more quickly. Although weight loss isn't as dramatic as with gastric bypass surgery, the risks are fewer.

Gastric bypass drastically decreases how much food a person can eat and absorb. Results are fast and dramatic, but there are many risks, including blood clots in the legs, a leak in a staple line in the stomach, pneumonia, infection, and death. The stomach pouch that remains after surgery is small (about the size of a lime), so the person can eat or drink only a tiny amount at a time. Possible side effects include nausea and vomiting, vitamin and mineral deficiencies, and dehydration.

Research has shown unexpected results from gastric surgeries: complete remission of type 2 diabetes in the majority of cases, with drastic reductions in blood glucose levels in others.[46] Researchers are exploring surgical options for diabetes prevention in other populations.[47]

Liposuction is a cosmetic (not weight loss) surgical procedure in which fat cells are removed from specific areas of the body. Risks include severe scarring, and even death has resulted. In many cases, people who have liposuction regain fat or require multiple surgeries to repair lumpy, irregular surfaces.

check yourself

- **What measures can be taken when body weight poses a risk to health? What are their risks?**

2.11 Trying to Gain Weight

learning outcome

2.11 Describe healthy strategies for trying to gain weight.

For some people, trying to gain weight is a challenge for a variety of metabolic, hereditary, psychological, and other reasons. If you are one of these individuals, the first priority is to determine why you cannot gain weight.

Perhaps you're an athlete and you burn more calories than you manage to eat. Perhaps you're stressed out and skipping meals to increase study time. Or stress, depression, or other emotional issues may make it difficult to focus on food and take good care of your body. Among older adults, the senses of taste and smell may decline, which makes food taste different and therefore less pleasurable to eat. Visual problems and other disabilities may make meals more difficult to prepare, and dental problems may make eating more difficult.

People who engage in extreme energy-burning sports and exercise routines may be at risk for caloric and nutritional deficiencies, which can lead not only to weight loss, but to immune system problems and organ dysfunction; weakness, which leads to falls and fractures; slower recovery from diseases; and a host of other problems as well.

People who are too thin need to take the same kind of steps as those who are overweight or obese to find out what their healthy weight is and attain that weight.

The Skills for Behavior Change feature gives ideas and tips for gaining weight. Depending on your situation, you may aim to gain as much as a pound per week, which would mean adding up to 500 calories a day to your diet. It is important that these calories be added in the form of energy-dense, nutritious choices from a variety of foods. For example, you could choose to eat a thick slice of whole grain toast topped with peanut butter and a banana for breakfast or garnish a salad with olive oil, avocado, nuts, and sunflower seeds for lunch. One cup of whole-wheat flakes provides 128 calories, while a cup of granola is 464 calories. Similarly, plain low-fat yogurt is 154 calories per cup, while strawberry low-fat yogurt offers 238 calories per cup. Just be sure that the calories you add are coming from high-quality sources, not high-fat junk food.[48]

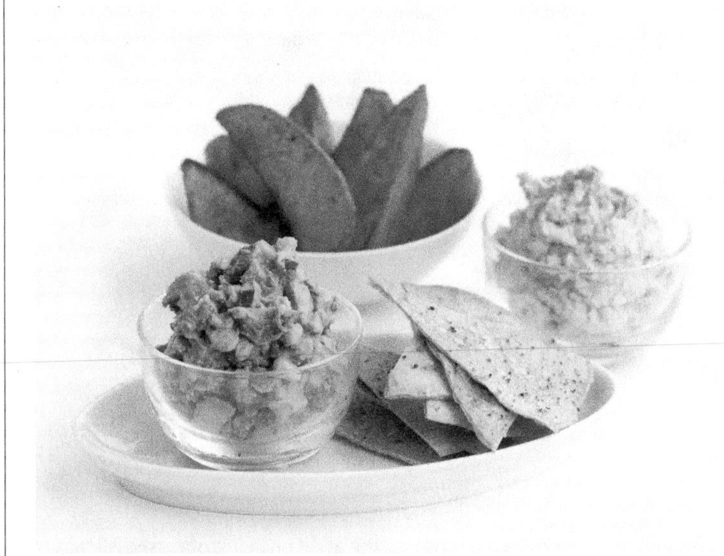

A snack of guacamole and whole-grain tortilla chips or hummus and baked potatoes is a healthy, nutrient-dense way to increase calorie intake.

Skills for Behavior Change

TIPS FOR GAINING WEIGHT

- Eat at regularly scheduled times.
- Eat more frequently, spend more time eating, eat high-calorie foods first if you fill up fast, and always start with the main course.
- Take time to shop, to cook, and to eat slowly.
- Put extra spreads such as peanut butter, cream cheese, or cheese on your foods. Make your sandwiches with extra-thick slices of bread and add more filling. Take seconds whenever possible, and eat high-calorie, nutrient-dense snacks such as nuts and cheese during the day.
- Supplement your diet. Add high-calorie drinks that have a healthy balance of nutrients, such as whole milk.
- Try to eat with people you are comfortable with. Avoid people who you feel are analyzing what you eat or make you feel as if you should eat less.
- If you are sedentary, be aware that moderate exercise can increase appetite. If you are exercising, or exercising to extremes, moderate your activities until you've gained some weight.
- Avoid diuretics, laxatives, and other medications that cause you to lose body fluids and nutrients.
- Relax. Many people who are underweight operate in high gear most of the time. Slow down, get more rest, and take steps to control stress and anxiety.

check yourself

- **What are some steps to be taken when weight needs to be gained? Do you think this is as difficult a task as trying to lose weight?**

2.12

Understanding and Improving Body Image

learning outcome

2.12 Identify the elements of the body image continuum, and list steps that can be taken to build a more positive body image.

When you look in the mirror, do you like what you see? If you feel disappointed, frustrated, or even angry, you're not alone. In a study, 93 percent of the women reported having negative thoughts about their appearance during the past week.[49] Negative feelings about one's body can contribute to behaviors that can threaten your health—and your life. In contrast, a healthy body image can contribute to reduced stress, an increased sense of personal empowerment, and more joyful living.

Body image includes several components:

- How you see yourself in your mind
- What you believe about your appearance
- How you feel about your body
- How you sense and control your body as you move

A *negative body image* is either a distorted perception of your shape or feelings of discomfort, shame, or anxiety about your body. A *positive body image* is a true perception of your appearance. You understand that everyone is different, and you celebrate your uniqueness. Figure 2.7 will help you identify whether your body image is positive, negative, or somewhere in between.

Factors Influencing Body Image

Images of celebrities in the media set the standard for what we find attractive, leading some people to go to dangerous extremes to have the biggest biceps or fit into size zero jeans. Though most of us think of this obsession with appearance as a recent phenomenon, it has long been part of American culture.

Social media has also increased concerns regarding negative body images.[50] Many sites actively warn against posts promoting self-harm, but images of unrealistically thin bodies—coupled with catch phrases telling young people to get "thin"—can still be hard to avoid.[51]

Body hate/ disassociation	Distorted body image	Body preoccupied/ obsessed	Body acceptance	Body is not an issue
I often feel separated and distant from my body—as if it belonged to someone else. I hate my body, and I often isolate myself from others. I don't see anything positive or even neutral about my body shape and size. I don't believe others when they tell me I look okay. I hate the way I look in the mirror.	I spend a significant amount of time exercising and dieting to change my body. My body shape and size keeps me from dating or finding someone who will treat me the way I want to be treated. I have considered changing (or have changed) my body shape and size through surgical means. I wish I could change the way I look in the mirror.	I weigh and measure myself a lot. I spend a significant amount of time viewing myself in the mirror. I compare my body to others. I have days when I feel fat. I accept society's ideal body shape and size as the best body shape and size. I'd be more attractive if I were thinner, more muscular, etc.	I pay attention to my body and my appearance because it is important to me, but it only occupies a small part of my day. I would like to change some things about my body, but I spend most of my time highlighting my positive features. My self-esteem is based on my personality traits, achievements, and relationships—not just my body image.	I feel fine about my body. I don't worry about changing my body shape or weight. I never weigh or measure myself. My feelings about my body are not influenced by society's concept of an ideal body shape. I know that the significant others in my life will always love me for who I am, not for how I look.

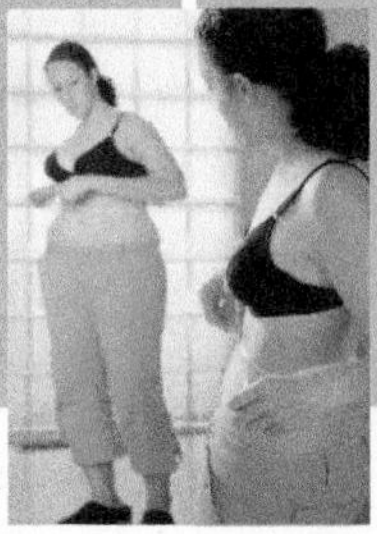

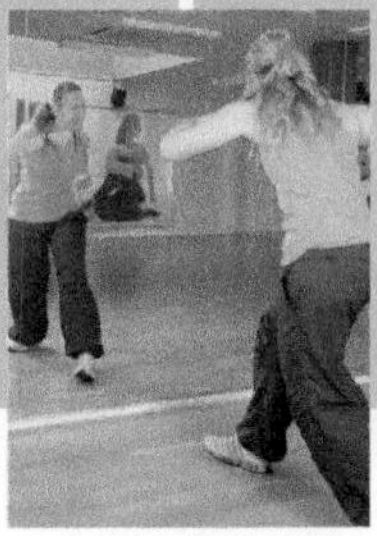

VIDEO TUTOR
Body Image Continuum

Figure 2.7 Body Image Continuum

This continuum shows a range of attitudes and behaviors toward body image. Functioning at either extreme—not caring at all or being obsessed—leads to problems. When you are functioning in the "body acceptance" area, you are taking care of your body and emotions.

Source: Adapted from Smiley/King/Avery, "Eating Issues and Body Image Continuum," Campus Health Service 1996. Copyright © 1997 Arizona Board of Regents for University of Arizona.

Today, as more than 69 percent of Americans are overweight or obese, a significant disconnect exists between idealized images of male and female bodies and the typical American body.[52] At the same time, the media bombards us with messages telling us that we just don't measure up.

Others strongly influence how we see ourselves. Parents are especially influential in body image development. For instance, fathers who validate the acceptability of their daughters' appearance throughout puberty and mothers who model body acceptance can help their daughters maintain a positive body image.

Interactions with others outside the family—for instance, teasing and bullying from peers—can contribute to negative body image. Moreover, associations within one's cultural group appear to influence body image. For example, European American females experience the highest rates of body dissatisfaction; as a minority group becomes more acculturated into the mainstream, the body dissatisfaction levels of women in that group increase.[53]

People diagnosed with a body image disorder show differences in the brain's ability to regulate *neurotransmitters* linked to mood,[54] in a way similar to that of depression and anxiety disorders, including obsessive-compulsive disorder. One magnetic resonance imaging (MRI) study linked distortions in body image to malfunctions in the brain's visual processing region.[55]

See It! Videos

What does a "real" woman look like? Watch **A Real Look at Real Women** in the Study Area of MasteringHealth.

Building a Positive Body Image

If you want to develop a more positive body image, your first step might be to bust some toxic myths and challenge some commonly held attitudes in contemporary society:[56]

- **Myth 1: How you look is more important than who you are.** Is your weight important in defining who you are? How much does it matter to you to have friends who are thin? How important do you think being thin is in attracting a partner?
- **Myth 2: Anyone can be slender and attractive if they work at it.** When you see someone who is thin, or obese, what assumptions do you make? Have you ever berated yourself for not having the "willpower" to change some aspect of your body?
- **Myth 3: Extreme dieting is an effective weight-loss strategy.** Do you believe in fad diets or "quick-weight-loss" products? How far would you go to attain the "perfect" body?
- **Myth 4: Appearance is more important than health.** How do you evaluate whether a person is healthy? Is your desire to change your body motivated by health or appearance?

Body Image Disorders

Although most Americans are dissatisfied with some aspect of their appearance, only a few have a true body image disorder. Approximately 1 percent of people in the United States suffer from **body dysmorphic disorder (BDD)**.[57] Persons with BDD are obsessively concerned with their appearance and have a distorted view of their own body shape, body size, and so on. Although the precise cause of BDD isn't known, an anxiety disorder such as obsessive-compulsive disorder is often present. Contributing factors may include genetic susceptibility, childhood teasing, physical or sexual abuse, low self-esteem, and rigid sociocultural expectations of beauty.[58]

People with BDD may try to fix their perceived flaws through excessive bodybuilding, repeated cosmetic surgeries, or other appearance-altering behaviors. It is estimated that 10 percent of people seeking dermatology or cosmetic treatments have BDD.[59] Psychotherapy and/or antidepressant medications are often successful in treating BBD.

In **social physique anxiety (SPA)**, the desire to "look good" is so strong that it has a destructive effect on one's ability to function effectively in interactions with others. People suffering from SPA may spend a disproportionate amount of time fixating on their bodies, working out, and performing tasks that are ego centered and self-directed.[60] Experts speculate that this anxiety may contribute to disordered eating behaviors.

Skills for Behavior Change

STEPS TO A POSITIVE BODY IMAGE

One list cannot create a positive body image, but it can help you think about new ways of looking more healthfully and happily at yourself and your body.

- **Step 1. Celebrate all of the amazing things your body does for you—running, dancing, breathing, laughing, dreaming.**
- **Step 2. Keep a list of things you like about yourself—things unrelated to how much you weigh or how you look. Read your list often, and add to it regularly.**
- **Step 3. Remind yourself that true beauty is not simply skin deep. When you feel good about who you are, you carry yourself with confidence, self-acceptance, and openness that makes you beautiful.**
- **Step 4. Surround yourself with people who are supportive and who recognize the importance of liking yourself as you are.**
- **Step 5. Shut down voices in your head that tell you your body is not "right" or that you are a "bad" person. You can overpower those negative thoughts with positive ones.**
- **Step 6. Become a critical viewer of social and media messages. Identify and resist images, slogans, or attitudes that make you feel bad about yourself or your body.**
- **Step 7. Do something that lets your body know you appreciate it. Take a bubble bath, make time for a nap, or find a peaceful place outside to relax.**
- **Step 8. Use the time and energy you might have spent worrying about your appearance to do something to help others.**

Source: Adapted with permission from the National Eating Disorders Association, www.nationaleatingdisorders.org.

check yourself

- **Where do you place yourself on the body image continuum?**
- **Are there steps that you may take to improve your body image?**

2.13

What Is Disordered Eating?

learning outcome

2.13 Identify the elements of the eating issues continuum.

The eating issues continuum in Figure 2.8 identifies thoughts and behaviors associated with disordered eating.

Some people who exhibit disordered eating patterns progress to a clinical **eating disorder**—a diagnosis that can be applied only by a physician to a patient who exhibits severe disturbances in thoughts, behavior, and body functioning.

The American Psychiatric Association (APA) has defined several eating disorders: *anorexia nervosa, bulimia nervosa, binge-eating disorder,* and a cluster of conditions referred to as **Other Specified Feeding or Eating Disorder (OSFED).**[61]

In the United States, 10 percent or more of late adolescent and adult women report symptoms of eating disorders.[62] In 2013, 2.1 percent of college students reported dealing with either anorexia or bulimia.[63] Disordered eating and eating disorders are also common in college athletes in sports such as gymnastics, wrestling, swimming, and figure skating.[64] Eating disorders are on the rise among men, who represent up to 25 percent of anorexia and bulimia patients.[65]

Many people with these disorders feel disenfranchised in other aspects of their lives and try to gain a sense of control through food. Many are clinically depressed, suffer from obsessive-compulsive disorder, or have other psychiatric problems. Individuals with low self-esteem, negative body image, and a high tendency for perfectionism are most at risk.[66]

Eating disordered	Disruptive eating patterns	Food preoccupied/ obsessed	Concerned in a healthy way	Food is not an issue
I worry about what I will eat or when I will exercise all the time. I follow a very rigid eating plan and know precisely how many calories, fat grams, or carbohydrates I eat every day. I feel incredible guilt, shame, and anxiety when I break my diet. I regularly stuff myself and then exercise, vomit, or use laxatives to get rid of the food. My friends and family tell me I am too thin, but I feel fat. I am out of control when I eat. I am afraid to eat in front of others. I prefer to eat alone.	My food and exercise concerns are starting to interfere with my school and social life. I use food to comfort myself. I have tried diet pills, laxatives, vomiting, or extra time exercising in order to lose or maintain my weight. I have fasted or avoided eating for long periods of time in order to lose or maintain my weight. If I cannot exercise to burn off calories, I panic. I feel strong when I can restrict how much I eat. I feel out of control when I eat more than I wanted to.	I think about food a lot. I'm obsessed with reading books and magazines about dieting, fitness, and weight control. I sometimes miss school, work, and social events because of my diet or exercise schedule. I divide food into "good" and "bad" categories. I feel guilty when I eat "bad" foods or when I eat more than I feel I should be eating. I am afraid of getting fat. I wish I could change how much I want to eat and what I am hungry for.	I pay attention to what I eat in order to maintain a healthy body. Food and exercise are important parts of my life, but they only occupy a small part of my time. I enjoy eating, and I balance my pleasure with my concern for a healthy body. I usually eat three balanced meals daily, plus snacks, to fuel my body with adequate energy. I am moderate and flexible in my goals for eating well and being physically active. Sometimes I eat more (or less) than I really need, but most of the time I listen to my body.	I am not concerned about what or how much I eat. I feel no guilt or shame no matter what I eat or how much I eat. Exercise is not really important to me. I choose foods based on cost, taste, and convenience, with little regard to health. My eating is very sporadic and irregular. I don't worry about meals; I just eat whatever I can, whenever I can. I enjoy stuffing myself with lots of tasty food at restaurants, holiday meals, and social events.

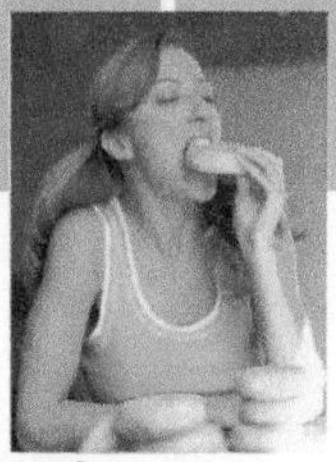

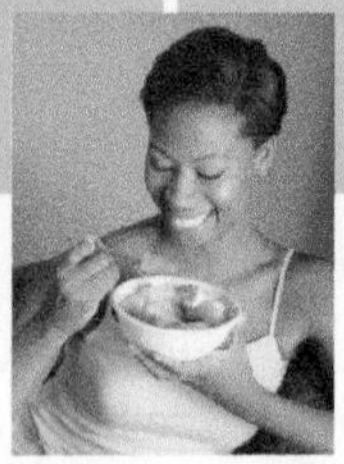

Figure 2.8 Eating Issues Continuum

This continuum shows progression from eating disorders to normal eating. The goal is to be concerned in a healthy way.

Source: Adapted from Smiley/King/Avery, "Eating Issues and Body Image Continuum," Campus Health Service 1996. Copyright © 1997 Arizona Board of Regents for University of Arizona.

check yourself

- **Where do you place yourself on the eating issues continuum?**

2.14 Eating Disorders: Anorexia Nervosa

learning outcome

2.14 List the criteria, effects, and treatment of anorexia nervosa.

Anorexia nervosa is a persistent, chronic eating disorder characterized by deliberate food restriction and severe, life-threatening weight loss. It involves self-starvation motivated by an intense fear of gaining weight along with an extremely distorted body image. Initially, most people with anorexia nervosa lose weight by reducing total food intake, particularly of high-calorie foods. Eventually, they progress to restricting their intake of almost all foods. The little they do eat, they may purge through vomiting or use of laxatives. Although they lose weight, people with anorexia nervosa never seem to feel thin enough.

An estimated 0.3 percent of females suffer from anorexia nervosa in their lifetime.[67] The American Psychiatric Association (APA) criteria for anorexia nervosa are:[68]

- Refusal to maintain body weight at or above a minimally normal weight for age and height
- Intense fear of gaining weight or becoming fat, even though considered underweight by all medical criteria
- Disturbance in the way in which one's body weight or shape is experienced, undue influence of body weight or shape on self-evaluation, or denial of the seriousness of the current low body weight

Physical symptoms and negative health consequences associated with anorexia nervosa are illustrated in Figure 2.9. Because it involves starvation and can lead to heart attacks and seizures, anorexia nervosa has the highest death rate (20%) of any psychological illness.[69]

The causes of anorexia nervosa are complex and variable. Many people with anorexia have other coexisting psychiatric problems, including low self-esteem, depression, an anxiety disorder such as obsessive-compulsive disorder, and substance abuse. Some people with anorexia nervosa have a history of being physically or sexually abused, and others have troubled interpersonal relationships with family members. Cultural norms that value people on the basis of their appearance and glorify thinness are of course a factor, as is weight-based teasing and weight bias.[70] Physical factors are thought to include an imbalance of neurotransmitters and genetic susceptibility.[71]

Once the patient is stabilized, treatment involves long-term therapy that focuses on the psychological, social, environmental, and physiological factors that have led to the problem. Through therapy, the patient works on adopting new eating behaviors, building self-confidence, and finding other ways to deal with life's problems. Support groups can also help.

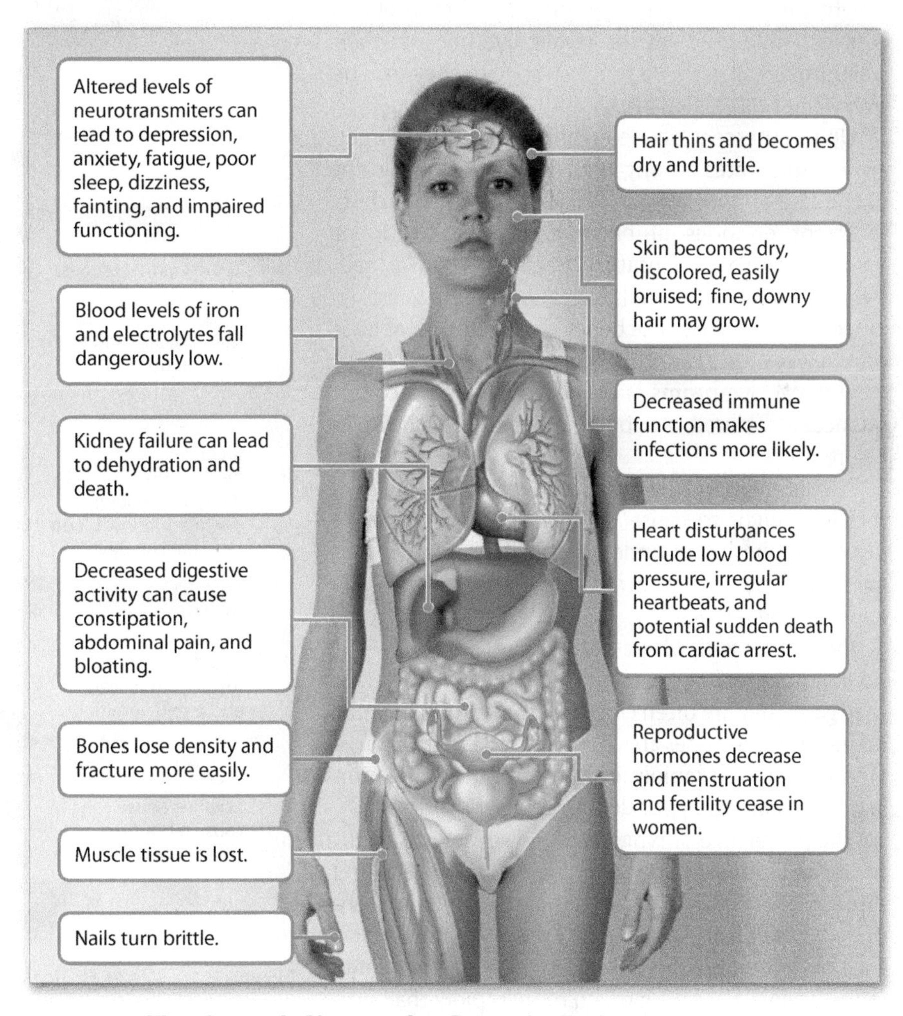

Figure 2.9 What Anorexia Nervosa Can Do to the Body

check yourself

- **What factors might put a person at risk for anorexia nervosa?**
- **How is anorexia nervosa treated?**

2.15 Eating Disorders: Bulimia Nervosa and Binge Eating

learning outcome

2.15 List the criteria, effects, and treatments for bulimia nervosa and binge eating.

Individuals with **bulimia nervosa** often binge on huge amounts of food and then engage in some kind of purging or "compensatory behavior," such as vomiting, taking laxatives, or exercising excessively, to lose the calories they have just consumed. People with bulimia are obsessed with their bodies, weight gain, and appearance, although their problem is often "hidden" from the public eye because their weight may fall within a normal range or they may be overweight.

Up to 3 percent of adolescents and young women are bulimic; rates among men are about 10 percent of the rate among women.[72] The APA criteria include recurrent episodes of binge eating and recurrent inappropriate compensatory behavior such as self-induced vomiting, use of laxatives or diuretics, fasting, or excessive exercise. The behavior must occur at least once a week for 3 months.[73]

Physical symptoms and negative health consequences associated with bulimia nervosa are shown in Figure 2.10.

A combination of genetic and environmental factors is thought to cause bulimia nervosa.[74] A family history of obesity, an underlying anxiety disorder, and an imbalance in neurotransmitters are all possible contributing factors.[75]

Individuals with **binge-eating disorder** gorge, but do not take excessive measures to lose the weight they gain; they are often clinically obese. As in bulimia, binge-eating episodes are characterized by eating large amounts of food rapidly, even when not feeling hungry, and feeling guilty or depressed after overeating.[76]

The prevalence of binge-eating disorder is thought to be 1.4 percent.[77] The APA criteria for binge-eating disorder are similar to those for bulimia nervosa, without compensatory behavior.[78] Those diagnosed with the condition also show three or more of the following behaviors: (1) eating much more rapidly than normal; (2) eating until uncomfortably full; (3) eating large amounts when not physically hungry; (4) eating alone because of embarrassment over how much one is eating; (5) feeling disgusted, depressed, or very guilty after overeating.

Without treatment, approximately 20 percent of people with a serious eating disorder will die from it; with treatment, long-term full recovery rates range from 44 to 76 percent.[79] Treatment for bulimia and binge eating is similar to treatment for anorexia. Support groups can help the family and the individual learn positive actions and interactions. Treatment of an underlying anxiety disorder or depression may also be a focus.

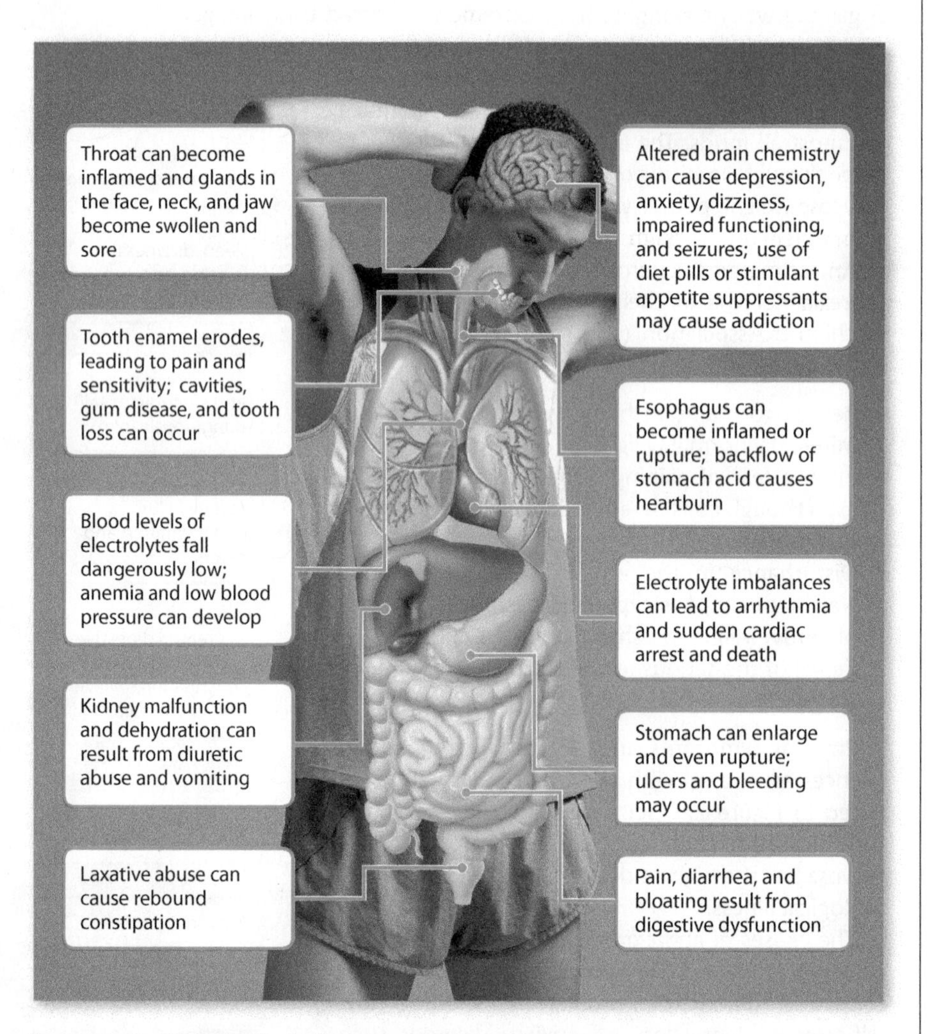

Figure 2.10 What Bulimia Nervosa Can Do to the Body

check yourself

- **What factors might put a person at risk for bulimia nervosa and binge-eating disorder?**
- **How are bulimia nervosa and binge-eating disorder treated?**

Exercise Disorders

learning outcome

2.16 List the criteria, effects, and treatment for exercise disorders.

Although exercise is generally beneficial to health, in excess it can be a problem. In addition to being a common compensatory behavior used by people with anorexia or bulimia, exercise can become a compulsion or contribute to muscle dysmorphia and the female athlete triad.

A recent study showed that participants used excessive exercise or compulsive exercise as a way to regulate their emotions.[80] **Compulsive exercise**, or *anorexia athletica*, is characterized not by a *desire* to exercise but a *compulsion* to do so, with guilt and anxiety if the person doesn't work out.

Compulsive exercise can contribute to injuries to joints and bones. It can also put significant stress on the heart, especially if combined with disordered eating. Psychologically, people who engage in compulsive exercise are often plagued by anxiety and/or depression.

Muscle Dysmorphia

Muscle dysmorphia appears to be a relatively new form of body image disturbance and exercise disorder in which a man believes that his body is insufficiently lean or muscular.[81] Men with muscle dysmorphia believe that they look "puny," when in reality they look normal or may even be unusually muscular. Behaviors characteristic of muscle dysmorphia include comparing oneself unfavorably to others, checking one's appearance in the mirror, and camouflaging one's appearance. Men with muscle dysmorphia also are likely to abuse anabolic steroids and dietary supplements.[82]

The Female Athlete Triad

Female athletes in competitive sports often strive for perfection. In an effort to be the best, they may put themselves at risk for a syndrome called the **female athlete triad**, with three interrelated problems (Figure 2.11): low energy intake, typically prompted by disordered eating; menstrual dysfunction such as amenorrhea; and poor bone density.[83]

How does the female athlete triad develop? First, a chronic pattern of low food intake and intensive exercise depletes nutrients essential to health. The body begins to burn stores of fat tissue for energy, reducing levels of the female reproductive hormone *estrogen*, and so stopping menstruation. Depletion of fat-soluble vitamins, calcium, and estrogen weakens the athlete's bones, leaving her at high risk for fracture.

See It! Videos

Can you go too far with extreme exercise? Watch **Young Boys Exercising to Extremes** in the Study Area of MasteringHealth.

The triad is particularly prevalent in athletes in highly competitive individual sports that emphasize leanness—gymnasts, figure skaters, cross-country runners, and ballet dancers.

Warning signs include dry skin; light-headedness/fainting; fine, downy hair covering the body; multiple injuries; and changes in endurance, strength, or speed. Associated behaviors include preoccupation with food and weight, compulsive exercising, use of weight-loss products or laxatives, self-criticism, anxiety, and depression. Treatment requires a multidisciplinary approach involving the athlete's coach or trainer, a psychologist, and family members and friends.

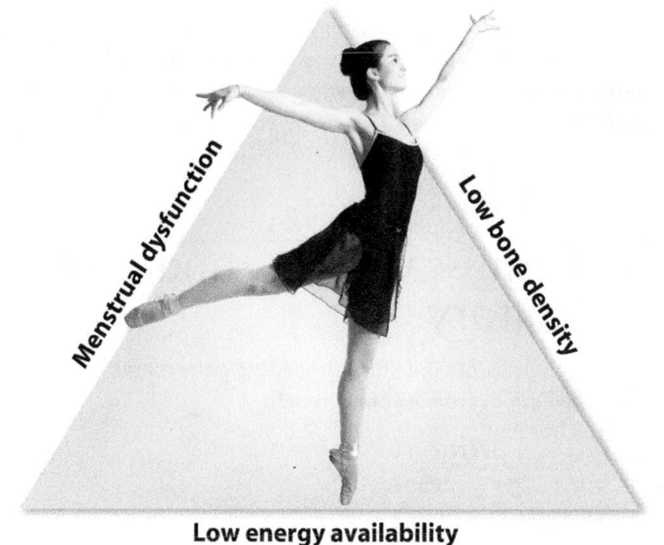

Figure 2.11 The Female Athlete Triad
The female athlete triad is a cluster of three interrelated health problems.

Men with muscle dysmorphia may have unusually muscular bodies but suffer from very low self-esteem.

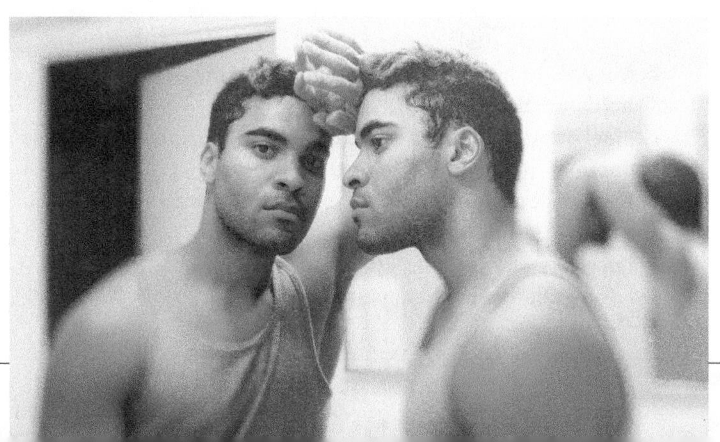

check yourself

- **What are the criteria, effects, and treatment for exercise disorders? How might these differ for men and women?**

Assessyourself

2.17

Are You Ready to Jump Start Your Weight Loss?

An interactive version of this assessment is available online in MasteringHealth.

If you are overweight or obese, complete each of the following questions by circling the response(s) that best represents your situation or attitudes, then total your points for each section. Section 1 indicates the factors that may predispose you to excess weight and make weight loss more challenging. Section 2 assesses how ready you are to begin losing weight right now.

1 Family, Weight, and Diet History

1. How many people in your immediate family (parents or siblings) are overweight or obese?

   a. No one is overweight or obese (0 points)
   b. One person (1 point)
   c. Two people (2 points)
   d. Three or more people (3 points)

2. During which periods of your life were you overweight or obese? (Circle all that apply.)

   a. Birth through age 5 (1 point)
   b. Ages 6 to 11 (1 point)
   c. Ages 12 to 13 (1 point))
   d. Ages 14 to 18 (2 points)
   e. Ages 19 to present (2 points)

3. How many times in the last year have you made an effort to lose weight but have had little or no success?

   a. None. I've never thought about it. (0 points)
   b. I've thought about it, but I've never tried hard to lose weight. (1 point)
   c. I have tried 2 to 3 times. (1 point)
   d. I have tried at least once a month. (2 points)
   e. I have tried so many times, I can't remember the number. (3 points)

4. How would you describe your weight right now?

   a. Normal and consistent (1 point)
   b. Normal but difficult to maintain (2 points)
   c. Overweight (3 points)
   d. Obese (4 points)

Total points: __________

Scoring

A score of 5 or higher suggests that you may have several challenges ahead as you begin a weight loss program. The higher your score, the greater the likelihood of challenges.

Your own weight problems may be related, at least in part, to the eating habits and preferences you learned at home, and it may take a conscious effort to change them. If in the past you tried repeatedly to lose weight but returned to your old behaviors, you may have to reframe your thinking.

2 Readiness to Change

Attitudes and Beliefs About Weight Loss

1. What is/are your main reason(s) for wanting to lose weight? (Circle all that apply.)

   a. I want to please someone I know or attract a new person. (0 points)
   b. I want to look great and/or fit into smaller size clothes for an upcoming event (wedding, vacation, date, etc.). (1 point)
   c. Someone I know has had major health problems because of being overweight/obese. (1 point)
   d. I want to improve my health and/or have more energy. (2 points)
   e. I was diagnosed with a health problem (pre-diabetes, diabetes, high blood pressure, etc.) because of being overweight/obese. (2 points)

2. What do you think about your weight and body shape? (Circle all that apply.)

   a. I'm fine with being overweight, and if others don't like it, tough! (0 points)
   b. My weight hurts my energy levels and my performance and holds me back. (1 point)
   c. I feel good about myself, but think I will be happier if I lose some of my weight. (1 point)
   d. I'm self-conscious about my weight and uncomfortable in my skin. (1 point)
   e. I'm really worried that I will have a major health problem if I don't change my behaviors now. (2 points)

Daily Eating Patterns

3. Which of the following statements describes you? (Circle all that apply.)

   a. I think about food several times a day, even when I'm not hungry. (0 point)

   b. There are some foods or snacks that I can't stay away from, and I eat them even when I'm not hungry. (0 point)

   c. I tend to eat more meat and fatty foods and never get enough fruits and veggies. (0 points)

   d. I've thought about the weaknesses in my diet and have some ideas about what I need to do. (1 point)

   e. I haven't really tried to eat a "balanced" diet, but I know that I need to start now. (1 point)

4. When you binge or eat things you shouldn't or too much at one sitting, what are you likely to do? (Circle all that apply.)

   a. Not care and go off of my diet. (0 points)

   b. Feel guilty for a while, but then do it again the next time I am out. (0 points)

   c. Fast for the next day or two to help balance the high consumption day. (0 points)

   d. Plan ahead for next time and have options in mind so that I do not continue to overeat. (1 point)

   e. Acknowledge that I have made a slip and get back on my program the next day. (1 point)

5. On a typical day, what are your eating patterns? (Circle all that apply.)

   a. I skip breakfast and save my calories for lunch and dinner. (0 point)

   b. I never really sit down for a meal. I am a "grazer" and eat whatever I find that is readily available. (0 point)

   c. I try to eat at least five servings of fruits and veggies and restrict saturated fats in my diet. (1 point)

   d. I eat several small meals, trying to be balanced in my portions and getting foods from different food groups. (1 point)

Commitment to Weight Loss and Exercise

6. How would you describe your current support system for helping you lose weight? (Circle all that apply.)

   a. I believe I can do this best by doing it on my own. (0 points)

   b. I am not aware of any sources that can help me. (0 points)

   c. I have two to three friends or family members I can count on to help me. (1 point)

   d. There are counselors on campus with whom I can meet to plan a successful approach to weight loss. (1 point)

   e. I have the resources to join Weight Watchers or other community or online weight loss programs. (1 point)

7. How committed are you to exercising? (Circle all that apply.)

   a. Exercise is uncomfortable, embarrassing, and/or I don't enjoy it. (0 points)

   b. I don't have time to exercise. (0 points)

   c. I'd like to exercise, but I'm not sure how to get started. (1 point)

   d. I've visited my campus recreation center or local gym to explore my options for exercise. (2 points)

   e. There are specific sports or physical activities I do already, and I can plan to do more of them. (2 points)

8. What statement best describes your motivation to start a weight loss/lifestyle change program?

   a. I don't want to start losing weight. (0 points)

   b. I am thinking about it sometime in the distant future. (0 points)

   c. I am considering starting within the next few weeks; I just need to make a plan. (1 point)

   d. I'd like to start in the next few weeks, and I'm working on a plan. (2 points)

   e. I already have a plan in place, and I'm ready to begin tomorrow. (3 points)

Total points: __________

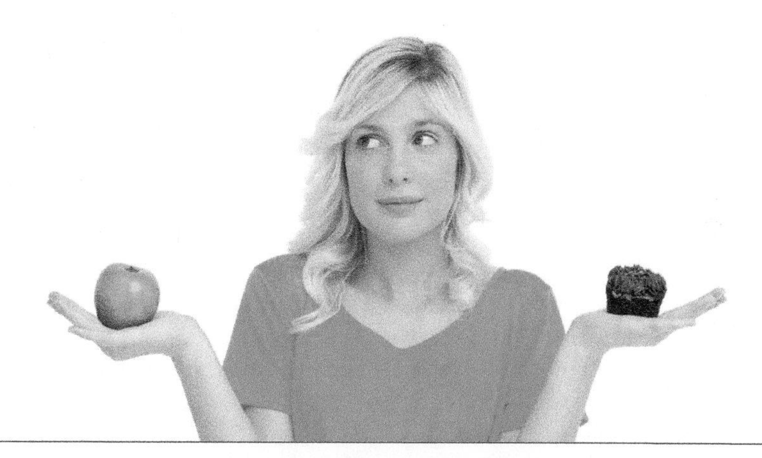

Scoring

A score higher than 8 indicates that you may be ready to change; the higher your score above 8, the more successful you may be. If you scored lower than 8, consider the following:

One of the first steps in making a plan to lose weight is to recognize your strengths and weaknesses and be ready to anticipate challenges. Think about the stages of change model to determine if your current thoughts and attitudes about weight loss reflect a good foundation for beginning a successful weight loss program. Which long-term motivations will you need to successfully lose weight? Which benefits of losing weight motivate you most strongly? Which behavioral changes are you ready to make to address your weight issues?

In order to lose weight, you will need to change your daily eating habits. Overeating (or eating poorly) may be a response to your food attitudes rather than to physical hunger. Poor eating may also reflect your emotional responses toward food, and/or unhealthy dietary choices. To increase your commitment to weight loss and exercise, think of friends or family who can support your efforts to stick to your plan. Also consider the wealth of available resources and where you can go for help. Having a plan and sticking to it will be crucial as you begin your weight loss journey!

Your Plan for Change

The Assess Yourself activity identifies areas of importance in determining your readiness for weight loss. If you wish to lose weight to improve your health, understanding your attitudes about food and exercise will help you succeed in your plan.

Today, you can:

◯ Set "SMART" goals for weight loss and give them a reality check: Are they specific, measurable, achievable, relevant, and time-oriented? For example, rather than aiming to lose 15 pounds this month (which probably wouldn't be healthy or achievable), set a comfortable goal to lose 5 pounds. Realistic goals will encourage weight-loss success by boosting your confidence in your ability to make lifelong healthy changes.

◯ Begin keeping a food log and identifying the triggers that influence your eating habits. Think about what you can do to eliminate or reduce the influence of your two most common food triggers.

Within the next 2 weeks, you can:

◯ Get in the habit of incorporating more fruits, vegetables, and whole grains in your diet and eating less fat. The next time you make dinner, look at the proportions on your plate. If vegetables and whole grains do not take up most of the space, substitute 1 cup of the meat, pasta, or cheese in your meal with 1 cup of legumes, salad greens, or a favorite vegetable. You'll reduce the number of calories while eating the same amount of food!

◯ Aim to incorporate more exercise into your daily routine. Visit your campus rec center or a local gym and familiarize yourself with the equipment and facilities that are available. Try a new machine or sports activity, and experiment until you find a form of exercise you really enjoy.

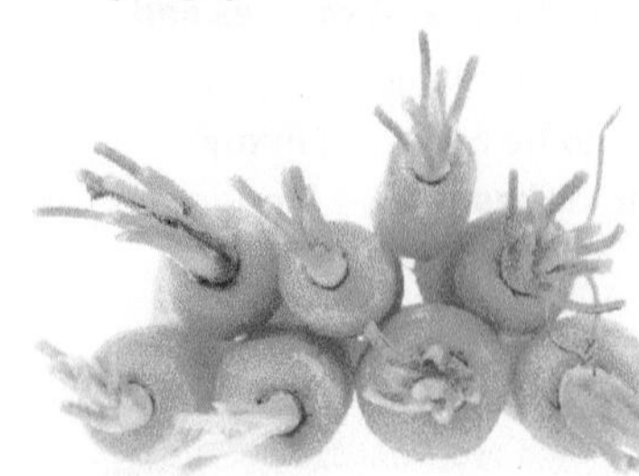

By the end of the semester, you can:

◯ Get in the habit of grocery shopping every week and buying healthy, nutritious foods while avoiding high-fat, high-sugar, or overly processed foods. As you make healthy foods more available and unhealthy foods less available, you'll find it easier to eat better.

◯ Chart your progress and reward yourself as you meet your goals. If your goal is to lose weight and you successfully take off 10 pounds, reward yourself with a new pair of jeans or other article of clothing (which will likely fit better than before!).

How Sensible Are Your Efforts to Be Thin?

An interactive version of this assessment is available online in MasteringHealth.

On one hand, just because you weigh yourself, count calories, or work out every day, don't jump to the conclusion that you have any of the health concerns discussed in this chapter. On the other hand, efforts to lose a few pounds can spiral out of control. To find out whether your efforts to be thin are harmful to you, take the following quiz from the National Eating Disorders Association (NEDA).

1. I constantly calculate numbers of fat grams and calories. T F
2. I weigh myself often and find myself obsessed with the number on the scale. T F
3. I exercise to burn calories and not for health or enjoyment. T F
4. I sometimes feel out of control while eating. T F
5. I often go on extreme diets. T F
6. I engage in rituals to get me through mealtimes and/or secretly binge. T F
7. Weight loss, dieting, and controlling my food intake have become my major concerns. T F
8. I feel ashamed, disgusted, or guilty after eating. T F
9. I constantly worry about the weight, shape, and/or size of my body. T F
10. I feel my identity and value are based on how I look or how much I weigh. T F

If any of these statements is true for you, you could be dealing with disordered eating. If so, talk about it! Tell a friend, parent, teacher, coach, youth group leader, doctor, counselor, or nutritionist what you're going through. Check out the NEDA's Sharing with EEEase handout at www.nationaleatingdisorders.org for help planning what to say the first time you talk to someone about your eating and exercise habits.

Source: Reprinted with permission from the National Eating Disorders Association, www.nationaleatingdisorders.org.

Your Plan for Change

The Assess Yourself activity gave you the chance to evaluate your feelings about your body, and to determine whether or not you might be engaging in eating or exercise behaviors that could undermine your health and happiness. Here are some steps you can take to improve your body image, starting today.

Today, you can:

◯ Talk back to the media. Write letters to advertisers and magazines that depict unhealthy and unrealistic body types. Boycott their products or start a blog commenting on harmful body image messages in the media.

◯ Visit www.choosemyplate.gov and create a personalized food plan. Just for today, eat the recommended number of servings from every food group at every meal, and don't count calories!

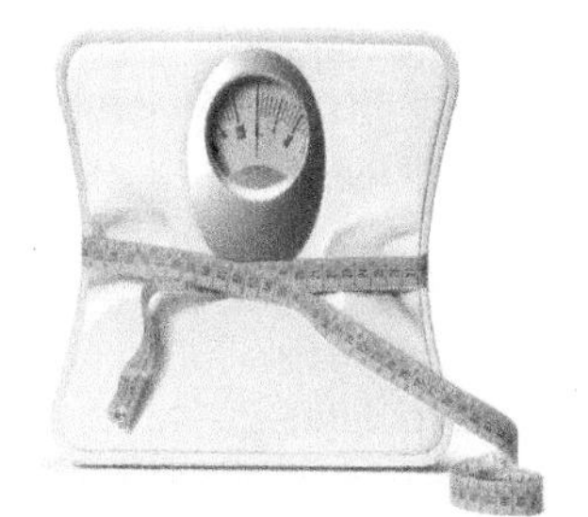

Within the next 2 weeks, you can:

◯ Find a photograph of a person you admire not for his or her appearance, but for his or her contribution to humanity. Paste it up next to your mirror to remind yourself that true beauty comes from within and benefits others.

◯ Start a journal. Each day, record one thing you are grateful for that has nothing to do with your appearance. At the end of each day, record one small thing you did to make someone's world a little brighter.

By the end of the semester, you can:

◯ Establish a group of friends who support you for who you are, not what you look like, and who get the same support from you. Form a group on a favorite social-networking site and keep in touch, especially when you start to feel troubled by self-defeating thoughts or have the urge to engage in unhealthy eating or exercise behaviors.

◯ Borrow from the library or purchase one of the many books on body image now available, and read it!

Summary

To hear an MP3 Tutor session, scan here or visit the Study Area in **MasteringHealth.**

LO 2.1 Overweight, obesity, and weight-related health problems have reached epidemic levels in the United States, largely due to obesogenic behaviors in an obesogenic environment.

LO 2.2 Societal costs from obesity include increased health care costs, lowered worker productivity, low self-esteem, and obesity-related stigma. Individual health risks from overweight and obesity include a variety of chronic diseases.

LO 2.3–2.4 Many factors contribute to risk for obesity, including environmental factors, poverty, education level, genetics, developmental factors, endocrine influences, psychosocial factors, eating cues, metabolic changes, and lifestyle.

LO 2.5–2.6 Percentage of body fat is a reliable indicator for levels of overweight and obesity. *Overweight* is most commonly defined as a BMI of 25 to 29 and *obesity* as a BMI of 30 or greater. Waist circumference is believed to be related to risk for several chronic diseases, particularly type 2 diabetes. Body mass index is one of the most commonly accepted measures of assessing body fat.

LO 2.7–2.9 Sensible eating and exercise offer the best options for weight loss and maintenance. The best diet programs allow you to make healthy choices in real-world settings without sacrificing everything enjoyable. Successful weight management includes making a plan and changing habits.

LO 2.10 Diet pills, surgery, and very-low-calorie diets are drastic measures for weight loss and may carry significant risks.

LO 2.11 To gain weight, increase intake of energy-dense, nutritious foods.

LO 2.12 Negative feelings about one's body can contribute to behaviors that can threaten health. In contrast, a healthy body image can contribute to reduced stress and personal empowerment. Body image disorders affect men and women of all ages. Body image can be affected by culture, media, and individual physiological and psychological factors.

LO 2.13–2.15 Disordered eating and eating disorders such as anorexia nervosa, bulimia nervosa, and binge-eating disorder can lead to serious health problems and even death.

LO 2.16 Although exercise is healthy in moderation, if it becomes a compulsion it can lead to disorders such as muscle dysmorphia and the female athlete triad.

Pop Quiz

Visit MasteringHealth to personalize your study plan with Chapter Review Quizzes and Dynamic Study Modules.

LO 2.3 1. The rate at which your body consumes food energy to sustain basic functions is your
a. basal metabolic rate.
b. resting metabolic rate.
c. body mass index.
d. set point.

LO 2.5 2. Which of the following statements is *false*?
a. A slowing basal metabolic rate may contribute to weight gain after age 30.
b. Hormones are implicated in hunger impulses and eating behavior.
c. The more muscles you have, the fewer calories you'll burn.
d. Overweight and obesity can have serious health consequences, even before middle age.

LO 2.6 3. Which of the following statements about BMI is *false*?
a. BMI is based on height and weight measurements.
b. BMI is accurate for everyone, including people with high muscle mass.
c. Children's BMIs are used to determine a percentile ranking among their age peers.
d. BMI stands for "body mass index."

LO 2.6 4. Which of the following BMI ratings is considered overweight?
a. 20
b. 25
c. 30
d. 35

LO 2.6 5. Which of the following body circumferences is most strongly associated with risk of heart disease and diabetes?
a. Hip circumference
b. Chest circumference
c. Waist circumference
d. Thigh circumference

LO 2.7 6. One pound of additional body fat is created through consuming how many extra calories?
a. 1,500 calories
b. 3,500 calories
c. 5,000 calories
d. 7,000 calories

LO 2.7 7. To lose weight, you must establish a(n)
a. negative caloric balance.
b. energy balance.
c. positive caloric balance.
d. set point.

LO 2.9 8. Successful, healthy weight loss is characterized by
a. a lifelong pattern of healthful eating and exercise.
b. cutting out fats and carbohydrates.
c. never eating foods considered bad for you.
d. a pattern of repeatedly losing and regaining weight.

LO 2.12 9. Which of the following is not a contributor to negative body image?
a. Idealized media images of celebrities
b. Increases in portion sizes
c. Cultural attitudes about body ideals
d. Neurotransmitter regulation in the brain

LO 2.15 10. Which of the following eating disorders includes compensatory behavior in its definition?
a. Anorexia nervosa
b. Bulimia nervosa
c. Binge-eating disorder
d. Muscle dysmorphia

Answers to these questions can be found on page A-1. If you answered a question incorrectly, review the module identified by the Learning Outcome. For even more study tools, visit MasteringHealth.

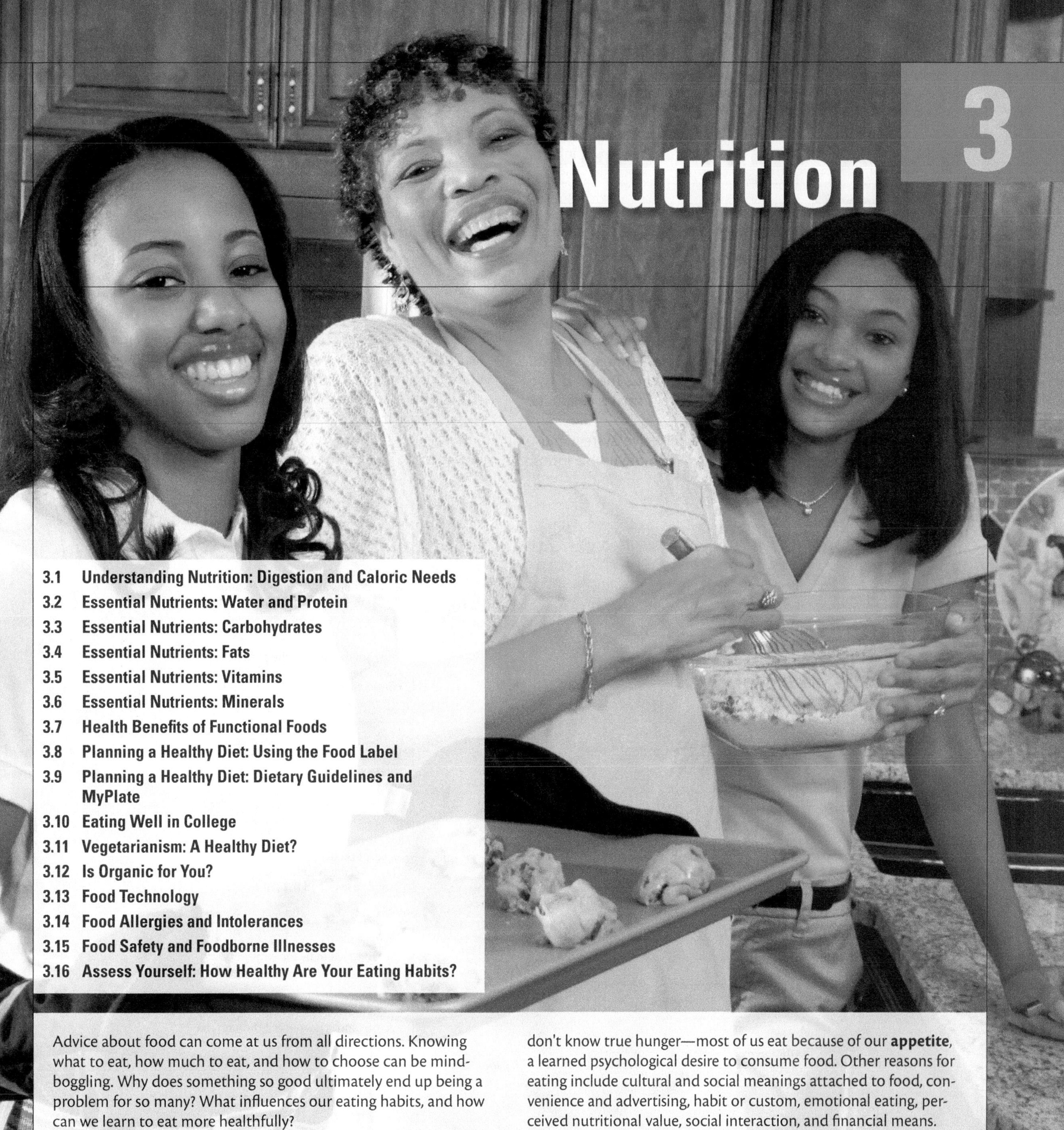

Nutrition 3

Advice about food can come at us from all directions. Knowing what to eat, how much to eat, and how to choose can be mind-boggling. Why does something so good ultimately end up being a problem for so many? What influences our eating habits, and how can we learn to eat more healthfully?

True **hunger** occurs when there is a lack of basic foods. When we're hungry, our brains initiate a physiological response that prompts us to seek food for the energy and **nutrients** our bodies need for proper functioning. Most people in the United States don't know true hunger—most of us eat because of our **appetite**, a learned psychological desire to consume food. Other reasons for eating include cultural and social meanings attached to food, convenience and advertising, habit or custom, emotional eating, perceived nutritional value, social interaction, and financial means.

Nutrition is the science that investigates the relationship between physiological function and the essential elements of the foods we eat. Your health largely depends on what and how much you eat.

3.1 Understanding Nutrition: Digestion and Caloric Needs

learning outcome

3.1 Describe the digestive process and identify daily calorie needs.

Food provides the chemicals we need for activity and body maintenance. Our bodies cannot synthesize certain *essential nutrients* (or cannot synthesize them in adequate amounts)—we must obtain them from the foods we eat. Of the six groups of essential nutrients, the four we need in the largest amounts—water, proteins, carbohydrates, and fats—are called *macronutrients*. The other two groups—vitamins and minerals—are needed in smaller amounts, so they are called *micronutrients*.

Before the body can use foods, the digestive system must break down larger food particles into smaller, more usable forms. The sequence of functions by which the body breaks down foods and either absorbs or excretes them is the digestive process (Figure 3.1).

Recommended Intakes for Nutrients

The recommended amounts of each nutrient group are known as the *Dietary Reference Intakes (DRIs)*. The DRIs are published by the Food and Nutrition Board of the Institute of Medicine, and they establish the amount of each nutrient needed to prevent deficiencies or reduce the risk of chronic disease, as well as identify maximum safe intake levels for healthy people. The DRIs are umbrella guidelines and include the following categories:

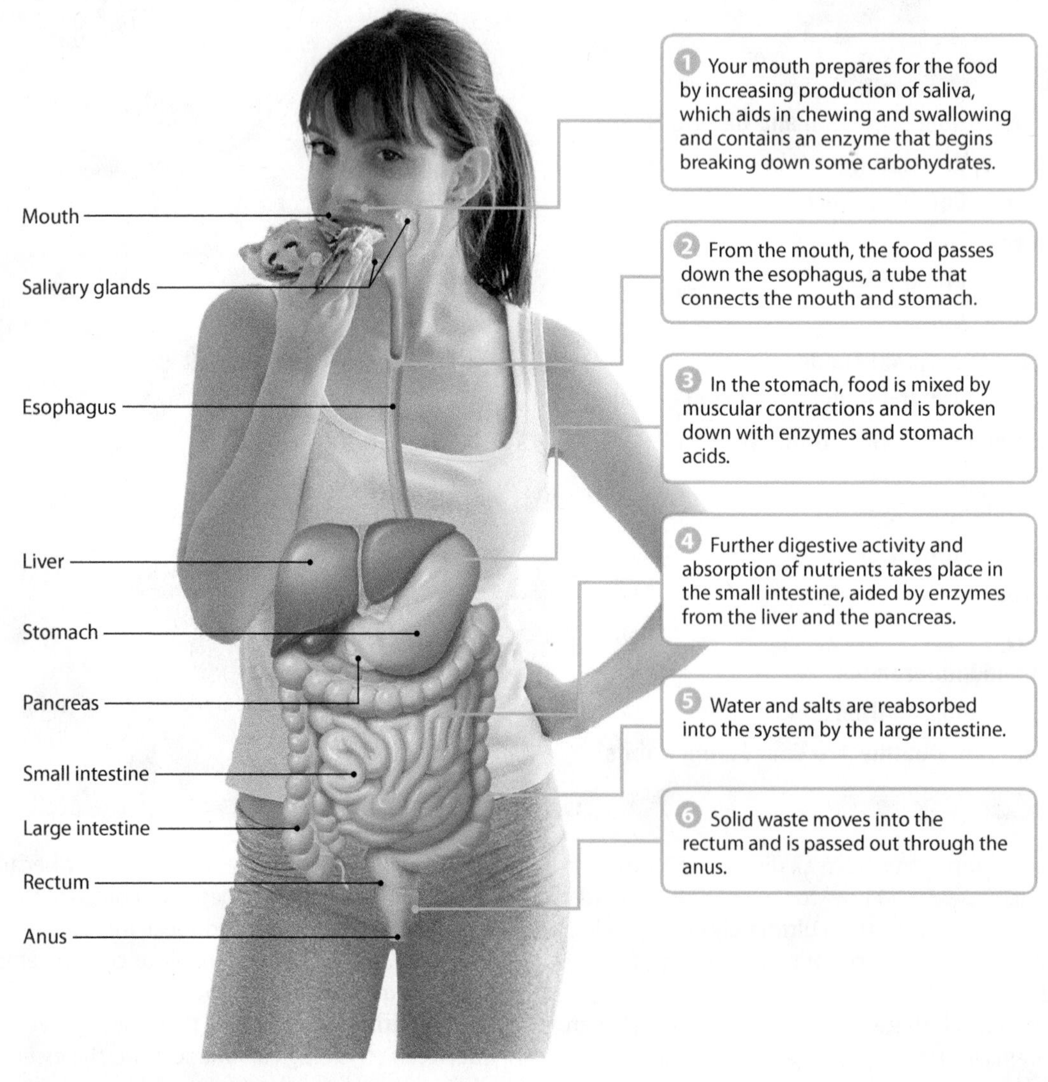

Figure 3.1 The Digestive Process
The entire digestive process takes approximately 24 hours.

- **Recommended Dietary Allowances (RDAs)** are daily nutrient intake levels meeting the nutritional needs of 97 to 98 percent of healthy individuals.
- **Adequate Intakes (AIs)** are daily intake levels assumed to be adequate for most healthy people. AIs are used when there isn't enough research to support establishing an RDA.
- **Tolerable Upper Intake Levels (ULs)** are the highest amounts of a nutrient that an individual can consume daily without risking adverse health effects.
- **Acceptable Macronutrient Distribution Ranges (AMDRs)** are ranges of protein, carbohydrate, and fat intake that provide adequate nutrition, and they are associated with a reduced risk for chronic disease.

Whereas the RDAs, AIs, and ULs are expressed as amounts—usually milligrams (mg) or micrograms (µg)—AMDRs are expressed as percentages. The AMDR for protein, for example, is 10 to 35 percent, meaning that no less than 10 percent and no more than 35 percent of the calories you consume should come from proteins. But that raises a new question: What are calories?

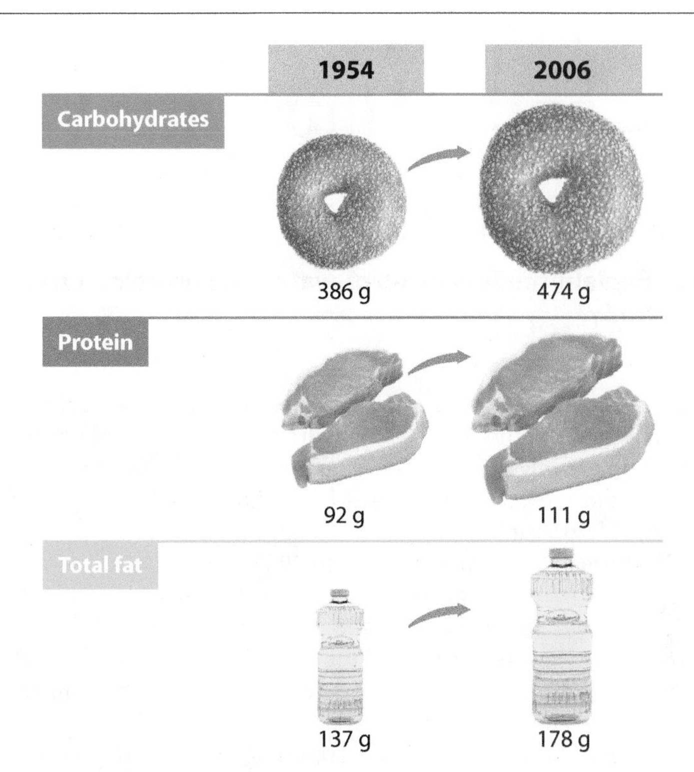

Figure 3.2 Trends in Per Capita Nutrient Consumption
Since 1954, Americans' daily caloric intake has increased by about 25 percent, as has daily consumption of carbohydrates and protein. Daily total fat intake has increased by 30 percent.
Source: Data from USDA Economic Research Service, "Nutrient Availability," Updated August 2012, www.ers.usda.gov.

TABLE 3.1 **Estimated Daily Calorie Needs**

	Calorie Range	
	Sedentary[a]	Active[b]
CHILDREN		
2–3 years old	1,000	1,400
FEMALES		
4–8 years old	1,200	1,800
9–13	1,400	2,200
14–18	1,800	2,400
19–30	1,800	2,400
31–50	1,800	2,200
51+	1,600	2,200
MALES		
4–8 years old	1,200	2,000
9–13	1,600	2,600
14–18	2,000	3,200
19–30	2,400	3,000
31–50	2,200	3,000
51+	2,000	2,800

[a] A lifestyle that includes only the light physical activity associated with typical day-to-day life.
[b] A lifestyle that includes physical activity equivalent to walking more than 3 miles per day at 3 to 4 miles per hour, in addition to the light physical activity associated with typical day-to-day life.

Source: U.S. Department of Agriculture and U.S. Department of Health and Human Services, *Dietary Guidelines for Americans, 2010*, 7th ed. (Washington, DC: U.S. Government Printing Office).

Calories

A *kilocalorie* is a unit of measure used to quantify the amount of energy in food. On nutrition labels and in consumer publications, the term is shortened to **calorie**. *Energy* is defined as the capacity to do work. We derive energy from the energy-containing nutrients in the foods we eat. These nutrients—proteins, carbohydrates, and fats—provide calories. Vitamins, minerals, and water do not. It's important to know your approximate caloric needs, based on your age, gender, and activity level. Table 3.1 shows the caloric needs for various individuals.

Overall, Americans today eat more food than ever before. From 1970 to 2008, average calorie consumption increased from 2,157 to 2,614 calories per day (see Figure 3.2).[1] In general, it isn't the actual amount of food, but the number of calories in the foods we choose to eat that has increased. When these trends are combined with our increasingly sedentary lifestyle, it is not surprising that we have seen a dramatic rise in obesity.[2] With an understanding of nutrition, you will be able to make more informed choices about your diet and lifestyle.

check yourself

- **Describe the digestive process, from mouth to excretion.**
- **What are your estimated daily calorie needs?**

3.2 Essential Nutrients: Water and Protein

learning outcome

3.2 Explain the functions of water and protein in the body.

Water

Humans can survive for several weeks without food but only for about 1 week without water. **Dehydration**, a state of abnormal depletion of body fluids, can develop within a single day, especially in a hot climate. Too much water—*hyponatremia*—can also pose a serious risk to your health.

The human body consists of 50 to 70 percent water by weight. The water in our system bathes cells, aids in fluid and electrolyte balance, maintains pH balance, and transports molecules and cells throughout the body. Water is the major component of blood, which carries oxygen and nutrients to the tissues, removes metabolic wastes, and keeps cells in working order.

Individual needs for water vary according to dietary factors, age, size, overall health, environmental temperature and humidity, and exercise. The latest DRIs suggest that most people can meet their hydration needs simply by eating a healthy diet and drinking in response to thirst. The general recommendations for women are approximately 9 cups of total water from all beverages and foods each day, and for men, an average of 13 cups.[3]

About 20 percent of our daily water needs are met through the food we eat. Fruits and vegetables are 80 to 95 percent water, meats more than 50 percent water, and bread and cheese about 35 percent water! Contrary to popular opinion, caffeinated drinks, including coffee, tea, and soda, also count toward total fluid intake for those who regularly consume them. Caffeinated beverages have not been found to dehydrate people whose bodies are used to caffeine.[4]

Of course, there are situations in which a person needs additional fluids to stay properly hydrated. It is important to drink extra fluids when you have a fever or an illness in which there is vomiting or diarrhea. People with kidney problems, diabetes, or cystic fibrosis may need more water, as may the elderly and very young. When the weather heats up or when you sweat profusely, extra water is needed to keep your core temperature within a normal range; visit the American College of Sports Medicine's website (www.acsm.org) to download its brochure, "Selecting and Effectively Using Hydration for Fitness."[5]

Protein

Next to water, **proteins** are the most abundant substances in the human body. Proteins are major components of nearly every cell; they've been called the "body builders" because of their role in developing and repairing bone, muscle, skin, and blood cells. They are the key elements of antibodies that protect us from disease, of enzymes that control chemical activities in the body, and of hormones that regulate body functions. Proteins help transport iron, oxygen, and nutrients to all body cells and supply another source of energy to cells when fats and carbohydrates are not available. Every gram of protein you eat provides 4 calories. Adequate amounts of protein in the diet are vital to many body functions and, ultimately, to survival.

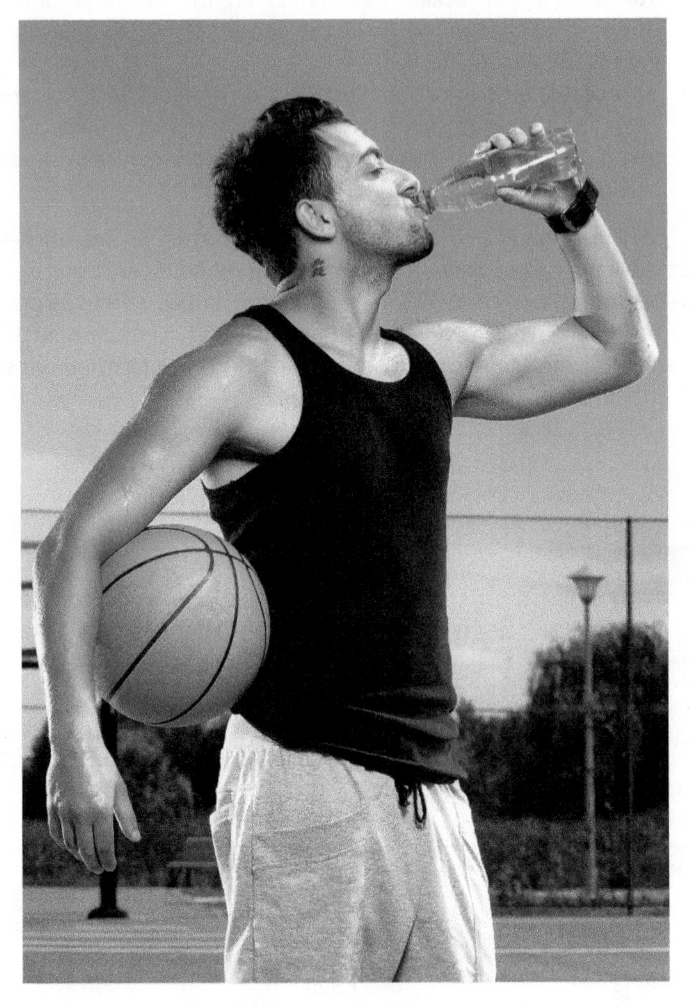

Drinking water is important to maintain normal body functioning. If you're exercising in hot weather or sweating profusely, it's crucial to stay adequately hydrated.

Your body breaks down proteins into smaller nitrogen-containing **amino acids**. Nine of the 20 amino acids are **essential amino acids**, which the body must obtain from the diet; the other 11 can be produced by the body. Dietary protein that supplies all the essential amino acids is called **complete protein.** Typically, protein from animal products is complete.

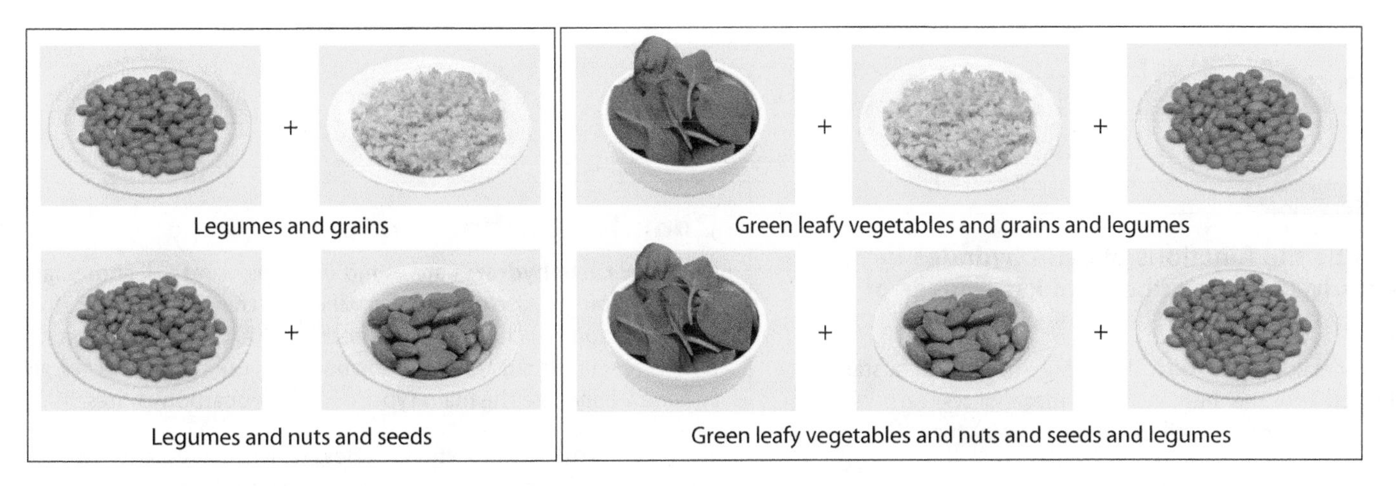

Figure 3.3 Complementary Proteins
Eaten in the right combinations, plant-based foods can provide complementary proteins and all essential amino acids.

Nearly all proteins from plant sources are **incomplete proteins** that lack one or more of the essential amino acids. However, it is easy to combine plant foods to produce a complete protein meal (Figure 3.3). Plant sources of protein fall into three general categories: *legumes* (e.g., beans, peas, peanuts, and soy products), *grains* (e.g., wheat, corn, rice, and oats), and *nuts and seeds.* Certain vegetables, such as leafy green vegetables and broccoli, also contribute valuable plant proteins. Consuming a variety of foods from these categories will provide all the essential amino acids.

Although protein deficiency poses a threat to the global population, few Americans suffer from protein deficiencies. In fact, the average American consumes more than 79 grams of protein daily, much of it from high-fat animal flesh and dairy products.[6] The AMDR for protein is 10 to 35 percent of calories. Adults should consume about 0.8 grams per kilogram of body weight.[7] To calculate your recommended protein intake per day, divide your body weight in pounds by 2.2 to get your weight in kilograms, then multiply by 0.8. For example, a woman who weighs 130 pounds should consume about 47 grams of protein each day. A 6-ounce steak provides 53 grams of protein—more than she needs!

A person might need extra protein if she is pregnant, fighting off a serious infection, recovering from surgery or blood loss, or recovering from burns. In these instances, proteins that are lost to cellular repair and development must be replaced. Athletes also require more protein to build and repair muscle fibers.[8] In addition, a sedentary person or one who gets little exercise may find it easier to stay in energy balance if more of his calories come from protein and fewer from carbohydrates. Why? Because proteins make a person feel full and satisfied for a longer period of time.

Toward Sustainable Seafood The U.S. Department of Agriculture (USDA) recommends consuming fish twice a week to reduce saturated fat and cholesterol levels and increase omega-3 fatty acid levels. However, the many environmental concerns surrounding the seafood industry today call into question the sustainability and safety of such consumption. More than 70 percent of the world's natural fishing grounds have been overfished, and whole stretches of the oceans are dead zones where fish and shellfish can no longer live.

To counteract the loss of wild fish populations, increasing numbers of fish are being farmed, which poses additional health risks and environmental concerns. Some farmed fish are laden with antibiotics, while highly concentrated levels of parasites and bacteria from fish farm runoff may enter the ocean and river fish populations through adjacent waterways. And some farmed fish are fed wild fish, resulting in a net loss of fish from the sea.

At the same time, high levels of chemicals, parasites, bacteria, and toxins are also found in many of the fish available on the market. Mercury, a waste product of many industries, binds to proteins and stays in an animal's body, accumulating as it moves up the food chain. In humans, mercury can damage the nervous system and kidneys and cause birth defects and developmental problems. Polychlorinated biphenyls (PCBs), chemicals that can build up in the fatty tissue of fish, are another cause of concern.

Purchasing seafood from regularly inspected, environmentally responsible sources will support fisheries and fish farms that are healthier for you and the environment. Several major environmental groups have developed guides to inform consumers of safe and sustainable seafood choices. The Monterey Bay Aquarium in California provides a national guide for seafood available for purchase in the United States; you can find the guide online at http://mobile.seafoodwatch.org or as a free smartphone application. Another great resource is the FishPhone service: Send a text message to 30644 with the word *FISH* and the type of fish you want to know about, and it will send you information about whether it is safe to eat.

check yourself

- **Why is water considered an essential nutrient?**
- **What are the functions of protein in the body?**

3.3 Essential Nutrients: Carbohydrates

learning outcome

3.3 Describe the functions of carbohydrates in the body, including fiber, and list sources of carbohydrates.

Carbohydrates supply us with the energy needed to sustain normal daily activity. The human body metabolizes carbohydrates more quickly and efficiently than it does proteins for a quick source of energy for the body. Carbohydrates are easily converted to glucose, the fuel for the body's cells. Carbohydrates also play an important role in the functioning of internal organs, the nervous system, and muscles. They are the best fuel for moderate to intense exercise because they can be readily broken down to glucose even when we're breathing hard and our muscle cells are getting less oxygen.

Like proteins, carbohydrates provide 4 calories per gram. The RDA for adults is 130 grams of carbohydrate per day.[9] There are two major types of carbohydrates: simple and complex.

Simple Carbohydrates

Simple carbohydrates, or *simple sugars*, are found naturally in fruits, many vegetables, and dairy. The most common form of simple carbohydrates is *glucose*. Fruits and berries contain *fructose* (commonly called *fruit sugar*). Glucose and fructose are **monosaccharides**. Eventually, the human body converts all types of simple sugars to glucose to provide energy to cells.

Disaccharides are combinations of two monosaccharides. Perhaps the best-known example is *sucrose* (granulated table sugar). *Lactose* (milk sugar), found in milk and milk products, and *maltose* (malt sugar) are other common disaccharides. Disaccharides must be broken down into monosaccharides before the body can use them.

Americans typically consume far too many refined carbohydrates (i.e., carbohydrates containing only sugars and starches, discussed below), which have few health benefits and are a major factor in our growing epidemic of overweight and obesity. Many of the simple sugars in these foods come from *added sugars*, sweeteners put in during processing to flavor foods, make sodas taste good, and ease our craving for sweets. A classic example is the amount of added sugar in one can of soda: more than 10 teaspoons per can! All that refined sugar can cause tooth decay and put on pounds.

Sugar is found in high amounts in a wide range of food products. Such diverse items as ketchup, barbecue sauce, and flavored coffee creamers derive 30 to 65 percent of their calories from sugar. Knowing what foods contain these sugars, considering the amounts you consume each day that are hidden in foods, and then trying to reduce these levels can be a great way to reduce excess weight. Read food labels carefully before purchasing. If *sugar* or one of its aliases (including *high fructose corn syrup* and *cornstarch*) appears near the top of the ingredients list, then that product contains a lot of sugar and is probably not your best nutritional bet. Also, most labels list the amount of sugar as a percentage of total calories.

Complex Carbohydrates

Complex carbohydrates are found in grains, cereals, legumes, and other vegetables. Also called *polysaccharides*, they are formed by long chains of monosaccharides. Like disaccharides, they must be broken down into simple sugars before the body can use them. *Starches, glycogen*, and *fiber* are the main types of complex carbohydrates.

Starches and Glycogen **Starches**, which make up the majority of the complex carbohydrate group, come from flours, breads, pasta, rice, corn, oats, barley, potatoes, and related foods. The body breaks down these complex carbohydrates into the monosaccharide glucose, which can be easily absorbed by cells and used as energy. Polysaccharides can also be stored in body muscles and the liver as **glycogen**. When the body requires a sudden burst of energy, it breaks down glycogen into glucose.

Fiber **Fiber**, sometimes referred to as "bulk" or "roughage," is the indigestible portion of plant foods that helps move foods through the digestive system, delays absorption of cholesterol and other nutrients, and softens stools by absorbing water. Dietary fiber is found only in plant foods, such as fruits, vegetables, nuts, and grains.

Fiber is either *soluble* or *insoluble*. Soluble fibers, such as pectins, gums, and mucilages, dissolve in water, form gel-like substances, and can be digested easily by bacteria in the colon. Major food sources

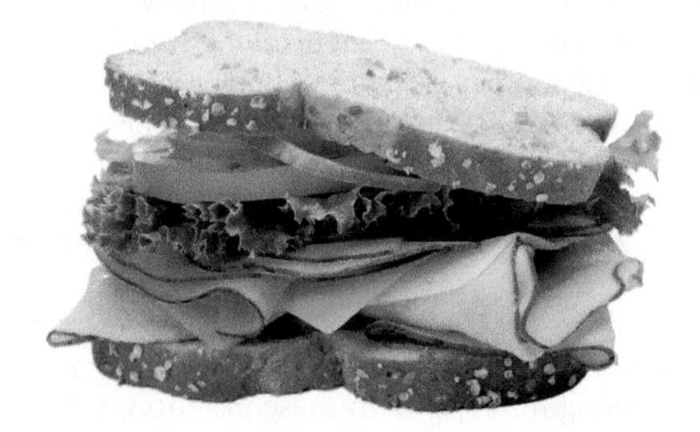

Why are whole grains better than refined grains?

Whole-grain foods contain fiber, a crucial form of carbohydrate that protects against some gastrointestinal disorders and reduces risk for certain cancers. Fiber is also associated with lowered blood cholesterol levels. Studies have shown that eating 2.5 servings of whole grains per day can reduce cardiovascular disease risk by as much as 21 percent. But are people getting the message? One nutrition survey showed that only 8 percent of U.S. adults consume three or more servings of whole grains each day, and 42 percent ate no whole grains at all on a given day.

Source: Dietary Guidelines Advisory Committee 2010, "What is the Relationship between Whole Grain Intake and Cardiovascular Disease?," *United States Department of Agriculture Nutrition Evidence Library*, 2010, www.nel.gov.

The average American consumes 15.9 grams of fiber daily—much less than the recommended

25 to 38

grams per day.

of soluble fiber include citrus fruits, berries, oat bran, dried beans (e.g., kidney, garbanzo, pinto, and navy beans), and some vegetables. Insoluble fibers, such as lignins and cellulose, are those that typically do not dissolve in water and that cannot be fermented by bacteria in the colon. They are found in most fruits and vegetables and in **whole grains**, such as brown rice, wheat, bran, and whole-grain breads and cereals (see Figure 3.4). The AMDR for carbohydrates is 45 to 60 percent of total calories, and heath experts recommend that the majority of this intake be fiber-rich carbohydrates.

Despite growing evidence supporting the benefits of whole grains and high-fiber diets, fiber intake among the general public remains low. Most experts believe that Americans should double their current consumption of dietary fiber. The AI for fiber is 25 grams per day for women and 38 grams per day for men.[10]

Research supports many benefits of fiber. Colorectal cancer, one of the leading causes of cancer deaths in the United States, is much less common in countries whose populations eat diets high in fiber and low in animal fat. A recent analysis found support for the hypothesis that high dietary fiber intake is associated with a reduced colorectal cancer risk.[11] Fiber also protects against constipation and *diverticulosis* (a condition in which tiny bulges form on the large intestinal wall and can become irritated under strain from constipation). Insoluble fiber helps reduce constipation and discomfort by absorbing moisture and producing softer stools. In addition, fiber helps delay or reduce the absorption of dietary cholesterol, a factor in heart disease.[12] Soluble fiber also improves control of blood sugar and can reduce the need for insulin or medication in people with type 2 diabetes.[13] And because most high-fiber foods are high in carbohydrates and low in fat, they help control caloric intake for those wishing to lose unhealthy weight. Fiber also stays in the digestive tract longer than other nutrients, making you feel full sooner.

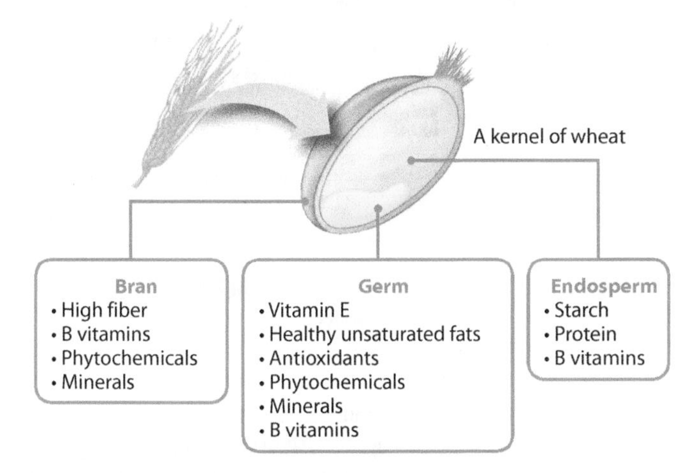

Figure 3.4 Anatomy of a Whole Grain

Whole grains are more nutritious than refined grains, because they contain the bran, germ, and endosperm of the seed—sources of fiber, vitamins, minerals, and beneficial phytochemicals (chemical compounds that occur naturally in plants).

Source: Adapted from Joan Salge Blake, Kathy D. Munoz, and Stella Volpe, *Nutrition: From Science to You*, 1st ed., © 2010. Reprinted by permission of Pearson Education, Inc., Upper Saddle River, New Jersey.

See It! Videos

Cut back on sugar while satisfying your sweet tooth! Watch **Ditching Sugar** in the Study Area of MasteringHealth.

To increase your fiber intake, eat fewer refined or processed carbohydrates in favor of more whole grains, fruits, vegetables, legumes, nuts, and seeds. If you haven't been eating enough fiber, however, make any such change gradually—in this case, too much of a good thing too quickly can pose problems. Sudden increases in dietary fiber may cause flatulence (intestinal gas), cramping, or bloating. Consume plenty of water or other (sugar-free!) liquids to reduce such side effects.

See It! Videos

Are whole grain product labels telling the truth? Watch **Grain Labels Do Not Reflect "Whole" Truth** in the Study Area of MasteringHealth.

Skills for Behavior Change

BULK UP YOUR FIBER INTAKE!

To increase your intake of dietary fiber:

- **Whenever possible, select whole-grain breads low in fat and sugars, with 3 or more grams of fiber per serving. Read labels—just because bread is brown doesn't mean it's better for you.**
- **Eat whole, unpeeled fruits and vegetables rather than drinking their juices. The fiber in whole fruit tends to slow blood sugar increases and helps you feel full longer.**
- **Substitute whole-grain pastas, bagels, and pizza crust for the refined, white flour versions.**
- **Add wheat crumbs or grains to meat loaf and burgers to increase fiber intake.**
- **Toast grains to bring out their nutty flavor and make foods more appealing.**
- **Sprinkle ground flaxseed on cereals, yogurt, and salads or add it to casseroles, burgers, and baked goods. Flaxseeds have a mild flavor and are also high in beneficial fatty acids.**

check yourself

- **What are the functions of carbohydrates in the body?**
- **What are the preferred sources of carbohydrates?**
- **Why is fiber important in the diet?**

3.4 Essential Nutrients: Fats

learning outcome

3.4 Describe the functions of fats in the body.

Fats, perhaps the most misunderstood nutrient, are the most energy dense, providing 9 calories per gram. Fats are a significant source of our body's fuel. The body can store only a limited amount of carbohydrate, so the longer you exercise, the more fat your body burns. Fats also play a vital role in maintaining healthy skin and hair, insulating body organs against shock, maintaining body temperature, and promoting healthy cell function. Fats make foods taste better and carry vitamins A, D, E, and K to cells. They also make you feel full after eating. So why are we constantly urged to cut back on fats? Because some fats are less healthy than others and because excessive consumption of fats can lead to weight gain.

Triglycerides, which make up about 95 percent of total body fat, are the most common form of fat circulating in the blood. When we consume too many calories from any source, the liver converts the excess into triglycerides, which are stored throughout our bodies.

Another oily substance in foods derived from animals is **cholesterol**. We don't need to consume any dietary cholesterol because our liver can make all that we need; the recommended intake for cholesterol is less than 300 milligrams a day (one egg contains about 215 milligrams).[14]

Neither triglycerides nor cholesterol can travel independently in the bloodstream. Instead, they are "packaged" inside protein coats to form compounds called lipoproteins. **High-density lipoproteins (HDLs)** are relatively high in protein and low in cholesterol and triglycerides. A high level of HDLs in the blood is healthful because HDLs remove cholesterol from dying cells and from plaques within blood vessels, eventually transporting cholesterol to the liver and eliminating it from the body. **Low-density lipoproteins (LDLs)** are much higher in both cholesterol and triglycerides than HDLs. They travel in the bloodstream delivering cholesterol to body cells; however, LDLs not taken up by cells degrade and release their cholesterol into the bloodstream. This cholesterol can then stick to the lining of blood vessels, contributing to the plaque that causes heart disease.

Types of Dietary Fats

Fat molecules include *fatty acid* chains of oxygen, carbon, and hydrogen atoms. Fatty acid chains that cannot hold any more hydrogen in their chemical structure are called **saturated fats**. These generally come from animal sources such as meat, dairy, and poultry and are solid at room temperature. **Unsaturated fats** have room for additional hydrogen atoms in their chemical structure and are liquid at room temperature. They come from plants and include most vegetable oils.

The terms *monounsaturated fatty acids (MUFAs)* and *polyunsaturated fatty acids (PUFAs)* refer to the relative number of hydrogen atoms missing in a fatty acid chain. Peanut and olive oils are high in monounsaturated fats. Corn, sunflower, and safflower oils are high in polyunsaturated fats.

There is controversy about which unsaturated fats are most beneficial. Monounsaturated fatty acids, such as olive oil, which seem to lower LDL levels and increase HDL levels, are currently preferred. Figure 3.5 shows fats in common vegetable oils.

Polyunsaturated fatty acids come in two forms: *omega-3 fatty acids* (in many fatty fish) and *omega-6 fatty acids* (in corn, soybean, and cottonseed oils). Both are classified as *essential fatty acids*—we must receive them from our diets. *Linoleic acid*, an omega-6 fatty acid, and alpha-linolenic acid, an omega-3 fatty acid, are needed to

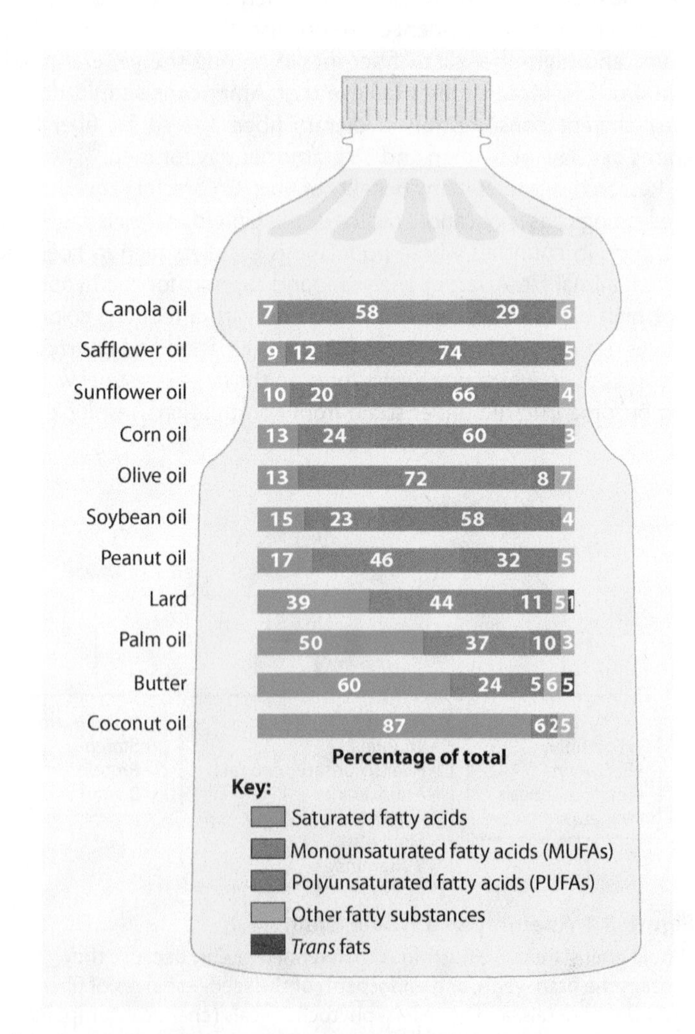

Figure 3.5 Percentages of Saturated, Polyunsaturated, Monounsaturated, and *Trans* Fats in Common Vegetable Oils

make hormone-like compounds that control immune function, pain perception, and inflammation and reduce cardiovascular disease (CVD) risks. EPA and DHEA, derivatives of alpha-linolenic acid that are found abundantly in oily fish such as salmon and tuna, are also associated with a reduced risk for heart disease.[15]

The AMDR for fats is 20 to 35 percent of calories, with 5 to 10 percent coming from essential fatty acids. Within this range, we should minimize our intake of saturated fats.

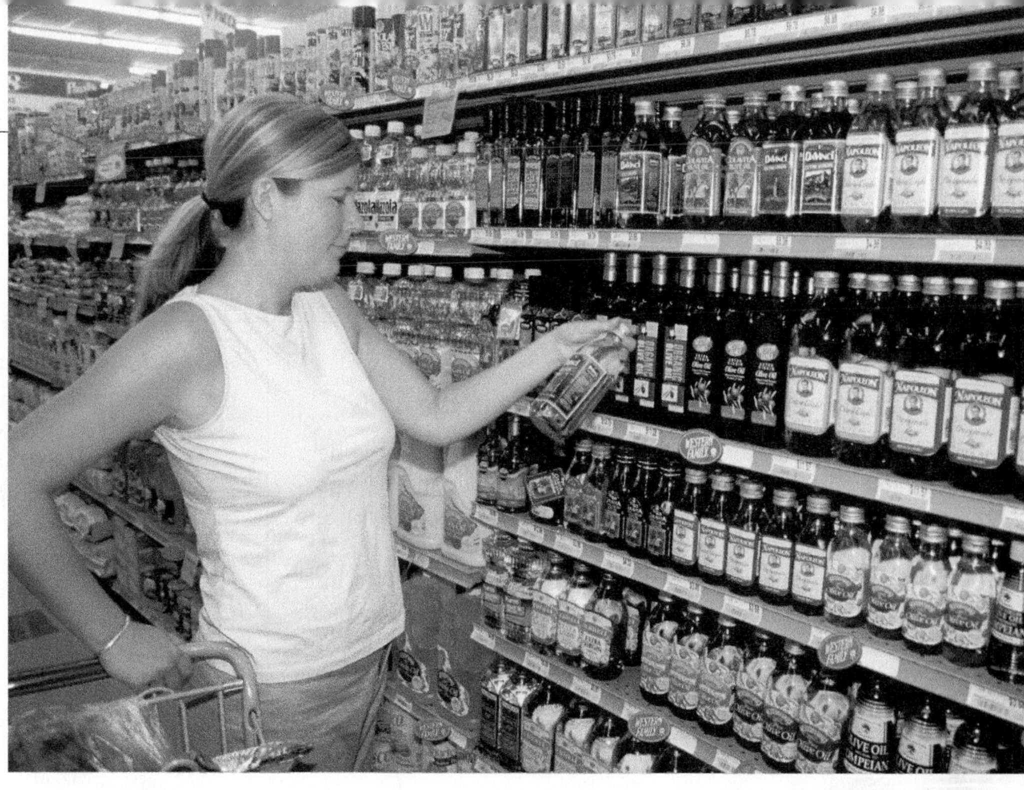

Are all fats bad for me?

All fats are not the same, and your body needs some fat to function healthily. Try to reduce saturated fats, those that come in meat, dairy, and poultry products; avoid *trans* fats, those that can come in stick margarine, commercially baked goods, and deep-fried foods; and replace these with monounsaturated fats, such as those in peanut and olive oils.

Avoiding *Trans* Fatty Acids

For decades, Americans shunned butter, red meat, and other foods because of their saturated fats. What they didn't know is that foods low in saturated fat, such as margarine, could be just as harmful because they contain ***trans* fatty acids**. Research shows that just a 2 percent caloric intake of these fats is associated with a 23 percent increased risk for heart disease and a 47 percent increased chance of sudden cardiac death.[16]

The great majority of *trans* fatty acids are found in processed foods made with partially hydrogenated oils (PHOs).[17] PHOs are produced when food manufacturers add hydrogen to a plant oil, solidifying it, helping it resist rancidity, and giving the food in which it is used a longer shelf life. This process straightens out the fatty acid chain so that it is more like a saturated fatty acid, and it has similar harmful effects, lowering HDLs and raising LDLs. *Trans* fats have been used in margarines, many commercial baked goods, and restaurant deep-fried foods.

In 2013, the U.S. Food and Drug Administration (FDA) issued a preliminary determination that PHOs are no longer recognized as safe for consumption. If it is finalized, foods containing PHOs will no longer be sold legally in the United States.[18] In the meantime, *trans* fats are being removed from most foods, and if they are present, they must be clearly indicated on food packaging. If you see the words *partially hydrogenated oils, fractionated oils, shortening, lard,* or *hydrogenation* on a food label, then *trans* fats are present.

Is More Fat Ever Better?

Despite all this, some studies have shown that balanced high-fat diets produce significant improvements in weight loss, blood fat, and blood glucose measures.[19]

Balance is the key. No more than 7 to 10 percent of your total calories should come from saturated fat, and no more than 35 percent should come from all forms of fat.[20] Follow these dietary guidelines to add more healthy fats to your diet:

- Eat sustainable fatty seafood (bluefish, herring, mackerel, salmon, sardines, or tuna) at least twice weekly.
- Use olive, peanut, soy, and canola oils instead of butter or lard.
- Add green leafy vegetables, walnuts, walnut oil, and ground flaxseed to your diet.
- Read the Nutrition Facts panel on food labels to find out how much fat is in your food.
- Chill meat-based soups and stews, scrape off any fat that hardens on top, then reheat to serve.
- Fill up on fruits and vegetables.
- Avoid all products with *trans* fatty acids. For healthy toppings on your bread, try vegetable spreads, bean spreads, nut butters, sugar-free jams, fat-free cheese, etc.
- Choose lean meats, fish, or skinless poultry. Broil, steam, poach, or bake whenever possible. Drain off fat after cooking.
- Choose fewer cold cuts, bacon, sausages, hot dogs, and organ meats.
- Select nonfat and low-fat dairy products, but remember that many nonfat and low-fat foods have higher amounts of carbohydrates and sugars. Choose wisely.

check yourself

- **What are the functions of fats in the body?**
- **What are more and less healthful sources of fats?**

3.5 Essential Nutrients: Vitamins

learning outcome

3.5 Describe the functions of vitamins in the body.

Vitamins are organic compounds that promote growth and help maintain life and health. They help maintain nerves and skin, produce blood cells, build bones and teeth, heal wounds, and convert food energy to body energy.

Vitamins can be *fat soluble* (absorbed through the intestinal tract with the help of fats) or *water soluble* (dissolvable in water). See Table 3.2 for the fat-soluble vitamins and Table 3.3 for the water-soluble vitamins. Vitamins A, D, E, and K are fat soluble; C- and B-complex vitamins are water soluble. Fat-soluble vitamins tend to be stored in the body; over-accumulation in the liver may cause cirrhosis-like symptoms. Water-soluble vitamins generally are excreted and cause few toxicity problems.

Vitamin D and folate are vitamins of special concern. Vitamin D is formed from a compound in the skin when exposed to the sun's ultraviolet rays. It's essential for the body's regulation of calcium, the primary mineral component of bone. An adequate amount of vitamin D can be synthesized with 5 to 30 minutes of sun on the body twice a week, without sunscreen,[21] or by consuming vitamin D–fortified milk, yogurt, soy milk, cereals, and fatty fish.

Folate is particularly important for proper cell division during embryonic development. Deficiencies during early pregnancy can

TABLE 3.2 Fat-Soluble Vitamins

Vitamin Name	Primary Functions	Recommended Intake[a]	Reliable Food Sources	Toxicity/Deficiency Symptoms
A (retinol, retinal, retinoic acid)	Required for ability of eyes to adjust to changes in light Protects color vision Assists cell differentiation Required for sperm production in men and fertilization in women Contributes to healthy bone Contributes to healthy immune system	RDA: Men: 900 µg Women: 700 µg UL: 3,000 µg/day	Preformed retinol: beef and chicken liver, egg yolks, milk Carotenoid precursors: spinach, carrots, mango, apricots, cantaloupe, pumpkin, yams	*Toxicity:* fatigue; bone and joint pain; spontaneous abortion and birth defects of fetuses in pregnant women; nausea and diarrhea; liver damage; nervous system damage; blurred vision; hair loss; skin disorders *Deficiency:* night blindness and xerophthalmia; impaired growth, immunity, and reproductive function
D (cholecalciferol)	Regulates blood calcium levels Maintains bone health Assists cell differentiation	RDA: Adult aged 19–70: 600 IU/day Adult aged >70: 800 IU/day UL: 4,000 IU/day	Canned salmon and mackerel, fortified milk and milk alternatives, fortified cereals	*Toxicity:* hypercalcemia *Deficiency:* rickets in children; osteomalacia and/or osteoporosis in adults
E (tocopherol)	As a powerful antioxidant, protects cell membranes, polyunsaturated fatty acids, and vitamin A from oxidation Protects white blood cells Enhances immune function Improves absorption of vitamin A	RDA: Men: 15 mg/day Women: 15 mg/day UL: 1,000 mg/day	Sunflower seeds, almonds, vegetable oils, fortified cereals	*Toxicity:* rare *Deficiency:* hemolytic anemia; impairment of nerve, muscle, and immune function
K (phylloquinone, menaquinone, menadione)	Serves as a coenzyme during production of specific proteins that assist in blood coagulation and bone metabolism	AI: Men: 120 µg/day Women: 90 µg/day	Kale, spinach, turnip greens, brussels sprouts	*Toxicity:* none known *Deficiency:* impaired blood clotting; possible effect on bone health

[a]Note: RDA, Recommended Dietary Allowance; UL, upper limit; AI, Adequate Intake.

TABLE **3.3** **Water-Soluble Vitamins**

Vitamin Name	Primary Functions	Recommended Intake[a]	Reliable Food Sources	Toxicity/Deficiency Symptoms
Thiamin (vitamin B1)	Required as enzyme cofactor for carbohydrate and amino acid metabolism	RDA: Men: 1.2 mg/day Women: 1.1 mg/day	Pork, fortified cereals, enriched rice and pasta, peas, tuna, legumes	*Toxicity:* none known *Deficiency:* beriberi; fatigue, apathy, decreased memory, confusion, irritability, muscle weakness
Riboflavin (vitamin B2)	Required as enzyme cofactor for carbohydrate and fat metabolism	RDA: Men: 1.3 mg/day Women: 1.1 mg/day	Beef liver, shrimp, milk and other dairy foods, fortified cereals, enriched breads and grains	*Toxicity:* none known *Deficiency:* ariboflavinosis; swollen mouth and throat; seborrheic dermatitis; anemia
Niacin, nicotinamide, nicotinic acid	Required for carbohydrate and fat metabolism Plays role in DNA replication and repair and cell differentiation	RDA: Men: 16 mg/day Women: 14 mg/day UL: 35 mg/day	Beef liver, most cuts of meat/fish/poultry, fortified cereals, enriched breads and grains, canned tomato products	*Toxicity:* flushing, liver damage, glucose intolerance, blurred vision differentiation *Deficiency:* pellagra; vomiting, constipation, or diarrhea; apathy
Pyridoxine, pyridoxal, pyridoxamine (vitamin B6)	Required as enzyme cofactor for carbohydrate and amino acid metabolism Assists synthesis of blood cells	RDA: Men and women aged 19–50: 1.3 mg/day Men aged >50: 1.7 mg/day Women aged >50: 1.5 mg/day UL: 100 mg/day	Chickpeas (garbanzo beans), most cuts of meat/fish/poultry, fortified cereals, white potatoes	*Toxicity:* nerve damage, skin lesions *Deficiency:* anemia; seborrheic dermatitis; depression, confusion, and convulsions
Folate (folic acid)	Required as enzyme cofactor for amino acid metabolism Required for DNA synthesis Involved in metabolism of homocysteine	RDA: Men: 400 μg/day Women: 400 μg/day UL: 1,000 μg/day	Fortified cereals, enriched breads and grains, spinach, legumes (lentils, chickpeas, pinto beans), greens (spinach, romaine lettuce), liver	*Toxicity:* masks symptoms of vitamin B12 deficiency, specifically signs of nerve damage *Deficiency:* macrocytic anemia; neural tube defects in a developing fetus; elevated homocysteine levels
Cobalamin (vitamin B12)	Assists with formation of blood Required for healthy nervous system function Involved as enzyme cofactor in metabolism of homocysteine	RDA: Men: 2.4 μg/day Women: 2.4 μg/day	Shellfish, all cuts of meat/fish/poultry, milk and other dairy foods, fortified cereals and other fortified foods	*Toxicity:* none known *Deficiency:* pernicious anemia; tingling and numbness of extremities; nerve damage; memory loss, disorientation, and dementia
Pantothenic acid	Assists with fat metabolism	AI: Men: 5 mg/day Women: 5 mg/day	Meat/fish/poultry, shiitake mushrooms, fortified cereals, egg yolk	*Toxicity:* none known *Deficiency:* rare
Biotin	Involved as enzyme cofactor in carbohydrate, fat, and protein metabolism	RDA: Men: 30 μg/day Women: 30 μg/day	Nuts, egg yolk	*Toxicity:* none known *Deficiency:* rare
Ascorbic acid (vitamin C)	Antioxidant in extracellular fluid and lungs Regenerates oxidized vitamin E Assists with collagen synthesis Enhances immune function Assists in synthesis of hormones, neurotransmitters, and DNA Enhances iron absorption	RDA: Men: 90 mg/day Women: 75 mg/day Smokers: 35 mg more per day than RDA UL: 2,000 mg	Sweet peppers, citrus fruits and juices, broccoli, strawberries, kiwi	*Toxicity:* nausea and diarrhea, nosebleeds, increased oxidative damage, increased formation of kidney stones in people with kidney disease *Deficiency:* scurvy; bone pain and fractures, depression, and anemia

[a]Note: RDA, Recommended Dietary Allowance; UL, upper limit; AI, Adequate Intake

prompt a neural tube defect, in which the primitive tube that eventually forms the brain and spinal cord fails to close properly. All bread, cereal, rice, and pasta products sold in the United States must be fortified with folic acid, the synthetic form of folate.

check yourself

- **What are some functions of vitamins in the body?**
- **What are key vitamins and some recommended food sources for them? Are there any that are difficult for you to eat in the recommended quantity?**

3.6 Essential Nutrients: Minerals

learning outcome

3.6 Describe the functions of minerals in the body.

Minerals are the inorganic, indestructible elements that aid physiological processes within the body. Without minerals, vitamins could not be absorbed.

Minerals are readily excreted and, with a few exceptions, are usually not toxic. **Major minerals** are the minerals that the body needs in fairly large amounts: sodium, calcium, phosphorus, magnesium, potassium, sulfur, and chloride. **Trace minerals** include iron, zinc, manganese, copper, fluoride, selenium, chromium, and iodine. Only very small amounts of trace minerals are needed, and serious problems may result if excesses or deficiencies occur (see Tables 3.4 and 3.5).

Sodium and calcium are two minerals of particular concern. Sodium enhances flavors and acts as a preservative, so it's often present in high quantities in the foods we eat—particularly processed foods. The average American consumes 3,463 milligrams of sodium per day,[22] much

TABLE 3.4 Major Minerals

Mineral Name	Primary Functions	Recommended Intake[a]	Reliable Food Sources	Toxicity/Deficiency Symptoms
Sodium	Fluid balance Acid–base balance Transmission of nerve impulses Muscle contraction	AI: Adults: 1.5 g/day (1,500 mg/day)	Table salt, pickles, most canned soups, snack foods, cured luncheon meats, canned tomato products	*Toxicity:* water retention, high blood pressure, loss of calcium *Deficiency:* muscle cramps, dizziness, fatigue, nausea, vomiting, mental confusion
Potassium	Fluid balance Transmission of nerve impulses Muscle contraction	AI: Adults: 4.7 g/day (4,700 mg/day)	Most fresh fruits and vegetables: potatoes, bananas, tomato juice, orange juice, melons	*Toxicity:* muscle weakness,vomiting, irregular heartbeat *Deficiency:* muscle weakness,paralysis, mental confusion,irregular heartbeat
Phosphorus	Fluid balance Bone formation Component of ATP, which provides energy for our bodies	RDA: UL: 1,100 μg/day	Milk/cheese/yogurt, soy milk and tofu, legumes (lentils, black beans), nuts (almonds, peanuts and peanut butter), poultry	*Toxicity:* muscle spasms, convulsions, low blood calcium *Deficiency:* muscle weakness, muscle damage, bone pain, dizziness
Calcium	Primary component of bone Acid–base balance Transmission of nerve impulses Muscle contraction	RDA: Adults aged 19 to 50 and men aged 51–70: 1,000 mg/day Women aged 51–70 and adults aged >70: 1,200 mg/day UL for adults 19–50: 2,500 mg/day UL for adults aged 51 and above: 2,000 mg/day	Milk/yogurt/cheese (best-absorbed form of calcium), sardines, collard greens and spinach, calcium fortified juices and milk alternatives	*Toxicity:* mineral imbalances, shock, kidney failure, fatigue, mental confusionw *Deficiency:* osteoporosis, convulsions, heart failure
Magnesium	Component of bone Muscle contraction Assists more than 300 enzyme systems	RDA: Men aged 19–30: 400 mg/day Men aged >30: 420 mg/day Women aged 19–30: 310 mg/day Women aged >30: 320 mg/day UL: 350 mg/day	Greens (spinach, kale, collard greens), whole grains, seeds, nuts, legumes (navy and black beans)	*Toxicity:* none known *Deficiency:* low blood calcium, muscle spasms or seizures, nausea, weakness, increased risk for chronic diseases, such as heart disease, hypertension, osteoporosis, and type 2 diabetes

[a]Note: RDA, Recommended Dietary Allowance; UL, upper limit; AI, Adequate Intake.

TABLE
3.5 Trace Minerals

Mineral Name	Primary Functions	Recommended Intake[a]	Reliable Food Sources	Toxicity/Deficiency Symptoms
Selenium	Required for carbohydrate and fat metabolism	RDA: Adults: 55 μg/day UL: 400 μg/day	Nuts, shellfish, meat/fish/poultry, whole grains	*Toxicity:* brittle hair and nails, skin rashes, nausea and vomiting, weakness, liver disease *Deficiency:* specific forms of heart disease and arthritis, impaired immune function, muscle pain and wasting, depression, hostility
Fluoride	Development and maintenance of healthy teeth and bones	RDA: Men: 4 mg/day Women: 3 mg/day UL: 2.2 mg/day for children aged 4–8; 10 mg/day for children aged >8	Fish, seafood, legumes, whole grains, drinking water (variable)	*Toxicity:* fluorosis of teeth and bones *Deficiency:* dental caries, low bone density
Iodine	Synthesis of thyroid hormones Temperature regulation Reproduction and growth	RDA: Adults: 150 μg/day UL: 1,100 μg/day	Iodized salt, saltwater seafood	*Toxicity:* goiter *Deficiency:* goiter, hypothyroidism, cretinism in infant of mother who is iodine deficient
Chromium	Glucose transport Metabolism of DNA and RNA Immune function and growth	AI: Men aged 19–50: 35 μg/day Men aged >50: 30 μg/day Women aged 19–50: 25 μg/day Women aged >50: 20 μg/day	Whole grains, brewer's yeast	*Toxicity:* none known *Deficiency:* elevated blood glucose and blood lipids, damage to brain and nervous system
Iron	Component of hemoglobin in blood cells Component of myoglobin in muscle cells Assists many enzyme systems	RDA: Adult men: 8 mg/day Women aged 19–50: 18 mg/day Women aged >50: 8 mg/day	Meat/fish/poultry (best-absorbed form of iron), fortified cereals, legumes, spinach	*Toxicity:* nausea, vomiting, and diarrhea; dizziness, confusion; rapid heartbeat, organ damage, death *Deficiency:* iron-deficiency microcytic (small red blood cells), hypochromic anemia
Zinc	Assists more than 100 enzyme systems Immune system function Growth and sexual maturation Gene regulation	RDA: Men: 11 mg/day Women: 8 mg/day UL: 40 mg/day	Meat/fish/poultry (best-absorbed form of zinc), fortified cereals, legumes	*Toxicity:* nausea, vomiting, and diarrhea; headaches, depressed immune function, reduced absorption of copper *Deficiency:* growth retardation, delayed sexual maturation, eye and skin lesions, hair loss, increased incidence of illness and infection

[a]Note: RDA, Recommended Dietary Allowance; UL, upper limit; AI, Adequate Intake.

more than the recommend AI, 500 milligrams.[23] High sodium intake is a major concern because a high-sodium diet increases blood pressure (hypertension), which contributes to heart disease and strokes.

The issue of calcium consumption has gained attention with the rising incidence of osteoporosis. Most Americans do not consume the recommended 1,000 to 1,200 milligrams of calcium per day.[24] For optimal absorption, consume calcium-rich foods (broccoli, collard greens, kale) and beverages (dairy products, calcium-fortified juices) throughout the day.

check yourself

- **What are some functions of minerals in the body?**
- **What are key minerals and some recommended food sources for them?**
- **Are there any key minerals that are difficult for you to eat in the recommended quantity? How could you incorporate more of these into your diet?**

3.7 Health Benefits of Functional Foods

learning **outcome**

3.7 Describe how functional foods impact health.

Increasingly, nutrition research is focusing on components of foods that interact with nutrients to promote human health, rather than solely as sources of macro- and micronutrients.[25] Foods that may confer health benefits beyond the nutrients they contribute to the diet—whole foods, fortified foods, enriched foods, or enhanced foods—are called **functional foods**. When functional foods are included as part of a varied diet, they have the potential to positively impact health.[26]

Some of the most popular functional foods today are those containing **antioxidants.** These substances appear to protect against oxidative stress, a complex process in which *free radicals* (atoms with unpaired electrons) destabilize other atoms and molecules, prompting a chain reaction that can damage cells, cell proteins, or genetic material in the cells. Free radical formation is a natural process that cannot be avoided, but antioxidants combat it by donating their electrons to stabilize free radicals, activating enzymes that convert free radicals to less damaging substances, or reducing or repairing the damage they cause.

Among the more commonly cited antioxidants are vitamins C and E, as well as the minerals copper, iron, manganese, selenium, and zinc. Other potent antioxidants are **phytochemicals**, compounds that occur naturally in plants and are thought to protect them against ultraviolet radiation, pests, and other threats. Common examples include the *carotenoids*, pigments found in red, orange, and dark green fruits and vegetables. Beta-carotene, the most researched carotenoid, is a precursor of vitamin A, meaning that vitamin A can be produced in the body from beta-carotene. Both vitamin A and beta-carotene have antioxidant properties. Phenolic phytochemicals, which include a group known as *flavonoids*, are found in an array of fruits and vegetables as well as soy products, tea, and chocolate. Like carotenoids, they are thought to have antioxidant properties that may prevent cardiovascular disease.[27]

To date, many such claims about the health benefits of antioxidant nutrients and phytochemicals have not been fully investigated. However, studies do show that individuals deficient in antioxidant vitamins and minerals have an increased risk for age-related diseases and that antioxidants consumed in whole foods, mostly fruits and vegetables, may reduce these individuals' risks. In contrast, antioxidants consumed as supplements do not confer such a benefit and may be harmful.[28]

Health Claims of Superfoods

In food advertisements, fitness and food magazines, and even among health care organizations, functional foods are increasingly being referred to as "superfoods." Do superfoods live up to their new name? Let's look at a few.

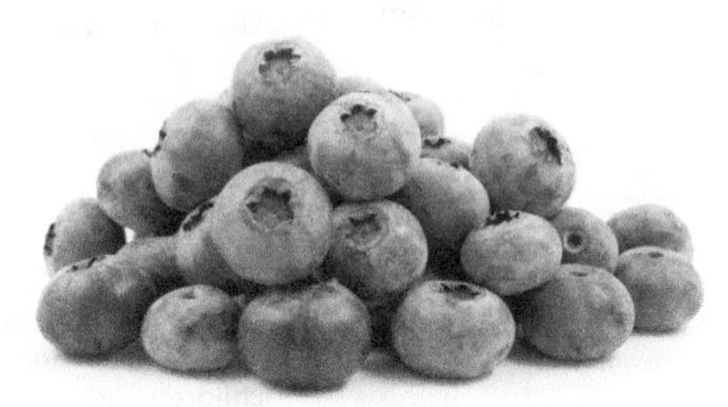

Blueberries are a great source of antioxidants.

Salmon is a rich source of the omega-3 fatty acids EPA and DHA, which combat inflammation, improve HDL/LDL blood profiles, and reduce the risk for cardiovascular disease. DHA may also promote a healthy nervous system, reducing the risk for age-related dementia.[29]

Yogurt makes it onto most superfood lists because, like other fermented milk products, it contains living, beneficial bacteria called probiotics. Probiotics colonize the large intestine, where they help complete digestion, produce certain vitamins, and are thought to reduce the risk of diarrhea and other bowel disorders, boost immunity, and help regulate body weight.[30]

Cocoa is particularly rich in a class of chemicals called flavonols that have been shown in many studies to reduce the risk for cardiovascular disease, diabetes, and even arthritis.[31] Dark chocolate is believed to have a higher level of flavonols than milk chocolate. However, while it is widely believed that dark chocolate contains the highest levels of flavonols, newer research indicates that processing can drastically reduce flavonal levels. Buying higher quality dark chocolate with a higher percentage of cocoa may be a good idea, but it isn't foolproof. When in doubt, your best bet is still dark over milk chocolate, but remember that moderation is key!

Given such claims, it's easy to get carried away by the idea that superfoods have superpowers. But eating a square of dark chocolate won't rescue you from the ill effects of a fast-food burger and fries. What matters is your whole diet. Focus on including superfoods as components of a varied diet rich in fresh fruits, legumes and other vegetables, whole grains, lean sources of protein, and nuts and seeds.

check yourself

- **How do functional foods benefit health?**
- **How can you incorporate more functional foods into your diet?**

3.8

Planning a Healthy Diet: Using the Food Label

learning outcome

3.8 Understand each component of the food label.

To help consumers evaluate the nutritional values of packaged foods, the FDA and the USDA developed the Nutrition Facts panel that is typically displayed on the side or back of packaged foods. One of the most helpful items on the panel is the **% daily values (%DVs)** list, which tells you how much of an average adult's allowance for a particular substance (fat, fiber, calcium, etc.) is provided by a serving of the food. The %DV is calculated based on a 2,000 calorie per day diet, so your values may be different from those listed on a label. The panel also includes information on the serving size and calories. In 2014, the FDA announced plans to make the data on the panel more helpful for consumers by identifying the calories per serving in much larger type, and adjusting the serving size so that it better reflects the amount of the food that people typically eat.[32] Figure 3.6 walks you through a typical Nutrition Facts panel.

Start here. The size of the serving on the food package influences the number of calories and all the nutrient amounts listed on the top part of the label. Pay attention to the serving size, especially how many servings there are in the food package. Then ask yourself, "How many servings am I consuming?"

Limit these nutrients. The nutrients listed first are the ones Americans generally eat in adequate amounts, or even too much of. Eating too much fat, saturated fat, *trans* fat, cholesterol, or sodium may increase your risk of certain chronic diseases, such as heart disease, some cancers, or high blood pressure.

Get enough of these nutrients. Most Americans don't get enough dietary fiber, vitamin A, vitamin C, calcium, and iron in their diets. Eating enough of these nutrients can improve your health and help reduce the risk of some diseases and conditions.

The footnote is not specific to the product. It shows recommended dietary advice for all Americans. The Percent Daily Values are based on a 2,000-calorie diet, but the footnote lists daily values for both a 2,000- and 2,500-calorie diet.

Sample Label for Macaroni and Cheese

Nutrition Facts

Serving size 1 cup (228g)
Servings Per Container 2

Amount Per Serving

Calories 250 | Calories from Fat 110

	% Daily Value*
Total Fat 12g	**18%**
Saturated Fat 3g	**15%**
Trans Fat 1.5g	
Cholesterol 30mg	**10%**
Sodium 470mg	**20%**
Total Carbohydrate 31g	**10%**
Dietary Fiber 0g	**0%**
Sugars 5g	
Protein 5g	
Vitamin A	4%
Vitamin C	2%
Calcium	20%
Iron	4%

* Percent Daily Values are based on a 2,000 calorie diet. Your Daily Values may be higher or lower depending on your calorie needs:

	Calories:	2,000	2,500
Total Fat	Less than	65g	80g
Sat Fat	Less than	20g	25g
Cholesterol	Less than	300mg	300mg
Sodium	Less than	2,400mg	2,400mg
Total Carbohydrate		300g	375g
Dietary Fiber		25g	30g

Pay attention to calories (and calories from fat). Many Americans consume more calories than they need. Remember: The number of servings you consume determines the number of calories you actually eat (your portion amount). Dietary guidelines recommend that no more than 30% of your daily calories consumed come from fat.

5% DV or less is low and 20% DV or more is high. The %DV helps you determine if a serving of food is high or low in a nutrient, whether or not you consume the 2,000-calorie diet it is based on. It also helps you make easy comparisons between products (just make sure the serving sizes are similar).

Note that a few nutrients—*trans* fats, sugars, and protein—do not have a %DV. Experts could not provide a reference value for *trans* fat, but it is recommended that you keep your intake as low as possible. There are no recommendations for the total amount of sugar to eat in one day, but check the ingredient list to see information on added sugars, such as high fructose corn syrup. A %DV for protein is required to be listed if a claim is made (such as "high in protein") or if the food is meant for infants and children under 4 years old. Otherwise, none is needed.

Figure 3.6 Reading a Food Label

Source: Center for Food Safety and Applied Nutrition, "A Key to Choosing Healthful Foods: Using the Nutrition Facts on the Food Label," Updated May 2009, www.fda.gov.

VIDEO TUTOR
Understanding Food Labels

check yourself

- **What are the key components of a food label? How can they help you make better food choices?**

3.9 Planning a Healthy Diet: Dietary Guidelines and MyPlate

learning outcome

3.9 Explain the principles for a healthy diet contained in the MyPlate food guidance system.

Now that you have some idea of your nutritional needs, let's discuss what a healthy diet looks like, how you can begin to meet your needs, and how you can meet the challenge of getting the foods you need on campus.

Dietary Guidelines for Americans

The *Dietary Guidelines for Americans* are a set of recommendations for healthy eating; they are revised every 5 years. The 2010 *Dietary Guidelines for Americans* are designed to help bridge the gap between the standard American diet and the key recommendations that aim to combat the growing obesity epidemic by balancing calories with adequate physical activity.[33] They provide advice about consuming fewer calories, making informed food choices, and being physically active to attain and maintain a healthy weight, reduce your risk for chronic disease, and improve your overall health. The 2010 *Dietary Guidelines for Americans* are presented as an easy-to-follow graphic and guidance system called MyPlate, found at www.choosemyplate.gov and illustrated in Figure 3.7.

The MyPlate Food Guidance System

The MyPlate food guidance system takes into consideration the dietary and caloric needs for a wide variety of individuals, such as pregnant or breast-feeding women, those trying to lose weight, and adults with different activity levels. When you visit the interactive website, you can create personalized dietary and exercise recommendations based on the information you enter.

MyPlate also encourages consumers to eat for health through three general areas of recommendation:

1. **Balance calories.** Find out how many calories you need for a day is a first step in managing your weight. Go to www.choosemyplate.gov to find your calorie level. Being physically active also helps you balance calories.
   - Enjoy your food, but eat less. Take time to fully enjoy your food as you eat it. Eating too fast or when your attention is elsewhere may lead to eating too many calories. Pay attention to hunger cues before, during, and after meals. Use them to recognize when to eat and when you've had enough.
   - Avoid oversized portions. Use a smaller plate, bowl, and glass. Portion out food before you eat. When eating out, choose a smaller size option, share a dish, or take home part of your meal.
2. **Increase some foods.** Eat more vegetables, fruits, whole grains, and fat-free or 1 percent milk and dairy products, These foods have the nutrients you need for health—including potassium, calcium, vitamin D, and fiber. Make them the basis for meals and snacks.
   - Make half your plate fruits and vegetables. Choose red, orange, and dark-green vegetables like tomatoes, sweet pota-

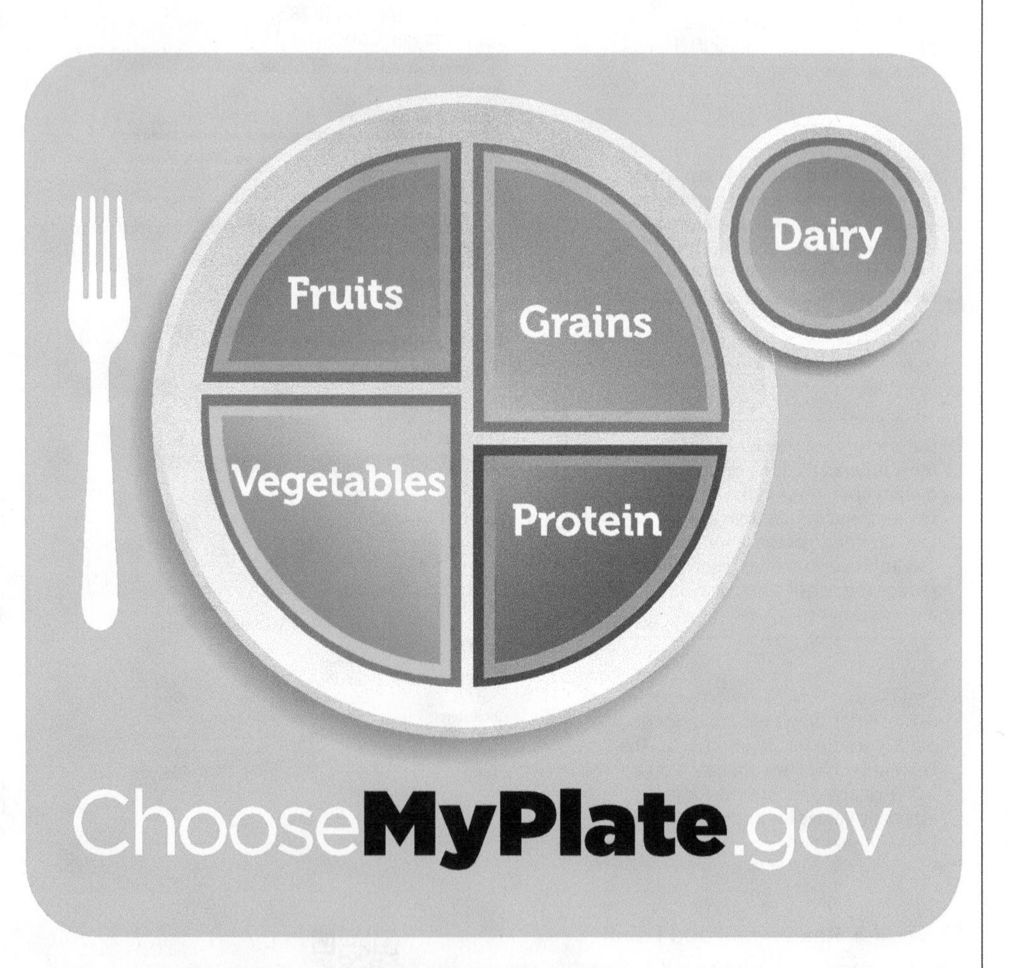

Figure 3.7 The MyPlate Food Guidance System
The USDA MyPlate food guidance system takes a new approach to dietary and exercise recommendations. Each colored section of the plate represents a food group. An interactive tool on www.choosemyplate.gov can provide individualized recommendations for users.
Source: U.S. Department of Agriculture, 2011, www.choosemyplate.gov.

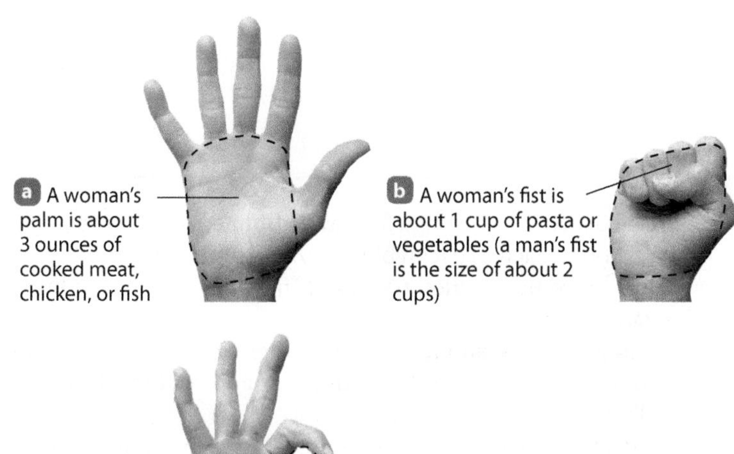

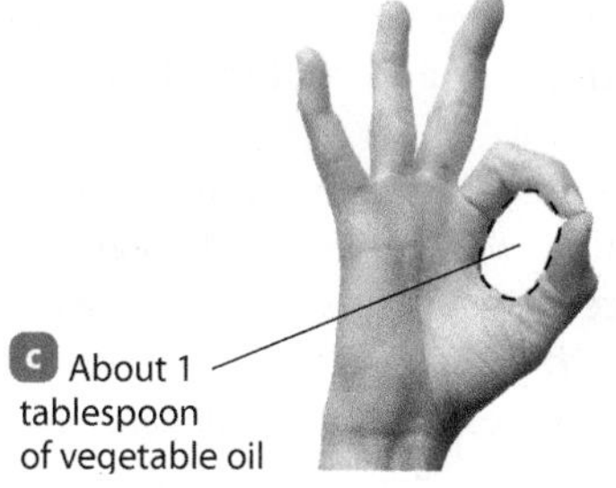

Figure 3.8 What's a Serving?
Your hands can guide you in estimating portion sizes.

toes, and broccoli. Add fruit to meals as part of main or side dishes or as dessert.
- Make at least half your grains whole grains. Substitute whole-wheat bread for white bread or brown rice for white rice.
- Switch to fat-free or 1 percent milk. They have the same amount of calcium and other essential nutrients as whole milk, but fewer calories and less saturated fat.
- Experiment with some spices and herbs. They have interesting flavors that can "spice up" food without the extra hit of sodium. Remember to replace them when they get old or lose flavor.

3. **Reduce some foods.** Cut back on foods high in solid fats, added sugars, and salt. Enjoy these foods as occasional treats, not every-day foods.
   - Compare sodium in foods like soup, bread, and frozen meals—and choose the foods with lower numbers. Look for "low sodium," "reduced sodium," or "no salt added" on the food label.
   - Drink water instead of sugary drinks. Cut calories by drinking water or unsweetened beverages. Soda, energy drinks, and sports drinks are a major source of added sugar and calories in American diets.

Understand Serving Sizes MyPlate presents personalized dietary recommendations in terms of numbers of servings of particular nutrients. But how much is one serving? Is it different from a portion? Although these two terms are often used interchangeably, they actually mean very different things. A *serving* is the recommended amount you should consume, whereas a *portion* is the amount you choose to eat at any one time. Many people select portions that are much bigger than recommended servings. See Figure 3.8 for an easy way to recognize serving sizes.

Unfortunately, we don't always get a clear picture from food producers and advertisers about what a serving really is. Consider a bottle of chocolate milk: The food label may list one serving size as 8 fluid ounces and 150 calories. However, note the size of the entire bottle. If it holds 16 ounces, drinking the whole thing serves up 300 calories.

Eat Nutrient-Dense Foods Although eating the proper number of servings from MyPlate is important, it is also important to recognize that there are large caloric, fat, and energy differences among foods within a given food group. For example, salmon and hot dogs provide vastly different nutrient levels per ounce. Salmon is rich in essential fatty acids and is considered nutrient dense. Hot dogs are loaded with saturated fats, cholesterol, and sodium—all substances we should limit. It is important to eat foods that have a high nutritional value for their caloric content.

Reduce Empty Calorie Foods Avoid *empty calories*, that is, calories that have little or no nutritional value. Sugar is sugar, but when you eat it in a piece of fruit, you're getting dietary fiber, lots of vitamins and minerals, and phytochemicals. In contrast, when you drink a 12-ounce soft drink, you're getting nearly 200 empty calories. Don't be fooled by fruit drinks, either. Unless the label states that they're 100 percent juice, they may also be loaded with added sugar. Even 100 percent fresh-squeezed orange juice has 20 grams (5 teaspoons!) of naturally occurring sugar in an 8-ounce serving. Bottled coffees, teas, and energy drinks usually are even higher in sugar and empty calories.

MyPlate recommends we limit our intake of sugary drinks as well as the following sugar- and fat-laden items:[34]

- **Cakes, cookies, pastries, and donuts:** One slice of chocolate cake contains 77 percent empty calories.
- **Cheese:** Switching from whole milk mozzarella cheese to non-fat mozzarella cheese saves you 76 empty calories per ounce.
- **Pizza:** One slice of pepperoni pizza adds 139 empty calories to your meal.
- **Ice cream:** More than 75 percent of the 275 calories in ice cream are empty calories.
- **Sausages, hot dogs, bacon, and ribs:** Adding a sausage link to your breakfast adds 96 empty calories.
- **Wine, beer, and all alcoholic beverages:** A whopping 155 empty calories are consumed with each 12 fluid ounces of beer.
- **Refined grains, including crackers, cookies, and white rice:** Switching to whole wheat versions can save you 25 fat-laden empty calories per serving.

Physical Activity Strive to be physically active for at least 30 minutes per day, preferably with moderate to vigorous activity levels on most days. Physical activity does not mean you have to go to the gym, jog 3 miles a day, or hire a personal trainer. Any activity that gets your heart pumping (e.g., gardening, playing basketball, heavy yard work, or dancing) is a good way to get moving. In addition to personalized recommendations on diet, MyPlate personalized plans will also offer recommendations for weekly physical activity.

check yourself

- **What are the main guidelines of the MyPlate food guidance system?**
- **Which parts of MyPlate can you most easily adopt in your diet? Which are the most challenging? Why?**

3.10 Eating Well in College

learning outcome

3.10 Provide examples of what college students can do to eat more healthfully.

Many college students may find it hard to fit a well-balanced meal into the day, but eating breakfast and lunch are important if you are to keep energy levels up and get the most out of your classes. Eating a complete breakfast that includes fiber-rich carbohydrates, protein, and healthy unsaturated fat (such as a banana, peanut butter, and whole-grain bread sandwich, or a bowl of oatmeal topped with dried fruit and nuts) is key. If you are short on time, bring a container of yogurt and some trail mix to your morning class.

If your campus is like many others, you've probably noticed a distinct move toward fast-food restaurants in your student unions. Generally speaking, you can eat more healthfully and for less money if you bring food from home or your campus dining hall. If you must eat fast food, follow the tips below to get more nutritional bang for your buck:

- Ask for nutritional analyses of items. Most fast-food chains now have them.
- Order salads, but be careful about what you add to them. Taco salads and Cobb salads are often high in fat, calories, and sodium. Ask for dressing on the side, and use it sparingly. Try the vinaigrette or low-fat dressings. Stay away from eggs and other high-fat add-ons, such as bacon bits, croutons, and crispy noodles.
- If you crave french fries, try baked "fries," which may be lower in fat.
- Avoid giant sizes, and refrain from ordering extra sauce, bacon, cheese, dressings, and other extras that add additional calories, sodium, carbohydrates, and fat.
- Limit sodas and other beverages that are high in added sugars.
- At least once per week, substitute a vegetable-based meat substitute into your fast-food choices. Most places now offer veggie burgers or similar products, which provide excellent sources of protein and often have considerably less fat and fewer calories.

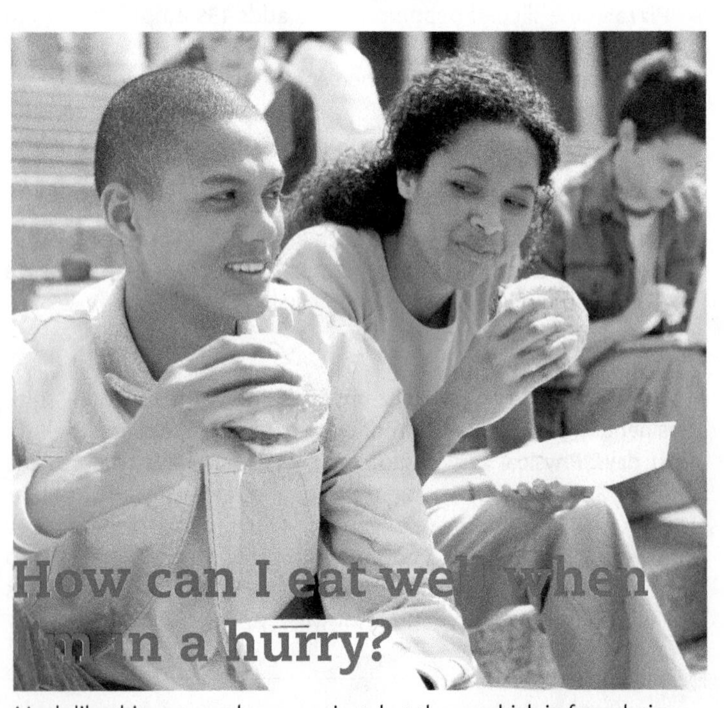

Meals like this one may be convenient, but they are high in fat, calories, sodium, and refined carbohydrates. Even when you are short on time and money, it is possible—and worthwhile—to make healthier choices. If you are ordering fast food, opt for foods prepared by baking, roasting, or steaming; ask for the leanest meat option; and request that sauces, dressings, and gravies be served on the side.

In the dining hall, try these ideas:

- Choose lean meats, grilled chicken, fish, or vegetable dishes. Avoid fried chicken, fatty cuts of red meat, or meat dishes smothered in creamy or oily sauce.
- Hit the salad bar and load up on leafy greens, beans, tuna, or tofu. Choose items such as avocado or nuts for a little "good" fat, and go easy on the dressing.
- When choosing items from a made-to-order food station, ask the preparer to hold the butter, oil, mayonnaise, sour cream, or cheese- or cream-based sauces.
- Avoid going back for seconds and consuming large portions.
- Pass on high-calorie, low-nutrient foods such as sugary cereals, ice cream, and other sweet treats. Choose fruit or low-fat yogurt to satisfy your sweet tooth.
- If there is something you'd like but don't see in your dining hall, speak to your food services manager and provide suggestions.

Between classes, avoid vending machines. Reach into your backpack for an apple, banana, some dried fruit and nuts, a single serving of unsweetened applesauce, or whole-grain crackers spread with peanut butter. Energy bars can be a nutritious option if you choose right. Check the Nutrition Facts panel for bars that are below 200 calories and provide at least 3 grams of dietary fiber. Cereal bars usually provide less protein than energy bars; however, they also tend to be much lower in calories and sugar, and high in fiber.

Many college students tend to think that fruits and vegetables are beyond their budget. Contrary to popular opinion, people on a tight budget can eat healthfully and spend less on food. Throughout the United States, five of the least expensive, perennially available fresh vegetables are carrots, eggplant, lettuce, potatoes, and summer squash. Five fresh fruit options are apples, bananas, pears, pineapple, and watermelon.[35] Additionally, choose fruits and veggies in season—they'll cost less. If you can freeze them, stock up. If not, enjoy them fresh while you can. Canned and frozen produce, especially when it's on sale, may also be less expensive than some fresh produce.

Maintaining a nutritious diet within the confines of student life can be challenging. However, if you take the time to plan healthy

College males spend an average of

$99.17

and college females spend an average of

$52.11

on fast food in a month.

meals, you will find that you are eating better, enjoying it more, and actually saving money.

What's Healthy on the Menu?

No matter what type of cuisine you enjoy, there will always be healthier and less healthy options on the menu. To help you order wisely, here are lighter options and high-fat pitfalls. "Best" choices contain fewer than 30 grams of fat, a generous meal's worth for an active, medium-sized woman. "Worst" choices have up to 100 grams of fat.

Breakfast

- Best: Hot or cold cereal with low fat milk; pancakes or French toast with syrup; scrambled eggs with hash browns and plain toast
- Worst: Belgian waffle with sausage; sausage and eggs with biscuits and gravy; ham-and-cheese omelet with hash browns and toast
- Tips: Ask for whole-grain cereal or shredded wheat with low-fat milk or whole wheat toast without butter or margarine. Order omelets without cheese, and order fried eggs without bacon or sausage.

Sandwiches

- Best: Ham and Swiss cheese; roast beef; turkey; hummus and red pepper
- Worst: Tuna salad; Reuben; submarine
- Tips: Ask for mustard; hold the mayonnaise and high-fat cheese. Load up sandwiches with veggies such as tomatoes, lettuce, cucumbers, sprouts, and bell peppers.

Seafood

- Best: Broiled bass, halibut, or snapper; grilled scallops; steamed crab or lobster
- Worst: Fried seafood platter; blackened catfish
- Tips: Order fish broiled, baked, grilled, or steamed—not panfried or sautéed. Ask for lemon instead of tartar sauce. Avoid creamy and buttery sauces.

Italian

- Best: Pasta with red or white clam sauce; spaghetti with marinara or tomato-and-meat sauce
- Worst: Eggplant parmigiana; fettuccine Alfredo; fried calamari; lasagna
- Tips: Stick with plain bread instead of garlic bread made with butter or oil. Avoid cream- or egg-based sauces. Try vegetarian pizza, and don't ask for extra cheese.

Mexican

- Best: Bean burrito (no cheese); chicken fajitas
- Worst: Beef chimichanga; quesadilla; chile relleno; refried beans
- Tips: Choose soft tortillas (not fried) with fresh salsa, not guacamole. Ask for beans made without lard or fat, and have cheeses and sour cream provided on the side or left out altogether.

See It! Videos

How accurate are restaurant calorie counts? Watch **Menu Calorie Counts** in the Study Area of MasteringHealth.

Skills for Behavior Change

HEALTHY EATING SIMPLIFIED

Messages from nutrition experts, marketing campaigns, and media blitzes may leave you scratching your head about how to eat healthfully. When it all starts to feel too complicated to be worthwhile, here are some simple tips to follow for health-conscious eating:

- **You don't need foods from fancy packages to improve your health. Fruits, vegetables, and whole grains should make up the bulk of your diet. Shop the perimeter of the store and the bulk foods aisle.**
- **Let the MyPlate method guide you. Your plate should be half vegetables, a quarter lean protein, and a quarter whole grains/bread. Have a serving of fruit for dessert.**
- **Limit processed and packaged foods. This will assist you in limiting added sodium, sugar, and fat. If you can't make sense of the ingredients, don't eat it.**
- **Eat natural snacks such as dried fruit, nuts, fresh fruits, string cheese, yogurt without added sugar, hard-boiled eggs, and vegetables.**
- **Be mindful of your eating. Eat until you are satisfied but not overfull.**
- **Bring healthful foods with you when you head out the door. Whether going to class, to work, or on a road trip, you *can* control the foods that are available. Don't put yourself in a position where you're forced to buy from a vending machine or convenience store.**

Source: M. Pollan, *Food Rules: An Eater's Manual* (New York, NY: Penguin Books, 2010).

check yourself

- **What challenges do you face when trying to eat more healthfully?**
- **What are some steps that you can take to eat more healthfully?**

3.11

Vegetarianism: A Healthy Diet?

learning outcome

3.11 Describe the benefits and drawbacks of a vegetarian diet.

More than 3 percent of U.S. adults, approximately 4 to 9 million people, are vegetarians.[36] Countless other Americans are heeding the advice of health, environmental, and animal ethics groups to reduce their meat consumption in favor of other "faceless" forms of protein. The word **vegetarian** can mean different things to different people—*vegans* eat no animal products at all, while many vegetarians eat dairy or other animal products but not animal flesh, and some eat seafood but not beef, pork, or poultry.

Common reasons for such eating choices include concern for animal welfare, improving health, environmental concerns, natural approaches to wellness, food safety, and weight loss or maintenance. Generally, people who follow a balanced vegetarian diet weigh less and have better cholesterol levels, less constipation and diarrhea, and a lower risk of heart disease than do nonvegetarians. Some studies suggest that vegetarianism may also reduce the risk of some cancers, particularly colon cancer.[37]

With proper meal planning, vegetarianism provides a healthful alternative to a high-fat, high-calorie, meat-based diet. Eating a variety of healthful foods throughout the day helps to ensure proper nutrient intake. Purely vegan diets may be deficient in some important vitamins and minerals, though many foods are fortified with these nutrients, or vegans can obtain them from supplements. Pregnant women, older adults, sick people, and children who are vegans or vegetarians need to take special care to ensure that their diets are adequate. In all cases, seek advice from a health care professional if you have questions.

Do Vegetarians Need to Take Supplements?

Dietary supplements are products intended to supplement existing diets. Ingredients range from vitamins, minerals, and herbs to enzymes, amino acids, fatty acids, and organ tissues. Supplement sales have skyrocketed in the last few decades. The FDA does not evaluate the safety and efficacy of supplements prior to their marketing; it can take action to remove a supplement from the market only after it has been proved harmful.

But do you really need any dietary supplements? That's a matter of some debate. The Office of Dietary Supplements, part of the National Institutes of Health, states that some supplements may help ensure that you get adequate amounts of essential nutrients if you don't consume a variety of foods, as recommended in the *Dietary Guidelines for Americans*. However, dietary supplements are not intended to prevent or treat disease, and recently the U.S. Preventive Services Task Force concluded that there is insufficient evidence to recommend that healthy people take multivitamin/mineral supplements to prevent cardiovascular disease or cancer.[38]

Taking high-dose supplements of the fat-soluble vitamins A, D, and E can be harmful or even fatal. Too much vitamin A, for example, can damage the liver, and excessive vitamin E increases the risk for a stroke.[39] Though some people—including vegans—benefit from taking supplements, The Academy of Nutrition and Dietetics recommends that a healthy diet is the best way to give your body what it needs.[40]

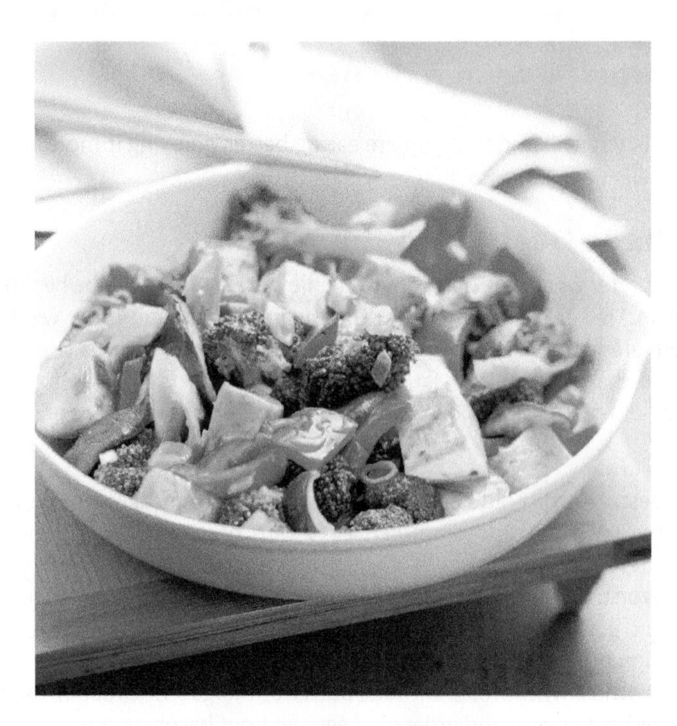

Are vegetarian diets healthy?

Adopting a vegan or vegetarian diet can be a very healthy way to eat. Take care to prepare your food healthfully by limiting the use of oils and avoiding added sugars and sodium. Make sure you get all the essential amino acids by eating meals like this tofu and vegetable stir fry. To further enhance it, add a whole grain such as brown rice.

check yourself

- **What are some of the benefits and drawbacks of a vegetarian diet?**
- **Should vegetarians supplement their diet in any way?**

3.12 Is Organic for You?

learning outcome

3.12 Explain the nature of organic foods.

Concerns about food safety, genetically modified foods, and the health impacts of chemicals used in the growth and production of food have led many people to turn to foods that are **organic**—foods and beverages developed, grown, or raised without the use of synthetic pesticides, chemicals, or hormones. Any food sold in the United States as organic has to meet criteria set by the USDA under the National Organic Rule and can carry a USDA seal verifying products as "certified organic."

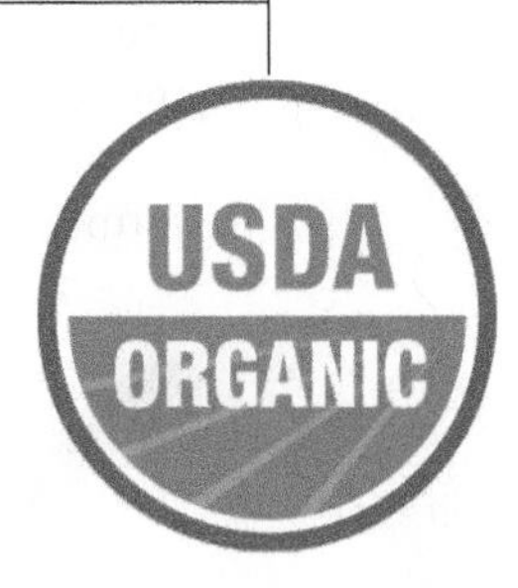

USDA label for certified organic foods.

Under the National Organic Rule, a product that is certified may carry one of the following terms: "100 percent Organic" (100% compliance with organic criteria), "Organic" (must contain at least 95% organic materials), "Made with Organic Ingredients" (must contain at least 70% organic ingredients), or "Some Organic Ingredients" (contains less than 70% organic ingredients—usually listed individually). Products that are labeled "all natural," "free-range," or "hormone free" are not necessarily organic. To be labeled with any of the above "organic" terms, the foods must be produced without hormones, antibiotics, herbicides, insecticides, chemical fertilizers, genetic modification, or germ-killing radiation. However, reliable monitoring systems to ensure credibility are still under development.

The market for organic foods has been increasing faster than food sales in general for many years. Whereas only a small subset of the population once bought organic, 81 percent of all U.S. families are now buying organic foods at least occasionally.[41] In 2010, annual organic food sales were estimated to be $31 billion.[42] Common reasons why people chose to buy organic include preferring the taste and wanting to limit exposure to pesticides and food additives. Some people purchase organics because of environmental concerns, since organic farming limits pesticide use and takes other measures to reduce pollution. One drawback is that organic foods are often more expensive than conventional foods, due in part to the higher costs associated with these organic farming practices.[43]

Is buying organic better for you? That all depends on what aspect of the food is being studied, and how the research is conducted. Two recent review studies, both of which examined decades of research into the nutrient quality of organic versus traditionally grown foods, reached opposite conclusions: One found organic foods more nutritious, and the other did not.[44] However, we do know that pesticide residues remain on conventionally grown produce. The U.S. Environmental Protection Agency warns that food pesticides can lead to health problems like cancer, nerve damage, and birth defects.[45] In 2013, the USDA reported that 3.7 percent of food samples harvested in 2011 had pesticide residues that exceeded the established tolerance level or for which no tolerance level has been established.[46] Both agencies advise consumers to wash fruits and vegetables before cooking or consuming them.

The word **locavore** has been coined to describe people who eat only food grown or produced locally, usually within close proximity to their homes. Farmers' markets or homegrown foods or those grown by independent farmers are thought to be fresher and to require far fewer resources to get them to market and keep them fresh for longer periods of time. Locavores believe that locally grown organic food is preferable to foods produced by large corporations or supermarket-based organic foods because they have a smaller impact on the environment and are believed to retain more of their nutritive value. Although there are many reasons organic farming is better for the environment, the fact that pesticides, herbicides, and other products are not used is perhaps the greatest benefit.

See It! Videos

Is organic produce better for you? Watch **Organic Produce** in the Study Area of MasteringHealth.

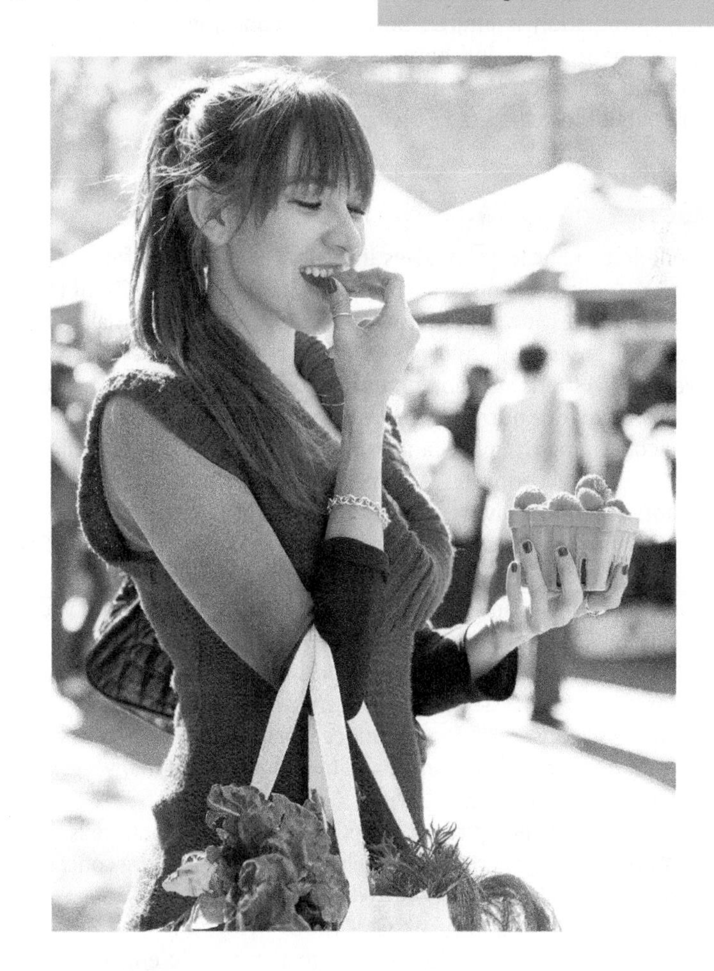

check yourself

- **What are organic foods?**
- **What are your reasons for buying or for not buying organic foods?**

3.13 Food Technology

learning outcome

3.13 Identify technologies being used in food production today.

Food Irradiation

Food irradiation involves exposing foods to low doses of radiation, or ionizing energy, which breaks chemical bonds in the DNA of harmful bacteria, destroying them or keeping them from reproducing. Essentially, the rays pass through the food without leaving any radioactive residue.[47]

Irradiation lengthens food products' shelf life and prevents spread of deadly microorganisms, particularly in high-risk foods such as ground beef and pork. Use of food irradiation is limited because of consumer concerns about safety and because irradiation facilities are expensive to build. Still, food irradiation is now common in over 40 countries. Irradiated foods are marked with the "radura" logo.

U.S. FDA label for irradiated foods.

Genetically Modified Food Crops

Genetic modification involves insertion or deletion of genes into the DNA of an organism. In the case of **genetically modified (GM) foods**, this is usually done to enhance production by making disease- or insect-resistant plants, improving yield, or controlling weeds. GM foods are sometimes created to improve foods' appearance or enhance nutrients; GM technology has been used to create rice containing vitamin A and iron, designed to help reduce disease in developing countries. Another use under development is the production and delivery of vaccines through GM foods.

The first genetically modified food crop was the FlavrSavr tomato, developed in 1996 to ripen without getting soft, increasing shipping capacity and shelf life. Since then, U.S. farmers have widely accepted GM crops.[48] Soybeans and cotton are the most common GM crops, followed by corn. On supermarket shelves, an estimated 75 percent of processed foods are genetically modified.[49]

Some scientists and food producers believe that GM crops could help address worldwide hunger and malnutrition, but many researchers and health advocates believe GM foods carry serious risks to humans and the ecosystem. Others are concerned about seeds being controlled by large corporations, while organic farmers are concerned about genetically modified seeds drifting into their fields.

The long-term safety of GM foods—for humans and other species—is still in question. Although the genetic engineering of insect-resistant crops has reduced the use of insecticides, it has simultaneously increased the use of herbicides (which kill weeds). This has not only led to the evolution of so-called "superweeds," but has also killed off beneficial weeds such as milkweed.[50] As a result, butterfly populations that depend on these weeds, particularly the monarch butterfly, have been decimated.[51] In addition, unintentional transfer of potentially allergy-provoking proteins has occurred, and although rigorous, validated tests of crops are performed to screen for known allergens, there is a potential for the transfer of new, unknown allergens.[52] However, the American Association for the Advancement of Science reports that foods containing genetically modified (GM) ingredients are no more a risk than are the same foods composed of crops modified over time with conventional plant breeding techniques, and the World Health Organization states that no adverse effects on human health have been shown from consumption of GM foods in countries that have approved their use.[53] Thus, the debate surrounding the risks and benefits of GM foods is not likely to end soon.

Arguments for the Development of GM Foods

- People have been manipulating food crops through selective breeding since the beginning of agriculture.
- Genetically modified seeds and products are tested for safety, and there has never been a substantiated claim for human illness resulting from their consumption.
- Insect- and weed-resistant GM crops allow farmers to use fewer chemical insecticides and herbicides.
- GM crops can be created to grow more quickly than conventional crops, increasing food yield. Nutrient-enhanced crops can address malnutrition.

Arguments against the Development of GM Foods

- Genetic modification is fundamentally different from and more problematic than selective breeding.
- There haven't been enough independent studies of GM products to confirm their safety. There are potential health risks if GM products approved for other uses are mistakenly or inadvertently used in production of food for human consumption.
- Inadvertent cross-pollination leads to "superweeds." Insect-resistant crops harm insect species that are not pests, and insect- and disease-resistant crops prompt evolution of even more virulent species, which then require aggressive control measures.
- Because corporations create and patent GM seeds, they control the market, forcing farmers worldwide to become reliant on these corporations.

check yourself

- **What are two technologies being used in our food?**
- **Are you more or less likely to buy foods that have been modified or irradiated? Why?**

3.14 Food Allergies and Intolerances

learning outcome

3.14 Define food allergies and intolerances.

About 33 percent of people today *think* they have a food allergy; however, it is estimated that only 5 percent of children and 4 percent of adults actually do.[54] Still, the prevalence of reported food allergies is on the rise. Data suggest the prevalence of peanut allergies among children tripled between 1997 and 2008.[55]

Food Allergies

A **food allergy**, or hypersensitivity, is an abnormal response to a food that is triggered by the immune system. Symptoms of an allergic reaction vary in severity and may include a tingling sensation in the mouth; swelling of the lips, tongue, and throat; difficulty breathing; hives; vomiting; abdominal cramps; diarrhea; drop in blood pressure; loss of consciousness; and death. Approximately 100 to 200 deaths per year occur from the *anaphylaxis* (the acute systemic immune and inflammatory response) that occurs with allergic reactions. These symptoms may appear within seconds to hours after eating the foods to which one is allergic.[56]

The Food Allergen Labeling and Consumer Protection Act (FALCPA) requires food manufacturers to label foods clearly to indicate the presence of (or possible contamination by) any of the eight major food allergens: milk, eggs, peanuts, wheat, soy, tree nuts (walnuts, pecans, etc.), fish, and shellfish. Although over 160 foods have been identified as allergy triggers, these 8 foods account for 90 percent of all food allergies in the United States.[57]

If you suspect that you have an actual allergic reaction to food, see an allergist to be tested to determine the source of the problem. Because there are several diseases that share symptoms with food allergies (ulcers and cancers of the gastrointestinal tract can cause vomiting, bloating, diarrhea, nausea, and pain), you should have persistent symptoms checked out as soon as possible. If particular foods seem to bother you consistently, look for alternatives or modify your diet. In true allergic instances, you may not be able to consume even the smallest amount of a substance safely.

Food Intolerance

In contrast to allergies, **food intolerance** can cause symptoms of gastric upset, but the upset is not the result of an immune system response. Probably the best example of a food intolerance is *lactose intolerance*, a problem that affects about 1 in every 10 adults. Lactase is an enzyme in the lining of the gut that degrades lactose, which is in dairy products. If you don't have enough lactase, you cannot digest lactose, and it remains in the gut to be used by bacteria. Gas is formed, causing bloating, abdominal pain, and sometimes diarrhea. Americans of European descent typically have rates of lactose intolerance as low as 2 to 3 percent, whereas 24 percent or more of minority populations are lactose intolerant.[58] Food intolerance also occurs in response to some food additives, such as the flavor enhancer MSG, certain dyes, sulfites, gluten, and other substances. In some cases, the food intolerance may have psychological triggers.

Celiac Disease

Celiac disease is an immune disorder that causes malabsorption of nutrients from the small intestine in genetically susceptible people. It is thought to affect over 2 million Americans, most of whom are undiagnosed.[59] When a person with celiac disease consumes gluten, a protein found in wheat, rye, and barley, the person's immune system attacks the small intestine and stops nutrient absorption. Pain, cramping, and other symptoms often follow in the short term. Untreated, celiac disease can lead to other health problems, such as osteoporosis, nutritional deficiencies, and cancer. Individuals diagnosed with celiac disease are encouraged to consult a dietitian for help designing a gluten-free diet. If you suspect you have celiac disease, see a doctor. Blood tests looking for specific antibodies or a small intestine biopsy can help determine whether you have celiac disease or other GI issues.

For those who need to achieve a gluten-free diet, there are increasing numbers of products available. Specially formulated gluten-free breads, pasta, and cereal products can allow people with celiac disease to enjoy meals similar to those without the disease. Reading food labels is particularly important, because many foods that seem safe may have hidden sources of gluten. Bouillon cubes, cold cuts, and soups are three examples of processed foods that may contain wheat, barley, or rye.

Peanuts are among the eight most common food allergens.

check yourself

- **What causes food allergies and intolerances?**
- **What is the difference between a food allergy and an intolerance?**

3.15 Food Safety and Foodborne Illnesses

learning outcome

3.15 Provide examples of food safety concerns and tips for reducing exposure to unsafe food.

Eating unhealthy food is one thing. Eating food that has been contaminated with a pathogen, toxin, or other harmful substance is quite another. As outbreaks of foodborne illness (commonly called food poisoning) make the news, the food industry has come under fire. The Food Safety Modernization Act, passed into law in 2011, included new requirements for food processors to take actions to prevent contamination of foods. The act gave the FDA greater authority to inspect food-manufacturing facilities and to recall contaminated foods.[60]

Are you concerned that the chicken you are buying doesn't look pleasingly pink or that your "fresh" fish smells a little *too* fishy? You may have good reason to be worried. In increasing numbers, Americans are becoming sick from what they eat, and many of these illnesses are life threatening. Scientists estimate that foodborne illnesses sicken 1 in 6 Americans (over 48 million people) and cause some 128,000 hospitalizations and 3,000 deaths in the United States annually.[61] Although the incidence of infection with certain microbes has declined, current data from the U.S. Centers for Disease Control and Prevention (CDC) shows a lack of recent progress in reducing foodborne infections and highlights the need for improved prevention.[62]

Most foodborne infections and illnesses are caused by several common types of bacteria and viruses; the following are some of the most common:[63]

- **Norovirus.** Transmitted through contact with the vomit or stool of infected people, norovirus is the most common cause of foodborne illness in the United States annually. Washing hands and all kitchen surfaces can help prevent transmission.
- ***Salmonella.*** Commonly found in the intestines of birds, reptiles, and mammals, the species *Salmonella* can spread to humans through foods of animal origin. Infection is more likely in people with poor underlying health or weakened immune systems.
- ***Clostridium perfringens.*** This is a bacterial species found in the intestinal tracts of humans and animals.
- ***Campylobacter.*** Most raw poultry has *Campylobacter* in it; bacterial infection most frequently results from eating undercooked chicken, raw eggs, or foods contaminated with juices from raw chicken. Shellfish and unpasteurized milk are also sources.
- ***Staphylococcus aureus.*** *Staph* lives on human skin, in infected cuts, and in the nose and throat.

Foodborne illnesses can also be caused by a toxin in food originally produced by a bacterium or other microbe in the food. These toxins can produce illness even if the microbes that produced them are no longer there. For example, botulism is caused by a deadly neurotoxin produced by the bacterium *Clostridium botulinum*. This bacterium is widespread in soil, water, plants, and intestinal tracts, but it can grow only in environments with limited or no oxygen. Potential food sources include improperly canned food and vacuum-packed or tightly wrapped foods. Though rare, botulism is fatal if untreated.

Signs of foodborne illnesses vary tremendously and usually include one or several symptoms: diarrhea, nausea, cramping, and vomiting. Depending on the amount and virulence of the pathogen, symptoms may appear as early as 30 minutes after eating contaminated food or as long as several days or weeks later. Most of the time, symptoms occur 5 to 8 hours after eating and last only a day or two. For certain populations, such as the very

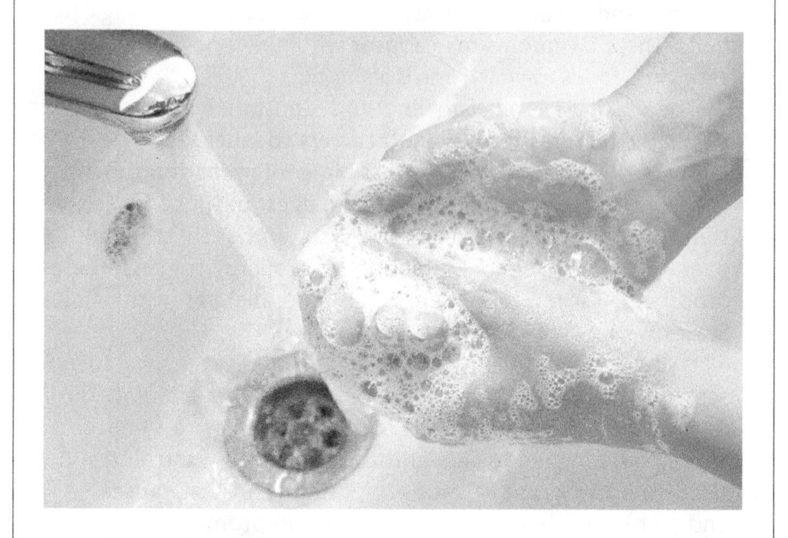

88% percent of college students said they understood the importance of hand washing in preventing foodborne illness. Yet only 49 percent of those surveyed actually washed their hands always or most of the time before meals.

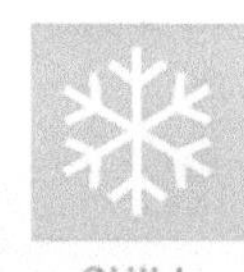

Figure 3.9 Education's Fight BAC!
This logo reminds consumers how to prevent foodborne illness.
Source: Partnership for Food Safety and Education, www.fightbac.org.

young; older adults; or people with severe illnesses such as cancer, diabetes, kidney disease, or AIDS, foodborne diseases can be fatal.

Several factors contribute to foodborne illnesses. Since fresh foods are not in season much of the year, the United States imports $18 billion in fresh fruits and vegetables from other countries, often from great distances. These countries include Mexico (36% of imports), several Central and South American countries (about 25%), and China (8%).[64] Although we are told when we travel to developing countries to "boil it, peel it, or don't eat it," we bring these foods into our kitchens at home and eat them, often without even washing them.

Food can become contaminated by being watered with tainted water, fertilized with animal manure, or harvested by people who have not washed their hands properly after using the toilet. Food-processing equipment, facilities, or workers may contaminate food, or it can become contaminated if not kept clean and cool during transport or on store shelves. To give you an idea of the implications, studies have shown that the bacterium *Escherichia coli* can survive in cow manure for up to 70 days and can multiply in foods grown with manure unless heat or additives such as salt or preservatives are used to kill the microbes.[65] No regulations prohibit farmers from using animal manure to fertilize crops. In addition, *E. coli* actually increases in summer months as factory-farmed cows await slaughter in crowded, overheated pens. This increases the chances of meat coming to market already contaminated.

Other key factors associated with the increasing spread of foodborne diseases include the inadvertent introduction of pathogens into new geographic regions and insufficient education about food safety. Globalization of the food supply, climate change, and global warming are also factors that may influence increasing spread.

Avoiding Risks in the Home

Part of the responsibility for preventing foodborne illness lies with consumers—more than 30 percent of all such illnesses result from unsafe handling of food at home. Fortunately, consumers can take several steps to reduce the likelihood of contaminating their food (see Figure 3.9). Among the most basic precautions is to wash your hands and wash all produce before eating it. Also, avoid cross-contamination in the kitchen by using separate cutting boards and utensils for meats and produce.

Temperature control is also important—refrigerators must be set at 40 degrees or less. Be sure to cook meats to the recommended temperature to kill contaminants before eating. Hot foods must be kept hot and cold foods kept cold in order to avoid unchecked bacterial growth. Eat leftovers within 3 days; if you're unsure how long something has been sitting in the fridge, don't take chances. When in doubt, throw it out. See Skills for Behavior Change for more tips about reducing risk of foodborne illness when shopping for and preparing food.

Skills for Behavior Change

REDUCE YOUR RISK FOR FOODBORNE ILLNESS

- When shopping, put perishable foods in your cart last. Check for cleanliness throughout the store, especially at the salad bar and at the meat and fish counters. Never buy dented cans of food. Check the "sell by" or "use by" date on foods.
- Once you get home, put dairy products, eggs, meat, fish, and poultry in the refrigerator immediately. If you don't plan to eat meats within 2 days, freeze them. You can keep an unopened package of hot dogs or luncheon meats for about 2 weeks.
- When refrigerating or freezing raw meats, make sure their juices can't spill onto other foods.
- Never thaw frozen foods at room temperature. Put them in the refrigerator to thaw or thaw in the microwave, following manufacturer's instructions.
- Wash your hands with soap and warm water before preparing food. Wash fruits and vegetables before peeling, slicing, cooking, or eating them—but not meat, poultry, or eggs! Wash cutting boards, countertops, and other utensils and surfaces with detergent and hot water after food preparation.
- Use a meat thermometer to ensure that meats are completely cooked. To find out proper cooking temperatures for different types of meat, visit http://foodsafety.gov.
- Refrigeration slows the secretion of bacterial toxins into foods. Never leave leftovers out for more than 2 hours. On hot days, don't leave foods out for longer than 1 hour.

check yourself

- **What are some current food safety concerns?**
- **Have you ever experienced a foodborne illness? If so, what were possible causes and how could you have avoided it?**

3.16 How Healthy Are Your Eating Habits?

An interactive version of this assessment is available online in MasteringHealth.

1 Keep Track of Your Food Intake

Keep a food diary for 5 days, writing down everything you eat or drink. Be sure to include the approximate amount or portion size. Add up the number of servings from each of the major food groups on each day and enter them into the chart below.

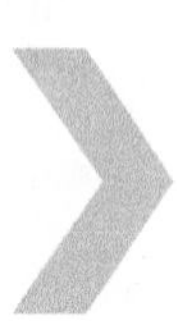

Number of Servings of:						
	Day 1	Day 2	Day 3	Day 4	Day 5	Average
Fruits						
Vegetables						
Grains						
Protein foods						
Dairy						
Fats and oils						
Sweets						

2A Does Your Diet Have Proportionality?

	Yes	No
1. Are grains the main food choice at all your meals?	○	○
2. Do you often forget to eat vegetables?	○	○
3. Do you typically eat fewer than three pieces of fruit daily?	○	○
4. Do you often have fewer than 3 cups of milk daily?	○	○
5. Is the portion of meat, chicken, or fish the largest item on your dinner plate?	○	○

Scoring 2A

If you answered yes to three or more of these questions, your diet probably lacks proportionality. Review the recommendations in this chapter, particularly the MyPlate guidelines, to learn how to balance your diet.

2 Evaluate Your Food Intake

Now compare your consumption patterns to the MyPlate recommendations. Visit www.choosemyplate.gov to evaluate your daily caloric needs and the recommended consumption rates for the different food groups. How does your diet match up?

	Less than the recommended amount	About equal to the recommended amount	More than the recommended amount
1. How does your daily fruit consumption compare to the recommendation for your age and activity level?	○	○	○
2. How does your daily vegetable consumption compare to the recommendation for your age and activity level?	○	○	○
3. How does your daily grain consumption compare to the recommendation for your age and activity level?	○	○	○
4. How does your daily protein food consumption compare to the recommendation for your age and activity level?	○	○	○
5. How does your daily fats and oils consumption compare to the recommendation for your age and activity level?	○	○	○

Scoring

If you found that your food intake is consistent with the MyPlate recommendations, congratulations! If, however, you are falling short in a major food group or overdoing it in certain categories, consider taking steps described in this chapter to adopt healthier eating habits.

2B Are You Getting Enough Fat-Soluble Vitamins in Your Diet?

	Yes	No
1. Do you eat at least 1 cup of deep yellow or orange vegetables, such as carrots and sweet potatoes, or dark green vegetables, such as spinach, every day?	○	○
2. Do you consume at least two glasses (8 ounces each) of milk daily?	○	○
3. Do you eat a tablespoon of vegetable oil, such as corn or olive oil, daily? (Tip: Salad dressings, unless they are fat free, count.)	○	○
4. Do you eat at least 1 cup of leafy green vegetables in your salad and/or put lettuce in your sandwich every day?	○	○

Scoring 2B

If you answered yes to all four questions, you are on your way to acing your fat-soluble vitamin needs! If you answered no to any of the questions, your diet needs some fine-tuning. Deep orange and dark green vegetables are excellent sources of vitamin A, and milk is an excellent choice for vitamin D. Vegetable oils provide vitamin E; if you put them on top of your vitamin K–rich leafy green salad, you'll hit the vitamin jackpot.

2C Are You Getting Enough Water-Soluble Vitamins in Your Diet?

	Yes	No
1. Do you consume at least 1/2 cup of rice or pasta daily?	○	○
2. Do you eat at least 1 cup of a ready-to-eat cereal or hot cereal every day?	○	○
3. Do you have at least one slice of bread, a bagel, or a muffin daily?	○	○
4. Do you enjoy a citrus fruit or fruit juice, such as an orange, a grapefruit, or orange juice, every day?	○	○
5. Do you have at least 1 cup of vegetables throughout your day?	○	○

Scoring 2C

If you answered yes to all of these questions, you are a vitamin B and C superstar! If you answered no to any of the questions, your diet could use some refinement. Rice, pasta, cereals, bread, and bread products are all excellent sources of B vitamins. Citrus fruits are a ringer for vitamin C. In fact, all vegetables can contribute to meeting your vitamin C needs daily.

Source: Adapted from J. Blake, *Nutrition and You*, 2nd ed. (San Francisco, CA: Benjamin Cummings, 2011).

Your Plan for Change

The Assess Yourself activity gave you the chance to evaluate your current nutritional habits. Now that you have considered these results, you can decide whether you need to make changes in your daily eating for long-term health.

Today, you can:

○ Start keeping a more detailed food log. The easy-to-use SuperTracker at www.supertracker.usda.gov can help you keep track of your food intake and analyze what you eat. Take note of the nutritional information of the various foods you eat and write down particulars about the number of calories, grams of fat, grams of sugar, milligrams of sodium, and so on of each food. Try to find specific weak spots: Are you consuming too many calories or too much salt or sugar? Do you eat too little calcium or iron? Use the SuperTracker to plan a healthier food intake to overcome these weak spots.

○ Take a field trip to the grocery store. Forgo your fast-food dinner and instead spend some time in the produce section of the supermarket. Purchase your favorite fruits and vegetables, and try something new to expand your tastes.

Within the next 2 weeks, you can:

○ Plan at least three meals that you can make at home or in your dorm room, and purchase the ingredients you'll need ahead of time. Something as simple as a chicken sandwich on whole-grain bread will be more nutritious, and probably cheaper, than heading out for a fast-food meal.

○ Start reading labels. Be aware of the amount of calories, sodium, sugars, and fats in prepared foods; aim to buy and consume those that are lower in all of these and are higher in calcium and fiber.

By the end of the semester, you can:

○ Get in the habit of eating a healthy breakfast every morning. Combine whole grains, proteins, and fruit in your breakfast—for example, eat a bowl of cereal with milk and bananas or a cup of yogurt combined with granola and berries. Eating a healthy breakfast will jump-start your metabolism, prevent drops in blood glucose levels, and keep your brain and body performing at their best through those morning classes.

○ Commit to one or two healthful changes to your eating patterns for the rest of the semester. You might resolve to eat five servings of fruits and vegetables every day, to switch to low-fat or nonfat dairy products, to stop drinking soft drinks, or to use only olive oil in your cooking. Use your food diary to help you spot places where you can make healthier choices on a daily basis.

Summary

To hear an MP3 Tutor session, scan here or visit the Study Area in **MasteringHealth**.

LO 3.1 Recognizing that we eat for more reasons than just survival is the first step toward improving our nutritional habits.

LO 3.1–3.7 The essential nutrients include water, proteins, carbohydrates, fats, vitamins, and minerals. Water makes up 50 to 60 percent of our body weight and is necessary for nearly all life processes. Proteins are major components of our cells and are key elements of antibodies, enzymes, and hormones. Carbohydrates are our primary sources of energy. Fats play important roles in maintaining body temperature and cushioning and protecting organs. Vitamins are organic compounds, and minerals are inorganic compounds. We need both in relatively small amounts to maintain healthy body function. Functional foods may provide health benefits in addition to the nutrients they contribute to the diet.

LO 3.8 Food labels provide information on serving size and number of calories in a food, as well as the amounts of various nutrients and the percentage of recommended daily values those amounts represent.

LO 3.9 A healthful diet is adequate, moderate, balanced, varied, and nutrient dense. The *Dietary Guidelines for Americans* and the MyPlate food guidance system provide guidelines for healthy eating. These recommendations, developed by the USDA, place emphasis on balancing calories and making appropriate food choices.

LO 3.10 College students face unique challenges in eating healthfully. Learning to make better choices at restaurants, to eat healthfully on a budget, and to eat nutritionally in the dorm are all possible when you use the information in this chapter.

LO 3.11 Vegetarianism can provide a healthy alternative for people wishing to eat less or no meat.

LO 3.12 Organic foods are grown and produced without the use of synthetic pesticides, chemicals, or hormones. The USDA offers certification of organics. These foods have become increasingly available and popular, as people take a greater interest in eating healthfully and sustainably.

LO 3.11–3.15 Foodborne illnesses, food irradiation, allergies, food intolerances, GM foods, and other food safety and health concerns are becoming increasingly important to health-wise consumers. Recognizing potential risks and taking steps to prevent problems are part of a sound nutritional plan.

Pop Quiz

Visit MasteringHealth to personalize your study plan with Chapter Review Quizzes and Dynamic Study Modules.

LO 3.2 1. What is the most crucial nutrient for life?
a. Water
b. Fiber
c. Minerals
d. Protein

LO 3.2 2. Which of the following nutrients is required for the repair and growth of body tissue?
a. Carbohydrates
b. Proteins
c. Vitamins
d. Fats

LO 3.3 3. Which of the following nutrients moves food through the digestive tract?
a. Water
b. Fiber
c. Minerals
d. Starch

LO 3.4 4. What substance plays a vital role in maintaining healthy skin and hair, insulating body organs against shock, maintaining body temperature, and promoting healthy cell function?
a. Fats
b. Fibers
c. Proteins
d. Carbohydrates

LO 3.4 5. Triglycerides make up about ________ percent of total body fat.
a. 5
b. 35
c. 55
d. 95

LO 3.4 6. Which of the following is a healthier fat to include in the diet?
a. *Trans* fat
b. Saturated fat
c. Unsaturated fat
d. Hydrogenated fat

LO 3.5 7. Which vitamin maintains bone health?
a. B_{12}
b. D
c. B_6
d. Niacin

LO 3.6 8. Which of the following is a trace mineral?
a. Calcium
b. Sodium
c. Potassium
d. Iron

LO 3.9 9. Which of the following foods would be considered a healthy, *nutrient-dense* food?
a. Nonfat milk
b. Celery
c. Soft drink
d. Potato chips

LO 3.14 10. Lucas's doctor diagnoses him with celiac disease. Which of the following foods should Lucas cut out of his diet to eat gluten-free?
a. Shellfish
b. Eggs
c. Peanuts
d. Wheat

Answers to these questions can be found on page A-1. If you answered a question incorrectly, review the module identified by the Learning Outcome. For even more study tools, visit MasteringHealth.

Stress 4

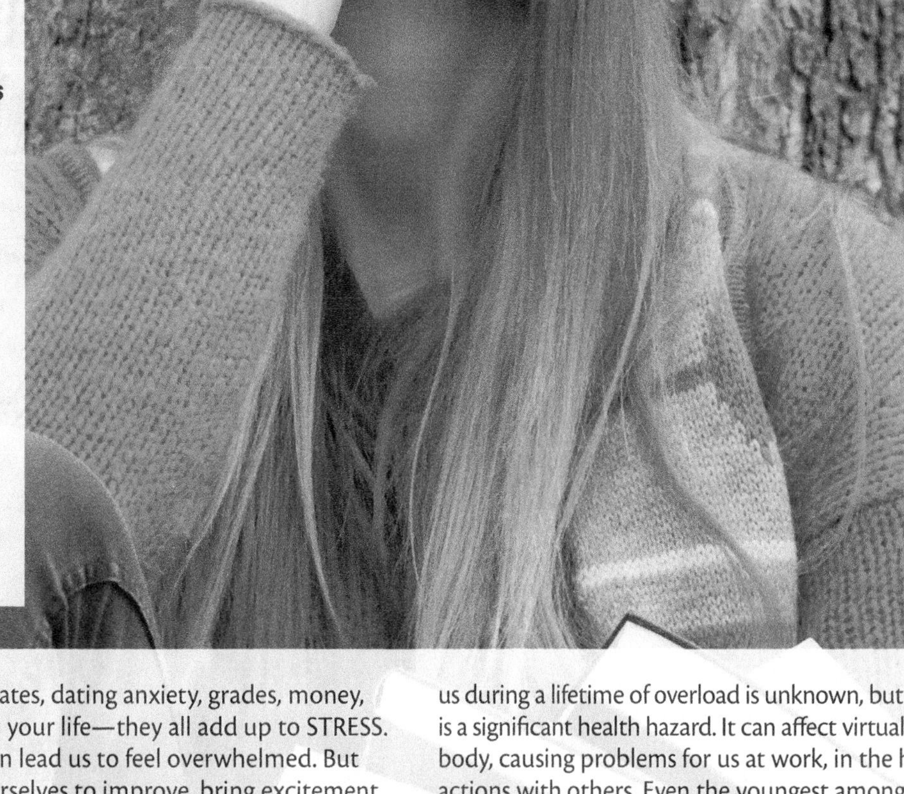

Rising tuition, difficult roommates, dating anxiety, grades, money, worries about what to do with your life—they all add up to STRESS. In today's 24/7 world, stress can lead us to feel overwhelmed. But it can also cause us to push ourselves to improve, bring excitement into an otherwise humdrum life, and leave us exhilarated. While we work, play, socialize, and sleep, stress affects us in myriad ways, many of which we may not even notice.

According to a recent American Psychological Association poll, Americans consistently report high stress levels, and 20 percent report extreme stress.[1] Adults ages 18–46 report the highest levels of stress and the greatest increases in stress levels.[2] The exact toll stress exerts on us during a lifetime of overload is unknown, but we do know that stress is a significant health hazard. It can affect virtually every system of the body, causing problems for us at work, in the home, and in our interactions with others. Even the youngest among us suffer from stress-related headaches, stomachaches, and difficulty sleeping, and stress seems to be particularly threatening to youth who are overweight.[3]

Is too much stress inevitable? Fortunately, the answer is no. To tame stress, we can learn to anticipate and recognize personal stressors—and develop skills to reduce or manage those we cannot avoid or control. First, we must understand what stress is and what effects it has on the body.

4.1 What Is Stress?

learning outcome

4.1 Define stress-related key terms.

Most current definitions state that **stress** is the mental and physical response and adaptation by our bodies to the real or perceived changes and challenges in our lives. A **stressor** is any real or perceived physical, social, environmental, or psychological event or stimulus that strains our abilities to cope. Several factors influence one's response to stressors, including the *characteristics of the stressor* (Can you control it? Is it predictable? Does it occur often?); *biological factors* (e.g., your age or gender); and *past experiences or fears* (e.g., things that have happened to you, their consequences, and how you responded). Stressors may be *tangible*, such as a failing grade on a test, or *intangible*, such as the angst associated with meeting your significant other's parents for the first time.

Distress, or negative stress, is more likely to occur when you are tired, under the influence of alcohol or other drugs, or coping with an illness, financial trouble, or relationship problems. In contrast, **eustress**, or positive stress, presents the opportunity for personal growth and satisfaction and can actually improve health. It can energize you, motivate you, and raise you up when you are down. Getting married or winning a major competition can give rise to the pleasurable rush associated with eustress.

There are several types of stress. **Acute stress** is typically intense, flares quickly, and disappears quickly. Seeing your crush could cause your heart to race and your muscles to tense while you appear cool, calm, and collected. Or anticipating a class presentation could cause shaking hands, nausea, headache, cramping, or diarrhea, along with a galloping heartbeat, stammering, and forgetfulness. **Episodic acute stress** is the state of *regularly* reacting with wild, acute stress to various situations. Individuals experiencing episodic acute stress may complain about all they have to do and focus on negative events that may or may not occur. These "awfulizers" are often reactive and anxious, but their thoughts and behaviors can be so habitual that to them they seem normal.

Although **chronic stress** may not feel as intense, it can linger indefinitely and wreak silent havoc on your body's systems. Caregivers are especially vulnerable to prolonged physiological stress as they watch a loved one struggle with a major disease or disability. Upon a loved one's eventual death, survivors may struggle to balance the need to process anger, grief, loneliness, and guilt with the need to stay caught up in classes, work, and everyday life. Another type of stress, **traumatic stress**, is often a result of witnessing or experiencing events like major accidents, war, shootings, assault, or natural disasters. Effects of traumatic stress may be felt for years after the event and cause significant disability, potentially leading to *post-traumatic stress disorder (PTSD)*.[4]

On any given day, we all experience both eustress and distress, each triggered by a wide range of both obvious and not-so-obvious

10.4%

of college students report experiencing "tremendous stress" over the past 12 months.

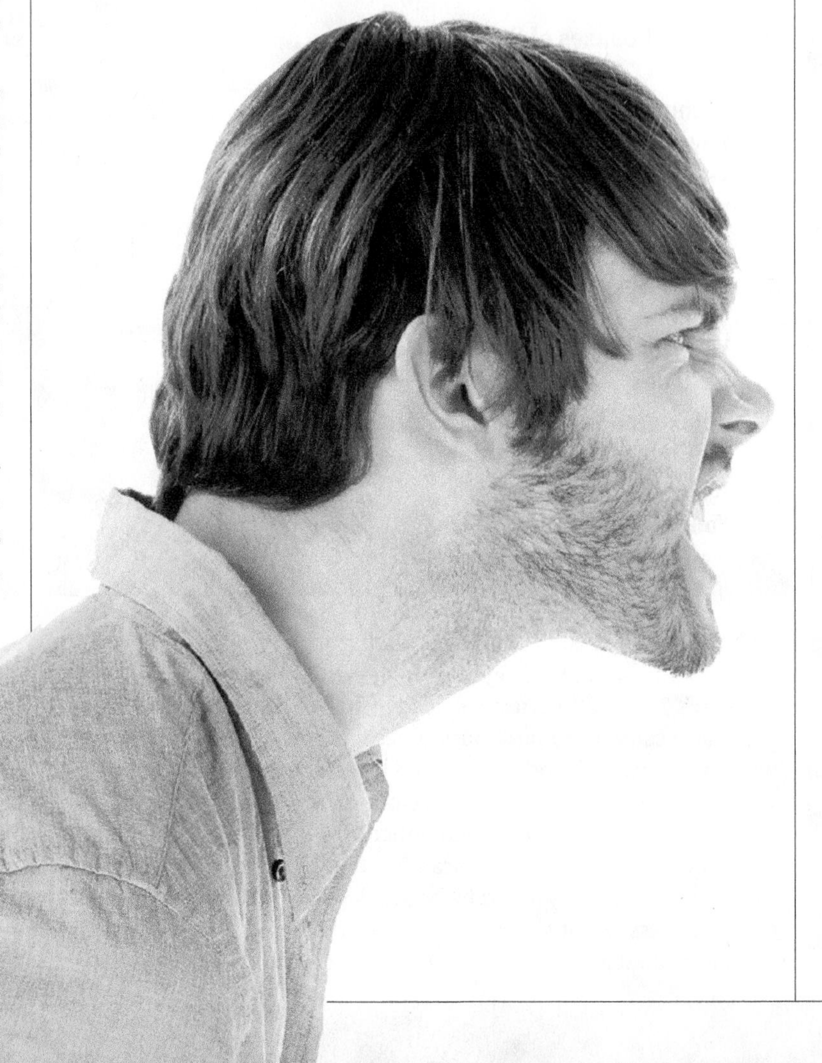

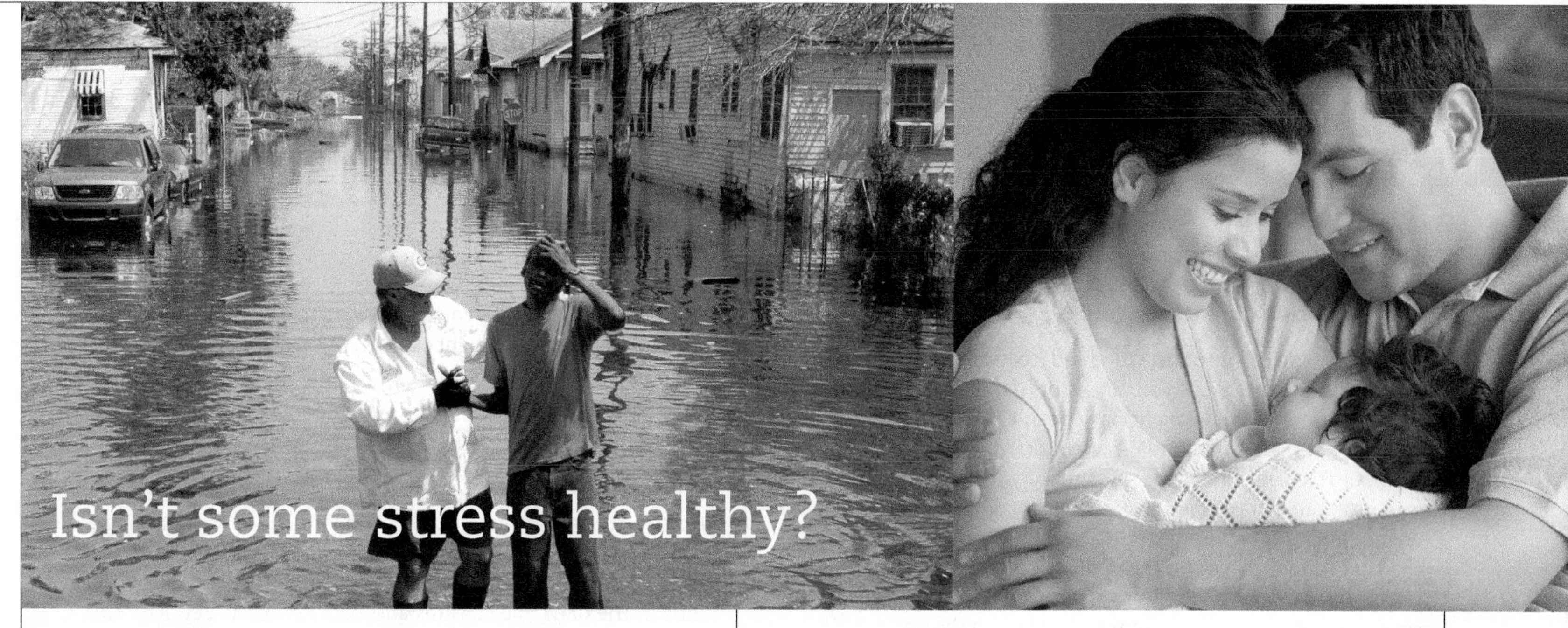

A moderate level of stress—especially eustress arising from new experiences—can actually help you live life to the fullest. Too much stress can affect your health for the worse, such as what is experienced by survivors of a natural disaster, but so can too little stress; we need change and challenge to keep us fulfilled and growing.

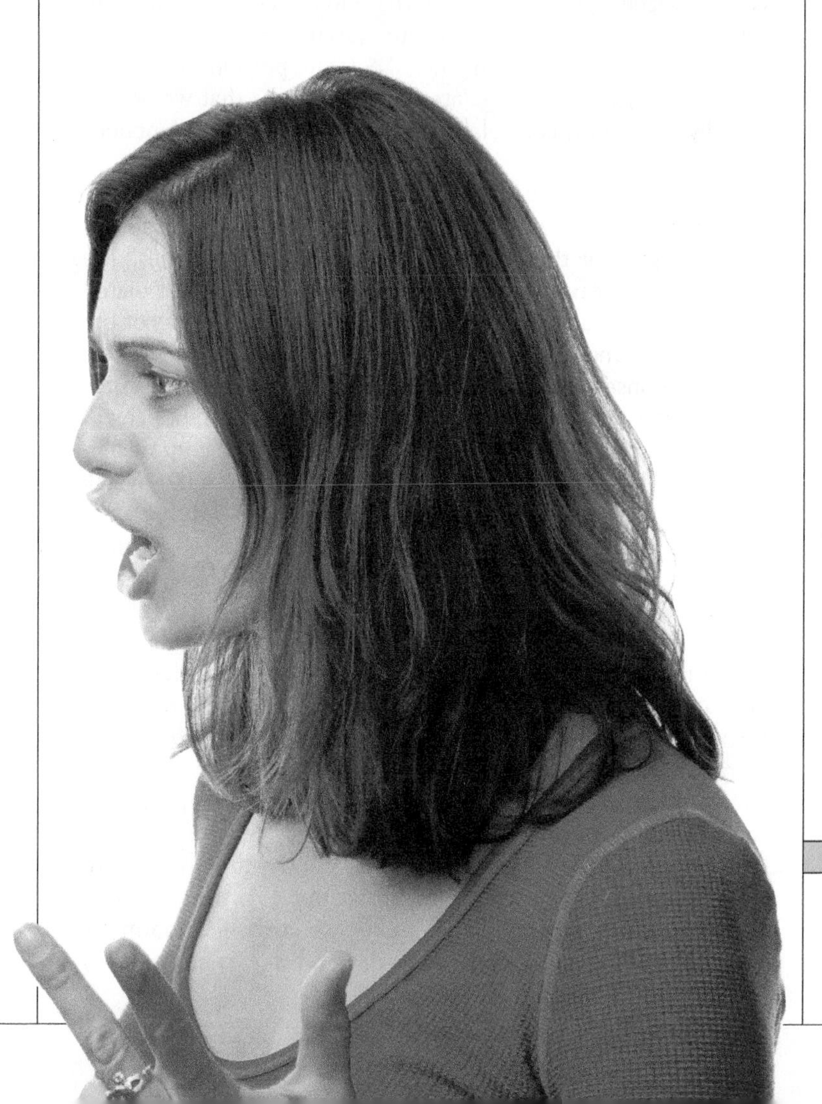

sources. Several studies in recent years have examined sources of stress among various populations in the United States and globally. One of the most comprehensive is conducted annually by the American Psychological Association; the 2013 survey found that the biggest sources of stress for adults ages 18–33 are work, money, and job stability, whereas individuals aged 67 and older were more likely to cite personal health concerns.[5] College students, in particular, face stressors that come from internal sources, as well as external pressures to succeed in a competitive environment that is often geographically far removed from the support of family and hometown friends.

While key sources of stress are similar for men and women (money, work, and the economy), huge gender differences exist in how people experience, report, and cope with stress. Both men and women report above average levels of stress, but women are more likely to report stress levels that are increasing and more extreme than those of their male counterparts.[6] Additionally, although men may recognize and report stress, they are much less likely to take action to reduce it.[7]

Awareness of the sources of the stress in your life can do much to help you develop a plan to avoid, prevent, and control the things that cause you stress.

check yourself

- **How do distress and eustress differ?**
- **Do you have more trouble managing acute stress or chronic stress? Why?**

4.2 Your Body's Response to Stress

learning outcome

4.2 Explain the purpose of the general adaptation syndrome, and the physiological changes that occur during each phase.

Our physiological responses evolved to protect us from harm. Thousands of years ago, if your ancestors didn't respond to stress by fighting or fleeing, they might have been eaten by a saber-toothed tiger or killed by a marauding enemy clan. Today when we face real or perceived threats, these same physiological responses kick into gear, but our instinctual reactions to fight, scream, or flee the enemy must be held in check. Restraining these responses rather than allowing them to run their course can make us physiologically charged for longer periods—sometimes chronically. Over time, a simmering stress response can wreak havoc on the body.

The General Adaptation Syndrome

When stress levels are low, the body is often in a state of **homeostasis**: All body systems are operating smoothly to maintain equilibrium. Stressors trigger a "crisis-mode" physiological response, after which the body attempts to return to homeostasis by means of an **adaptive response**. First characterized by Hans Selye in 1936, the internal fight to restore homeostasis in the face of a stressor is known as the **general adaptation syndrome (GAS)** (Figure 4.1). The GAS has three distinct phases: alarm, resistance, and exhaustion.[8]

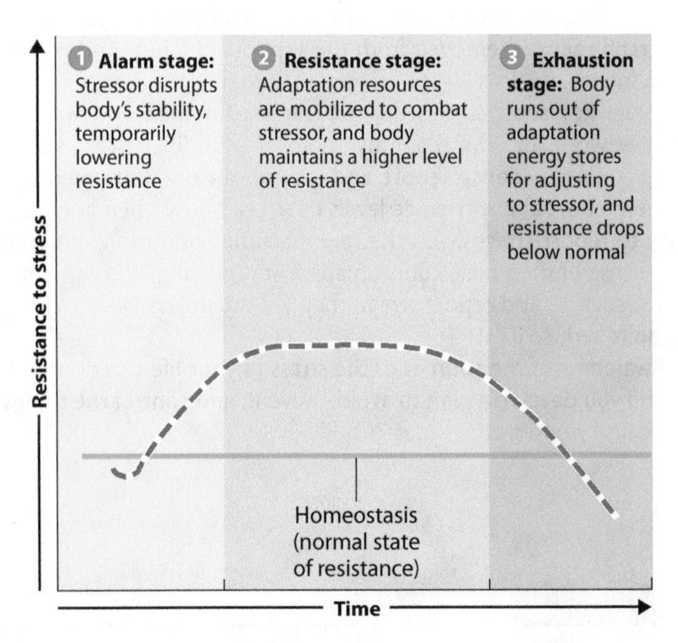

Figure 4.1 The General Adaptation Syndrome (GAS)
The GAS describes the body's method of coping with prolonged stress.

Regardless of whether you are experiencing distress or eustress, similar physiological changes occur.

Alarm Phase Suppose you are walking to your residence hall on a dimly lit campus after a night class. You hear someone cough behind you, and you sense someone approaching rapidly. You walk faster, only to hear the quickened footsteps of the other person. Your senses become increasingly alert, your breathing quickens, your heart races, and you begin to perspire. In desperation you stop, rip off your backpack, and prepare to fling it at your attacker to defend yourself. You turn around quickly and let out a blood-curdling yell. To your surprise, the only person you see is a classmate: She has been trying to stay close to you out of her own anxiety about walking alone in the dark. She screams and backs off the sidewalk into the bushes, and you both start laughing with startled embarrassment. You and your classmate have just experienced the alarm phase of the GAS. Also known as the **fight-or-flight response**, this physiological reaction is one of our most basic, innate survival instincts.[9]

When the mind perceives a real or imaginary stressor, the cerebral cortex, the region of the brain that interprets the nature of an event, triggers an **autonomic nervous system (ANS)** response that prepares the body for action. The ANS is the portion of the central nervous system that regulates body functions that we do not normally consciously control, such as heart and glandular functions and breathing.

The ANS has two branches: sympathetic and parasympathetic. The **sympathetic nervous system** energizes the body for fight or flight by signaling the release of several stress hormones. The **parasympathetic nervous system** slows all the systems stimulated by the stress response; in effect, it counteracts the actions of the sympathetic branch.

The responses of the sympathetic nervous system to stress involve a series of biochemical exchanges between different parts of the body. The brain's **hypothalamus** functions as the control center of the sympathetic nervous system and determines the overall reaction to stressors. When the hypothalamus perceives that extra energy is needed to fight a stressor, it stimulates the adrenal glands, which are located near the top of the kidneys, to release the hormone **epinephrine**, also called *adrenaline*. Epinephrine causes more blood to be pumped with each beat of the heart, dilates the airways in the lungs to increase oxygen intake, increases the breathing rate, stimulates the liver to release more glucose (which fuels muscular exertion), and dilates the pupils to improve visual sensitivity (see Figure 4.2).

In addition to the fight-or-flight response, the alarm phase can also trigger a longer-term reaction to stress. The hypothalamus uses chemical messages to trigger the pituitary gland within the brain to release a powerful hormone, *adrenocorticotropic hormone (ACTH)*. ACTH signals the adrenal glands to release **cortisol**, a hormone that makes stored nutrients more readily available to meet energy

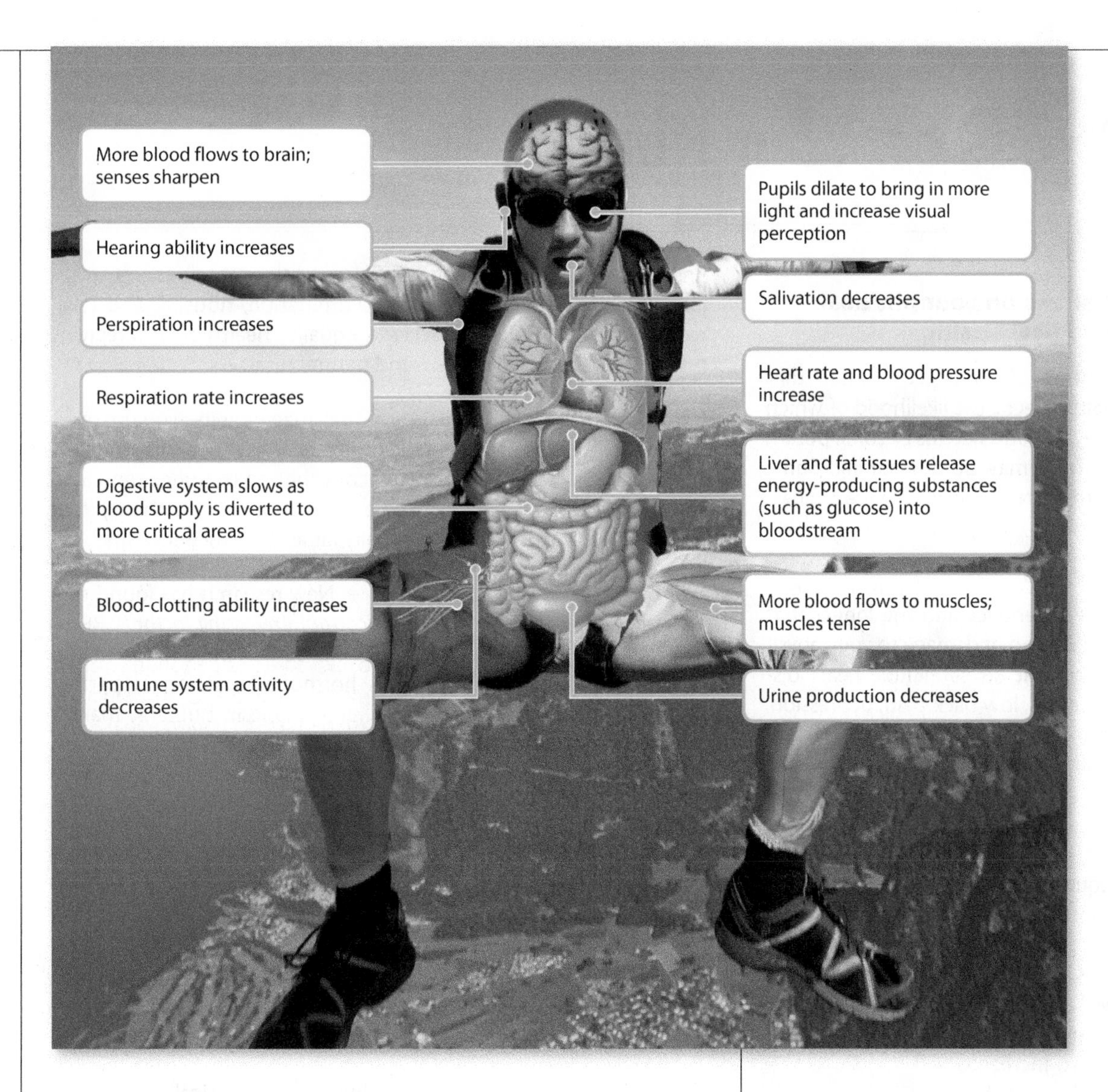

Figure 4.2 The Body's Acute Stress Response
Exposure to stress of any kind causes a complex series of involuntary physiological responses.

VIDEO TUTOR
Body's Stress Response

demands. Finally, other parts of the brain and body release endorphins, which relieve pain that a stressor may cause.

Resistance Phase In the resistance phase of the GAS, the body tries to return to homeostasis by resisting the alarm responses. However, because some perceived stressor still exists, the body does not achieve complete calm or rest. Instead, the body stays activated or aroused at a level that causes a higher metabolic rate in some organ tissues.

Exhaustion Phase In the exhaustion phase of the GAS, the hormones, chemicals, and systems that trigger and maintain the stress response are depleted, and the body returns to *allostasis*, or balance. You may feel tired or drained as your body returns to normal. In situations where stress is *chronic*, triggers may reverberate in the body, keeping body systems at a heightened arousal state. The prolonged effort to adapt to the stress response leads to **allostatic load**, or exhaustive wear and tear on the body. As the body adjusts to chronic unresolved stress, the adrenal glands continue to release cortisol, which remains in the bloodstream for longer periods of time as a result of slower metabolic responsiveness. Over time, cortisol can reduce **immunocompetence**, or the ability of the immune system to respond to attack. In turn, this increases the risk of diabetes, cardiovascular disease, and other chronic diseases.[10]

Men and Women Respond to Stress Differently

Ever since Walter Cannon's landmark studies in the 1930s, it's been thought that humans respond similarly to stressful events via the "fight-or-flight" response. However, several researchers now believe that men and women may respond differently to stressors. While men may be prone to fighting or fleeing, women may be more likely to "tend and befriend" by either trying to befriend the enemy or obtaining social support from others to ease stress-related reactions.[11] Additional studies point to the fact that one's mind-set may influence stress responses, and males and females may differ in their stress responses based on the way they perceive stressful events.[12]

check yourself

- **How does the general adaptation syndrome help us understand our reaction to stressors?**
- **How does the body react during each phase of the general adaptation syndrome?**
- **What are the differences between the *fight-or-flight* and the *tend-and-befriend* stress responses?**

4.3 Effects of Stress on Your Health

learning outcome

4.3 Describe the impact of stress on your physical, intellectual, and psychological health.

Stress is often described as a "disease of prolonged arousal" that leads to a cascade of negative health effects, the likelihood of which increases with ongoing stress. Nearly all body systems become potential targets, and the long-term effects may be devastating. Some warning symptoms of prolonged stress are shown in Figure 4.3.

Physical Effects of Stress

The higher the levels of stress you experience and the longer that stress continues, the greater the likelihood of damage to your physical health.[13] Ailments related to chronic stress include heart disease, diabetes, cancer, headaches, ulcers, low back pain, depression, and the common cold. Increases in rates of suicide, homicide, and domestic violence across the United States are additional symptoms of a nation under stress.

Stress and Cardiovascular Disease Perhaps the most documented health consequence of unresolved stress is cardiovascular disease (CVD). Research indicates that chronic stress plays a significant role in heart rate problems, high blood pressure, and atherosclerosis, as well as increased risk for a wide range of cardiovascular diseases.[14]

Chronic stress has been linked to increased arterial plaque buildup caused by elevated cholesterol, hardening of the arteries, increases in inflammatory responses in the body, alterations in heart rhythm, increased and fluctuating blood pressures, and other CVD risks.[15] Research has also shown direct links between CVD risks and social conditions, such as job strain, job instability, social isolation, discrimination, housing and environmental threats, lack of access to quality health care, caregiving responsibilities, bereavement, and natural disasters.[16]

Stress and Weight Gain You're not imagining it—you *are* more likely to gain weight when stressed. Higher stress levels may increase cortisol levels in the bloodstream, contributing to hunger and activating fat-storing enzymes; studies also support the theory that cortisol plays a role in increased belly fat and eating behaviors.[17]

Stress and Alcohol Dependence New research has found that a specific stress hormone, the *corticotropin-releasing factor* (CRF), is key to the development and maintenance of alcohol dependence in animals. CRF stimulates stress hormone secretion as part of the stress response. It may play a similar role in humans, making it harder for stressed alcoholics to abstain from alcohol. If proven, substances that diminish CRF receptor activity may help those dealing with the difficulties of abstaining from alcohol when stressed.[18]

Stress and Hair Loss The most common stress-induced hair loss is *telogen effluvium*. Often seen in individuals who have lost a loved one or experienced severe weight loss or other trauma, this condition pushes colonies of hair into a resting phase; over time, hair may begin to fall out. A similar condition, *alopecia areata*, occurs when stress triggers white blood cells to attack and destroy hair follicles.[19]

Stress and Diabetes Controlling stress is critical for preventing development of type 2 diabetes as well as for successful diabetes management.[20] People under severe stress often don't get enough sleep, don't eat well, and may drink or take other drugs. These behaviors can alter blood sugar levels and promote development of diabetes.

Stress and Digestive Problems Although stress may not directly cause digestive diseases or disorders, it is clearly related and may actually make

Why do I always get sick during finals week?

Prolonged stress can compromise your immune system, leaving you vulnerable to infection. If you spend exam week in a state of high stress—sleeping too little, studying too hard, and worrying a lot—chances are you'll reduce your body's ability to fight off any cold or flu bugs you may encounter.

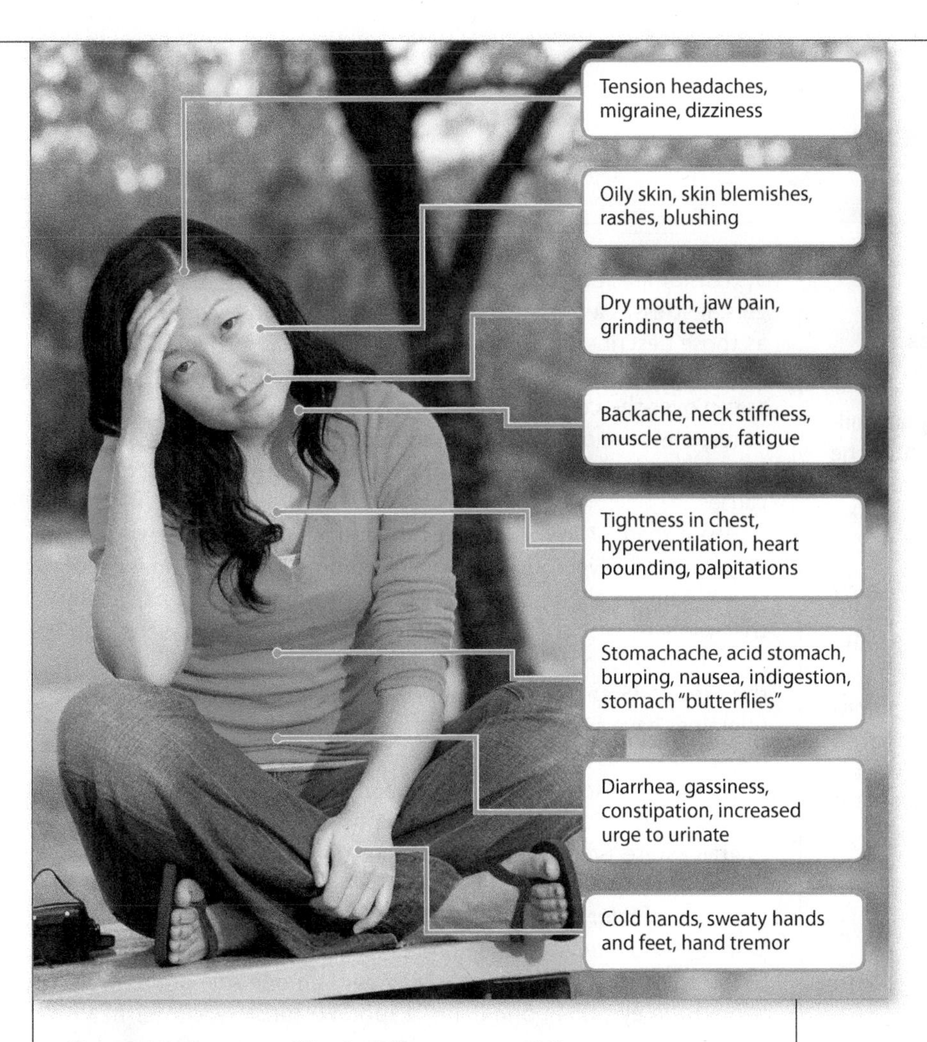

Figure 4.3 Common Physical Symptoms of Stress
You may not even notice how stressed you are until your body starts sending you signals. Do you frequently experience any of these physical symptoms of stress?

your risk of having symptoms worse.[21] Irritable bowel syndrome may be more likely, in part, because stress stimulates colon spasms by means of the nervous system. Relaxation techniques and mindfulness training may reduce the activity of the sympathetic nervous system, leading to decreases in heart rate, blood pressure, and other stress responses that trigger gastrointestinal tract flare-ups.[22]

Stress and Impaired Immunity A growing area of investigation known as **psychoneuroimmunology (PNI)** analyzes the relationship between stress and immune function. Research suggests that increased stress over time can affect cellular immune response. This increases risks for upper respiratory infections and certain chronic conditions, increases adverse birth outcomes and fetal development, and exacerbates problems for children and adults suffering from post-traumatic stress.[23]

Intellectual and Psychological Effects of Stress

In a recent national survey of college students, over half (51.8%) said they felt overwhelmed by all that they had to do within the past 2 weeks, with a similar number reporting they felt exhausted. Forty-two percent felt they had been under more than average stress in the past 12 months, with 10 percent reporting tremendous stress during that period. Not surprisingly, these same students rated stress as their number one impediment to academic performance, followed by anxiety and lack of sleep.[24] Stress can play a huge role in whether a student stays in school, gets good grades, and succeeds on a career path. It can also wreak havoc on a person's ability to concentrate, remember, and understand and retain complex information.

39% **of those ages 18–33 say their stress levels have increased in the last year, with 52 percent saying their stress levels keep them awake at night.**

Stress, Memory, and Concentration Animal studies provide compelling indicators of how *glucocorticoids*—stress hormones released from the adrenal cortex—affect memory. In humans, acute stress has been shown to impair memory—affecting the way we think, decide, and respond in stressful situations.[25] Prolonged exposure to *cortisol* (a key stress hormone) has been linked to shrinking of the hippocampus, the brain's major memory center.[26] Other research indicates that prolonged exposure to high levels of stress hormones may actually predispose women, in particular, to Alzheimer's disease.[27]

Stress and Mental Disorders Stress is an enormous contributor to mental disability and emotional dysfunction in industrialized nations. Studies have shown that the rates of mental disorders, particularly depression and anxiety, are associated with various environmental stressors from childhood through adulthood, including violence and abuse, marital and relationship conflict, poverty, and other stressful life events.[28]

See It! Videos
Can a test identify your risk for stress-related illnesses? Watch **Stress Can Damage Women's Health** in the Study Area of MasteringHealth.

check yourself

- **What are four possible effects of stress on your physical and psychological health?**
- **Give an example of an instance in which psychological stress had a physical effect on you.**

4.4 Stress and Headaches

learning outcome

4.4 Describe common types of headaches, and explain possible connections between stress and headaches.

Millions of people see their doctors for headaches each year; millions more put up with the pain or take pain relievers to blunt the symptoms. The good news: Most headaches are not a sign of serious diseases or underlying conditions. The vast majority are tension headaches and migraines.

Nearly 80 percent of adults (slightly more women than men) get the most common type of headache, a *tension-type headache*.[29] Symptoms may include dull pain; a sensation of tightness; and tender scalp, neck, and shoulder muscles.[30]

Tension headaches are generally caused by muscle contractions or tension and pain in the neck or head, forehead, or temples; they can last for as little as 30 minutes or as long as a week.[31] Possible triggers include red wine, lack of sleep, fasting, muscle overuse, stress, anger, and menstruation.

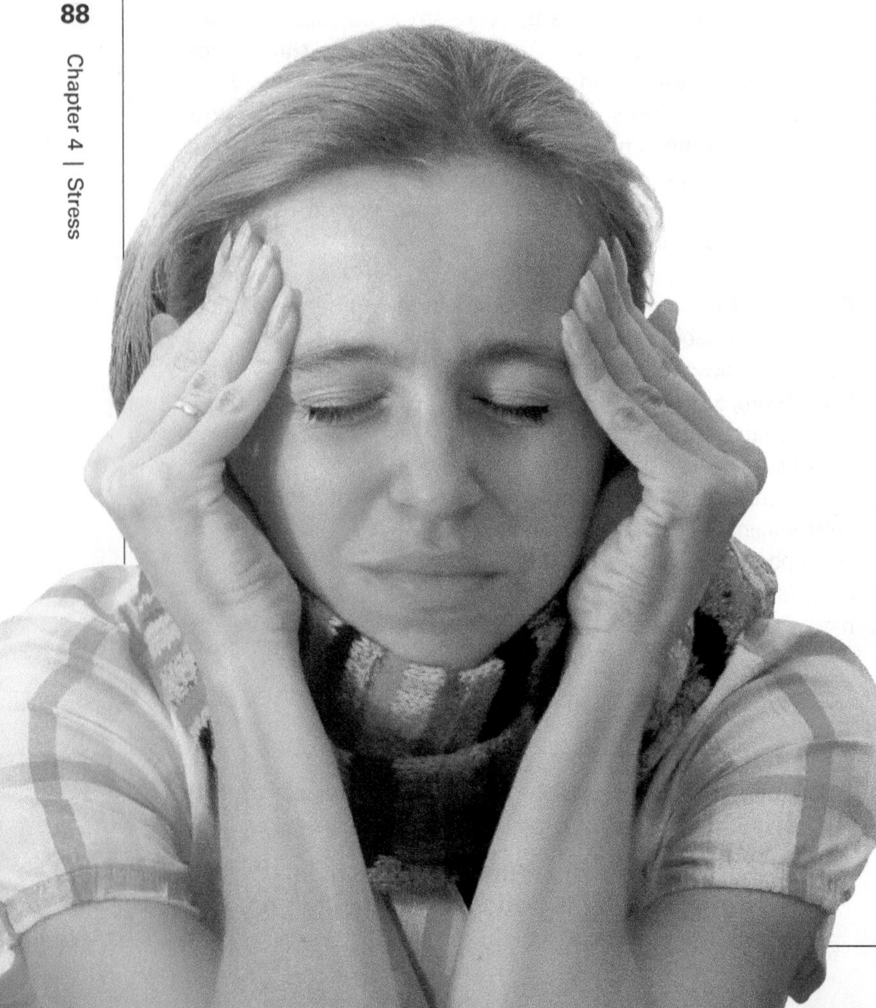

Tension headaches are most often helped by reducing triggers. If stress is a trigger, try a range of relaxation techniques, such as those described later in the module "Relaxation Techniques for Stress Management." Exercise can relieve some tension headaches, as can over-the-counter pain relievers. Frequent headaches that are unresponsive to over-the-counter medications are probably *chronic tension headaches*; these warrant a doctor visit to assess underlying causes.

More than 37 million Americans suffer from **migraines**, headaches whose severe, debilitating symptoms include moderate to severe pain on one or both sides of the head, throbbing pain, pain that worsens with or interferes with activity, nausea, and sensitivity to light and sound.[32] Usually, migraine incidence peaks between the ages of 15 and 55, and 70 to 80 percent of those experiencing migraines have a family history of these headaches.[33] Three times as many women as men suffer from migraines.[34]

Migraine symptoms vary greatly for each individual, and attacks can last anywhere from 4 to 72 hours. In about 20 percent of cases, migraines are preceded by a warning sign called an *aura*—most often flickering vision, blind spots, tingling in the arms or legs, or a sensation of odor or taste.[35] Prescription drugs and over-the-counter pain relievers often help migraine sufferers.

Cluster headaches cause stabbing pain on one side of the head, behind the eye, or in one defined spot. Fortunately, cluster headaches are among the more rare forms of headache, affecting less than 1 percent of people, usually men. Young adults in their twenties tend to be particularly susceptible.[36]

Cluster headaches can last for weeks and disappear quickly. More commonly, they last for 40 to 90 minutes during rapid eye movement (REM) sleep. Oxygen therapy, drugs, and even surgery have been used to treat severe cases.

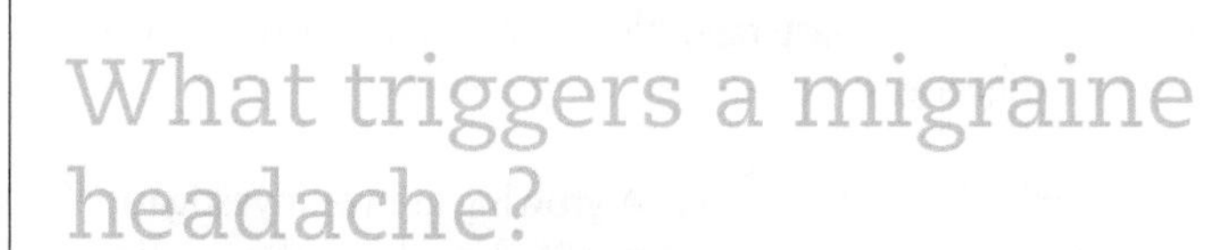

Patients report that migraines can be triggered by emotional stress, too much or not enough sleep, fasting, caffeine, alcohol, hormonal changes, altitude, weather, chocolate or other foods, and a litany of other causes. There is tremendous variability, and what triggers a migraine in one person may relieve it in another.

check yourself

- **What are three common types of headaches?**
- **How could effective stress management contribute to headache reduction?**

4.5

Stress and Sleep Problems

learning **outcome**

4.5 Describe the importance of sleep to good health, and list strategies for ensuring restful sleep.

In a recent survey, over 60 percent of students said they felt tired, dragged out, or sleepy for 3 or more days in the past week.[37] Sleep deficiencies have been linked to a host of student issues, including poor academic performance, weight gain, increased alcohol abuse, accidents, daytime drowsiness, relationship issues, depression, and other problems.[38]

Sleep is much more important than most people realize. Sleep conserves body energy and restores you physically and mentally. Sleep also contributes to healthy metabolism, which helps you maintain a healthy body weight.

Colds, flu, and many other ailments are more common when your immune system is depressed by lack of sleep. Recent studies found that poor sleep quality and shorter sleep duration increased susceptibility to the common cold.[39] Sleep disruption can also disrupt overall immune function.[40]

High blood pressure is more common in people who get fewer than 7 hours of sleep a night.[41] Short-duration sleep increases the risk of developing and/or dying from cardiovascular disease.[42]

Restricting sleep can cause attention lapses, slow or poor memory, reduced cognitive ability, and a tendency for thinking to get "stuck in a rut."[43] Your ability not only to remember facts but also to integrate those facts, make meaningful generalizations about them, and consolidate what you've learned requires adequate sleep.[44]

Sleep also has a restorative effect on motor function, affecting one's ability to perform tasks such as driving a car.[45] Researchers contend that a night without sleep impairs motor skills and reaction time as much as driving drunk.[46]

Certain brain regions, including the cerebral cortex (your "master mind"), achieve some form of essential rest only during sleep. You're also more likely to feel stressed out, worried, or sad when you're sleep deprived. Stress and sleep problems can reinforce or exacerbate each other.

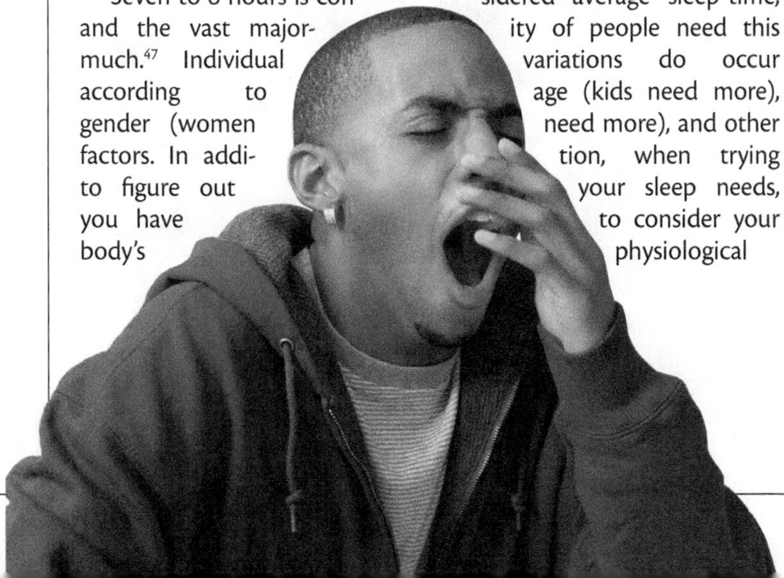

Seven to 8 hours is considered "average" sleep time, and the vast majority of people need this much.[47] Individual variations do occur according to age (kids need more), gender (women need more), and other factors. In addition, when trying to figure out your sleep needs, you have to consider your body's physiological need plus your **sleep debt**—the total hours of missed sleep you're carrying. The good news is that you can catch up, if you do it sensibly over time. Ways to ensure a good night's sleep include the following:

People aged

13 to 29

are the sleepiest members of the U.S. population.

- **Let there be light.** Stay in sync with your circadian rhythm by spending time in the daylight.
- **Stay active.** Exercisers are much more likely to feel rested than those who are sedentary.
- **Sleep tight.** Comfortable pillows, bedding, and mattress can help you sleep more soundly.
- **Create a sleep "cave."** As bedtime approaches, keep your bedroom quiet, cool, dark, and free of technology.
- **Condition yourself into better sleep.** Go to bed and get up at the same time each day.
- **Avoid foods and drinks that keep you awake.** Large meals, nicotine, energy drinks, caffeine, and alcohol close to bedtime can affect your ability to fall asleep and stay asleep. It takes your body about 6 hours to clear just *half* of a caffeinated drink from your system.[48]
- **Don't drink large amounts of liquid before bed.** This prevents having to get up in the night to use the bathroom.
- **Don't toss and turn.** If you're not asleep after 20 minutes, read or listen to gentle music. Once you feel sleepy, go back to bed.
- **Don't nap in the late afternoon or evening.** Also, don't nap for longer than 30 minutes.
- **Don't read, study, watch TV, use your laptop, talk on the phone, eat, or smoke in bed.** Emotionally intense phone conversations can also make it hard to calm yourself enough to sleep.
- **Don't take sleeping pills.** Don't take sleep aids unless prescribed by your health care provider. Over-the-counter sleep aids can interfere with progression through the stages of sleep.

See It! Videos

What kind of sleep keeps your memory sharp? Watch **How Sleep Affects Your Memory** in the Study Area of MasteringHealth.

check yourself

- **Why is it important for your health to sleep well?**
- **What are three common reasons for poor sleep, and how can you overcome them?**

4.6 Psychosocial Causes of Stress

learning outcome

4.6 Discuss and classify psychosocial sources of stress.

Psychosocial stressors refer to the factors in our daily routines and in our social and physical environments that cause us to experience stress (Figure 4.4). Which of these are most common in your life?

Adjustment to Change Any change, whether good or bad, occurring in your normal routine can result in stress. The more changes you experience and the more adjustments you must make, the greater the chances are that stress will have an impact on your health. The enormous changes associated with starting college, while exciting, can also be among the most stressful you will face in your life. Moving away from home, trying to fit in and make new friends from diverse backgrounds, adjusting to a new schedule, learning to live with strangers in housing that is often lacking in the comforts of home—all of these things can cause sleeplessness and anxiety and keep your body in a continual fight-or-flight mode.

Hassles Some psychologists have proposed that little stressors, frustrations, and petty annoyances, known collectively as *hassles*, can be just as stressful as major life changes.[49] Listening to classmates who talk too much during lectures, being near people chatting on the phone and texting while you are trying to study, not finding parking on campus, and a host of other small but bothersome situations can trigger frustration, anger, and fight-or-flight responses.[50]

Technostress Technostress is stress created by a dependence on technology and the constant state of connection, which can include a perceived obligation to always respond or be ever present. Research supports the concept that being "wired" 24/7 can lead to anxiety, obsessive compulsive disorder, narcissism, sleep disorders, frustration, time pressures, and guilt—some of the negative consequences known as iDisorders.[51] According to a new study, college students who can't keep their hands off their mobile devices are reporting higher levels of anxiety, less satisfaction with life, and lower grades than peers who use their devices less often. The average student surveyed spent nearly 5 hours per day using his or her cell phone for everything from calling and texting to Facebook, e-mails, gaming, and more.[52]

To reduce technostress, set limits on your technology use, and make sure that you devote sufficient time to face-to-face interactions with people you care about, cultivating and nurturing your relationships. You don't always need to answer your phone or respond to a text or e-mail immediately. Leave your devices at home or turn them off when you are out with others or on vacation. Tune in to your surroundings, your loved ones and friends, your job, and your classes.

The Toll of Relationships Relationships can trigger enormous fight-or-flight reactions—whether we're talking about the exhilaration of new love or the pain of a breakup, the result is often lack of focus, lack of sleep, and an inability to focus on anything but the love interest. And although we may think first of love relationships, even relationships with friends, family members, and coworkers can be the sources of overwhelming struggles, just as they can be sources of strength and support. These relationships can make us strive to be the best that we can be and give us hope for the future, or they can diminish our self-esteem and leave us reeling from a destructive interaction.

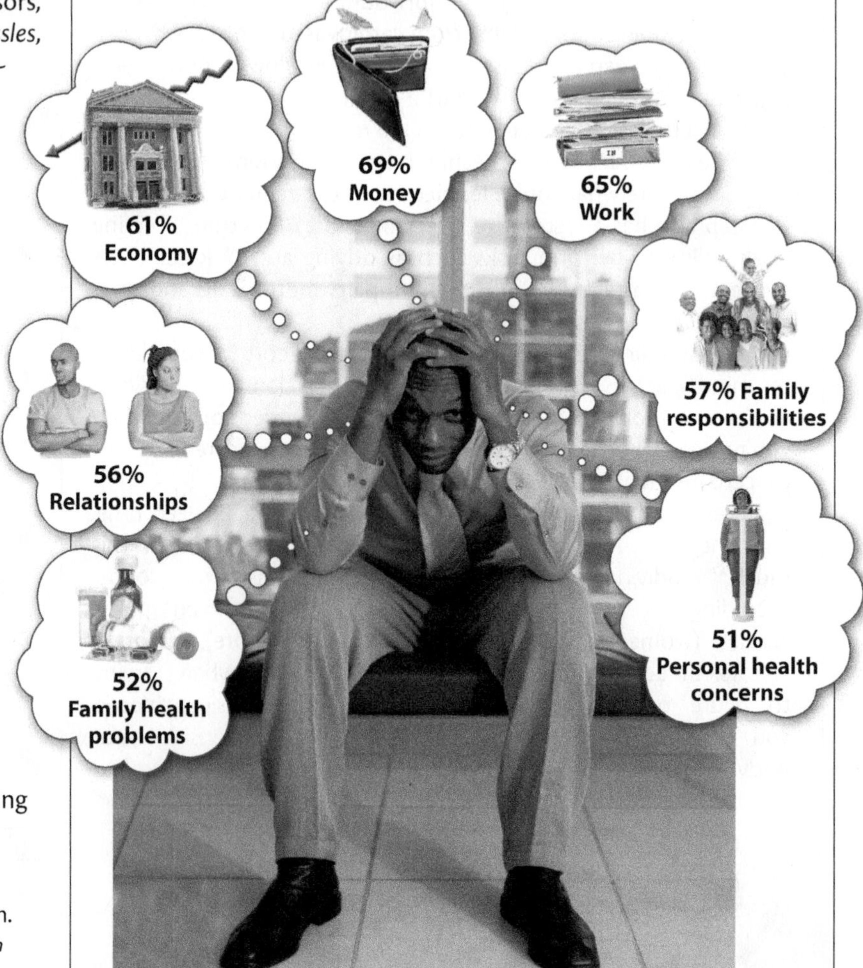

Figure 4.4 What Stresses Us?
Respondents indicated the events and issues that cause stress for them.
Source: Data are from the American Psychological Association, *2012 Stress in America, Key Findings*, 2013, www.apa.org.

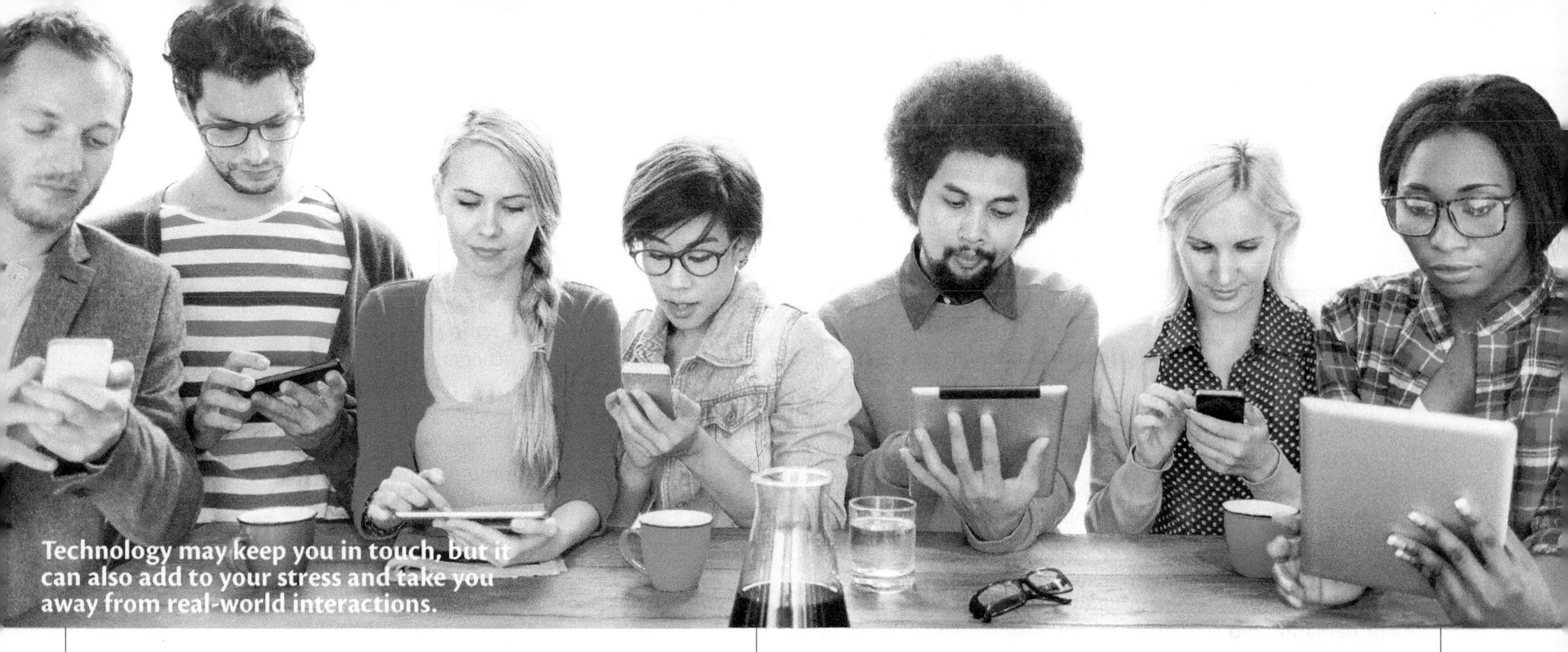
Technology may keep you in touch, but it can also add to your stress and take you away from real-world interactions.

Academic and Financial Pressure It isn't surprising that today's college and university students face mind-boggling amounts of pressure competing for grades, athletic positions, internships, and jobs. Challenging classes can be tough enough, but many students must also juggle work in order to pay bills. When economic conditions become strained, the effects on people with limited resources (particularly students) can be significant. An economic downturn can even make student dreams seem unattainable. Increasing reports of mental health problems on college campuses may be one of the results of too much stress.

Frustrations and Conflicts Disparity between our goals (what we hope to obtain in life) and our behaviors (actions that may or may not lead to these goals) can trigger frustration. Conflicts occur when we are forced to decide among competing motives, impulses, desires, and behaviors, or to face demands incompatible with our own values and sense of importance. College students away from their families and familiar communities for the first time may face conflicts among parental values, their own beliefs, and the beliefs of those different from themselves.

Overload We've all experienced times when the combined demands of work, responsibilities, and relationships seem to be pulling us under—and our physical, mental, and emotional reserves are insufficient to deal with it all. Students suffering from **overload** may experience depression, sleeplessness, mood swings, frustration, and anxiety. Unrelenting overload can lead to a state of physical and mental exhaustion known as *burnout*.

Stressful Environments For many students, the environment around them can cause significant stress. Perhaps you cannot afford safe, healthy housing, a bad roommate constantly makes life uncomfortable, or loud neighbors keep you up at night.

Unexpected natural disasters—such as flooding, earthquakes, hurricanes, blizzards, and tornadoes—can cause tremendous stress at the time and for years later. Often equally damaging are environmental **background distressors**—including noise, air, and water pollution; allergy-aggravating pollen and dust; and secondhand smoke—that trigger a constant resistance phase.

Bias and Discrimination Diversity of students, faculty members, and staff enriches everyone's educational experience. It also challenges us to examine our attitudes and biases. Those perceived as dissimilar due to race, ethnicity, religious affiliation, age, or sexual orientation—or differences in viewpoint, appearance, behavior, or background—may become victims of subtle and not-so-subtle bigotry, insensitivity, harassment, or hostility, or may simply be ignored.[53]

Evidence of the health effects of excessive stress in minority groups abounds. For example, African Americans suffer higher rates of hypertension, CVD, and most cancers than do whites.[54] Although poverty and socioeconomic status have been blamed for much of the spike in hypertension rates for African Americans and other marginalized groups, this chronic, physically debilitating stress may reflect real and perceived effects of institutional racism even more than it reflects poverty. While more research is necessary to show a direct link, racism may influence stress-related hypertension and make it difficult for those affected to engage in healthy lifestyle behaviors.[55]

International students experience unique adjustment issues such as language barriers, financial issues, cultural barriers, and a lack of social support. Academic stress may pose a particular problem for the more than 765,000 international students who have left family and friends in their native countries to study in the United States. Yet many international students refrain from seeking emotional support from others because of cultural norms, feelings of shame, or the belief that seeking support is a sign of weakness. These factors, coupled with language barriers, cultural conflicts, and other stressors, can lead international students to suffer significantly more stress-related illnesses than their American counterparts.[56]

check yourself

- **What are five sources of psychosocial stress?**
- **Which psychosocial sources of stress do you encounter most frequently?**

4.7 Internal Causes of Stress

learning outcome

4.7 Discuss and classify internal causes of stress.

Although stress can come from the environment and other external sources, it can result from internal factors as well. Internal stressors such as negative appraisal, low self-esteem, and low self-efficacy can cause unsettling thoughts or feelings and can ultimately affect your health. It is important to address and manage these internal stressors.

Appraisal and Stress Throughout life, we encounter many different demands and potential stressors—some biological, some psychological, and others sociological. In any case, it is our **appraisal** of these demands, rather than the demands themselves, that results in our experiencing stress. Appraisal is defined as the interpretation and evaluation of information provided to the brain by the senses. As new information becomes available, appraisal helps us recognize stressors, evaluate them on the basis of past experiences and emotions, and decide whether or not we have the ability to cope with them. When you feel that the stressors of life are overwhelming and you lack control, you are more likely to feel strain and distress.

Self-Esteem and Self-Efficacy *Self-esteem* refers to how you feel about yourself. Self-esteem varies; it can and does continually change.[57] When you feel good about yourself, you are less likely to view certain events as stressful and more likely to be able to cope.[58]

Of particular concern, research with high school and college students has found that low self-esteem and stressful life events significantly predict **suicidal ideation**, a desire to die and thoughts about suicide. On a more positive note, research has also indicated that it is possible to increase an individual's ability to cope with stress by increasing self-esteem.[59]

Self-efficacy, or confidence in one's skills and ability to cope with life's challenges, appears to be a key buffer in preventing negative stress effects. Research has shown that people with high levels of self-efficacy tend to feel more in control of stressful situations and, as such, report fewer stress effects.[60] Self-efficacy is considered one of the most important personality traits that influence psychological and physiological stress responses.[61]

Developing self-efficacy is also vital to coping with and overcoming academic pressures and worries. For example, by learning to handle anxiety around testing situations, you improve your chances of performing well; the more you feel yourself capable of handling testing situations, the greater will be your sense of academic self-efficacy.

Type A and Type B Personalities It should come as no surprise to you that personality can have an impact on whether you are happy and socially well-adjusted or sad and socially isolated. However, your personality may affect more than just your social interactions: It may be a critical factor in your stress level, as well as in your risk for CVD, cancer, and other chronic and infectious diseases.

In 1974, physicians Meyer Friedman and Ray Rosenman published a book indicating that type A individuals had a greatly increased risk of heart disease.[62] *Type A* personalities are defined as hard-driving, competitive, time-driven perfectionists. In contrast, *type B*

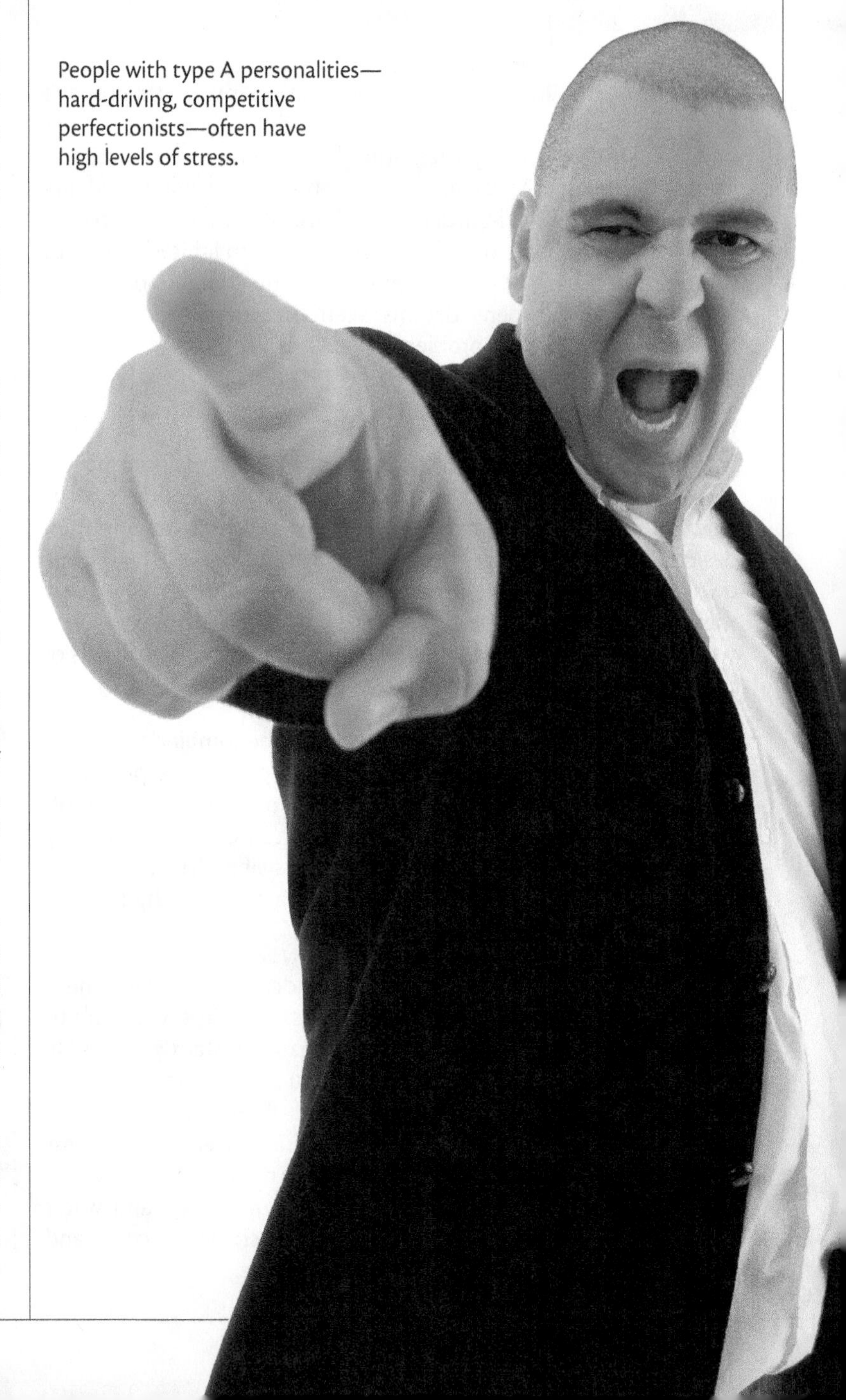

People with type A personalities—hard-driving, competitive perfectionists—often have high levels of stress.

personalities are described as being relaxed, noncompetitive, and more tolerant of others.

Today, most researchers recognize that none of us will be wholly type A or type B all of the time, and we may exhibit either type in selected situations. In addition, recent research indicates that not all type A people experience negative health consequences; in fact, some hard-driving individuals seem to thrive on their supercharged lifestyles. Only those type A individuals who exhibit a "toxic core"—who have disproportionate amounts of anger, are distrustful of others, and have a cynical, glass-half-empty approach to life; in total, a set of characteristics referred to as **hostility**—are at increased risk for heart disease.[63]

How daunting that pile of books and homework is all depends on your own appraisal of it.

Type C and Type D Personalities In addition to CVD risks, personality types have been linked to increased risk for a variety of illnesses ranging from asthma to cancer. *Type C* personality is one such type, characterized as stoic, with a tendency to stuff feelings down and conform to the wishes of others (or be "pleasers"). Preliminary research suggests that type C individuals may be more susceptible to illnesses such as asthma, multiple sclerosis, autoimmune disorders, and cancer; however, more research is necessary to support this relationship.[64]

A more recently identified personality type is *type D* (distressed), characterized by a tendency toward excessive negative worry, irritability, gloom, and social inhibition. Several recent studies have shown that type D people may be up to eight times more likely to die of a heart attack or sudden cardiac death.[65]

Psychological Hardiness and Resilience According to psychologist Susanne Kobasa, **psychological hardiness** may negate self-imposed stress associated with type A behavior. Psychologically hardy people are characterized by control, commitment, and willingness to embrace challenge.[66] People with a sense of control are able to accept responsibility for their behaviors and change those that they discover to be debilitating. People with a sense of commitment have good self-esteem and understand their purpose in life. Those who embrace challenge see change as a stimulating opportunity for personal growth. Today, the concept of hardiness has evolved to include a person's overall ability to cope with stress and adversity.[67] In recent years, it has become common for people to think of this general hardiness concept in terms of **psychological resilience**—our capacity to maintain or regain psychological well-being in the face of challenge.[68]

Shift and Persist An emerging body of research proposes that in the midst of extreme, persistent adversity, youth—often with the help of positive role models in their lives—are able to reframe appraisals of current stressors more positively (*shifting*), while *persisting* in focusing on a positive future. These youth are able to endure the present by adapting, holding on to meaningful things in their lives, and staying optimistic and positive. These "**shift-and-persist**" strategies are among the most recently identified factors that protect against the negative effects of too much stress in our lives.[69]

Skills for Behavior Change

OVERCOMING TEST-TAKING ANXIETY

Here are helpful hints to increase your self-efficacy and reduce your stress levels in a familiar situation: an academic exam.

Before the Exam

- Manage your study time. Start studying at least a week before your test to reduce anxiety. Do a limited review the night before, get a good night's sleep, and arrive for the exam early.
- On an index card, write down three reasons you will pass the exam. Keep the card with you and review it whenever you study. When you get the test, write your three reasons on the test or on a piece of scrap paper.
- Eat a balanced meal before the exam. Avoid sugar and rich or heavy foods, as well as foods that might upset your stomach. You want to feel your best.
- Think about how much time you might need to answer different types of test questions. Make a general strategy before the test to efficiently use the time allotted. Wear a watch to class on the day of the test.

During the Test

- Manage your time during the test. Look at how many questions there are and what each is worth. Prioritize the high-point questions, allow a certain amount of time for each, and make sure that you leave some time for the rest. Hold to this schedule.
- Slow down and pay attention. Focus on one question at a time. Check off each part of multipart questions to make sure your answers are complete.

check yourself

- **What are five causes of internal stress?**
- **Which internal causes of stress do you experience most frequently?**

4.8 Stress Management Techniques: Mental and Physical Approaches

learning outcome

4.8 Examine mental and physical approaches to stress management.

Being on your own in college may pose challenges, but it also lets you take control of and responsibility for your life and take steps to reduce negative stressors. **Coping** is the act of managing events or conditions to lessen the physical or psychological effects of excess stress.[70] One of the most effective ways to combat stressors is to build coping strategies and skills, known collectively as *stress-management techniques.*

Practicing Mental Work to Reduce Stress

Your perceptions often contribute to your stress, so assessing your "self-talk," beliefs, and actions are good first steps. Here's how:

- Make a list of things you're worried about.
- Examine the causes of your problems and worries.
- Consider the size of each problem. What are the consequences of doing nothing versus taking action?
- List your options, including ones you may not like much.

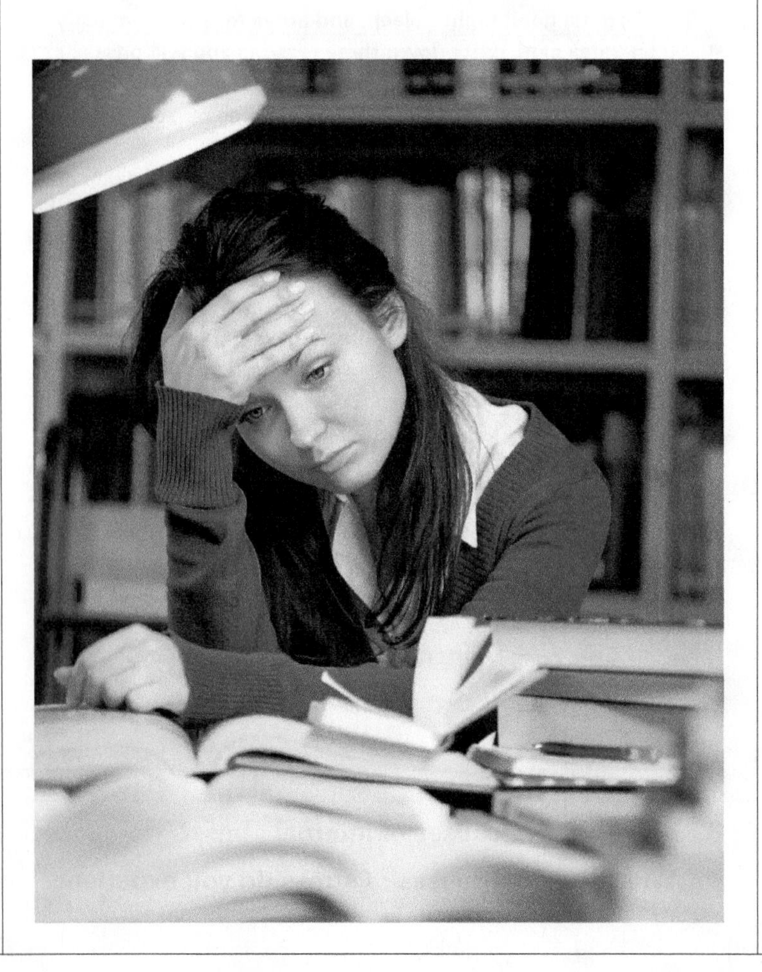

- Outline a plan, then act. Even little things can make a big difference.
- After you act, evaluate. How did you do? Do you need to change your actions to achieve a better outcome next time? How?

One way to anticipate and prepare for specific stressors is a technique known as **stress inoculation**. Suppose speaking in front of a class scares you. To prevent freezing up during a presentation, practice in front of friends or a video camera.

Negative self-talk can take the form of *pessimism*, or focusing on the negative; *perfectionism*, or expecting superhuman standards; *should-ing*, or reprimanding yourself for things you should have done; *blaming* yourself or others for circumstances and events; and *dichotomous thinking*, in which everything is seen as either entirely good or bad. To combat negative self-talk, become aware of an irrational or overreactive thought, interrupt it by saying "stop" (under your breath or out loud), then replace it with positive thoughts—a process called **cognitive restructuring**.

People fall into patterns and ways of thinking that can cause stress and increase their levels of anxiety. The fact is, your thought patterns can be your own worst enemy. If you can become aware of the internal messages you are giving yourself, you can recognize them and work to change them. Some strategies for doing this include the following:

- **Reframe a distressing event from a positive perspective.** For example, if you feel perpetually frustrated that you can't be the best in every class, reframe the issue to highlight your strengths.
- **Break the worry habit.** If you are preoccupied with "what if's" and worst case scenarios, doubts and fears can sap your strength and send your stress levels soaring.
  - If you must worry, create a "worry period"—a 20-minute time period each day when you can journal or talk about it. After that, move on.
  - Focus on the many things that are going right, rather than the one thing that might go wrong.
- **Look at life as being fluid.** If you accept that change is a natural part of living and growing, the jolt of changes will become less stressful.

Are college students more stressed out than other groups?

The combination of a new environment, peer and parental pressure, and the demands of course work, campus activities, and social life contribute to above average stress levels in college students.

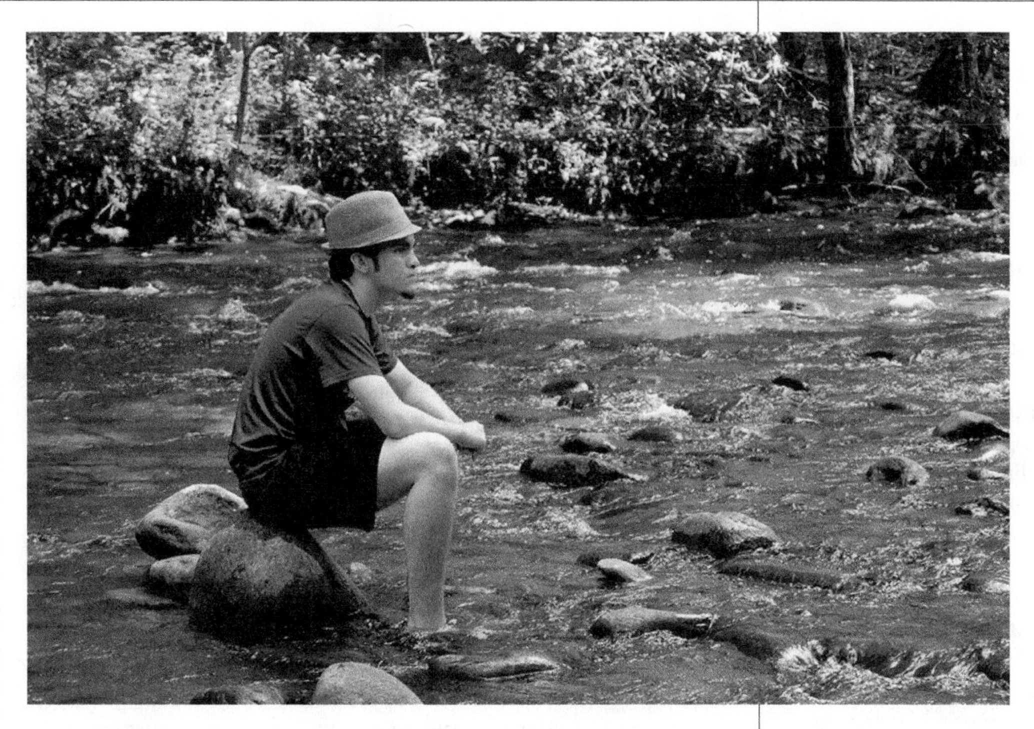

Practicing mindfulness means tuning in to the present, such as taking time to contemplate a scenic view. When you pay attention to the present, you can begin to let go of the stressful distractions in your life.

- **Moderate your expectations.** Aim high, but be realistic about your circumstances and motivation.
- **Weed out trivia.** Cardiologist Robert Eliot offers two rules for coping with life's challenges: "Don't sweat the small stuff," and remember, "It's all small stuff."
- **Tolerate mistakes by yourself and others.** Rather than getting angry or frustrated by mishaps, evaluate what happened and learn from it.

Mindfulness

Practicing *mindfulness*—by observing the present moment in a focused, nonjudgmental way—can help you increase awareness of your thinking patterns and refocus stressful thoughts. Try taking 10 minutes every day to pay focused attention to your senses and the world around you, without forming judgments. Rather than dwelling on the past or agonizing about the future, concentrate on the present. Recognize that your thoughts and emotions are fleeting, and they don't ultimately define who you are.

Cultivating Happiness

For decades, noted psychologist Martin Seligman has conducted research focused on positive psychology and authentic happiness. His work has been the framework for a new way of looking at life with a glass-half-full perspective. Research supports the idea that people who are optimistic and happier have fewer mental and physical problems.[71] Today, Seligman takes happiness a step further, focusing on the concept of *flourishing*. Flourishing consists of five elements, which positive psychologists believe will help you flourish in life, avoid stress, and be healthier:

- **Positive emotion.** Take time to get to know people's names. Share highs of the day rather than lows. Be active in complimenting others and verbalize their strengths.
- **Engagement.** Practice mindfulness: see, hear, touch, and feel the present moment. Make time to fully engage in the activities that bring you joy.
- **Relationships.** Listen to others and ask questions. Connect in person. Empower others to see their strengths, and check in to show that you care.
- **Meaning.** Think about how you want to be remembered. Read and explore new things. Learn about different cultures and history. Work to help others and to improve the world.
- **Achievement.** Consider the steps to achieve your goals in life, and view failure along the way as an opportunity. Celebrate accomplishments, both your own and those of others, and readily give praise.

Taking Physical Action

Physical activities can complement your strategies of stress management.

- **Exercise Regularly** The human stress response is intended to end in physical activity; exercise "burns off" stress hormones by directing them toward their intended metabolic function and can combat stress by raising levels of endorphins—mood-elevating, painkilling hormones—in the bloodstream.[72]
- **Get Enough Sleep** Adequate sleep allows you to cope with multiple stressors more effectively and to be more productive.
- **Practice Self-Nurturing** Find time each day for something fun—something that you enjoy and that calms you. Like exercise, relaxation can help you cope with stressful feelings, as well as preserve and refocus your energies.
- **Eat Healthfully** A balanced, healthy diet will help provide the stamina you need to get through problems while stress-proofing you in ways not yet fully understood. Undereating, overeating, and eating the wrong foods can create distress in the body. In particular, avoid **sympathomimetics**, foods that produce (or mimic) stresslike responses, such as caffeine.

check yourself

- **What are four effective mental or physical approaches to managing stress? Which might be best for you?**

4.9

Stress Management Techniques: Managing Emotional Responses

learning outcome

4.9 Explain how management of emotional responses contributes to stress management.

We often get upset not by realities, but by our faulty perceptions. Stress management requires examining your emotional responses to interactions with others—and remembering that you are responsible for the emotion and the resulting behaviors. Learning to identify emotions based on irrational beliefs, or expressed and interpreted in an over-the-top manner, can help you stop such emotions or express them in healthy and appropriate ways.

Learn to Laugh, Be Joyful, and Cry Smiling, laughing, and even crying can elevate mood, relieve stress, and improve relationships. In the moment, laughter and joy raise endorphin levels, increase blood oxygen, decrease stress, relieve pain, and enhance productivity. Additional evidence for long-term effects on immune function and protection against disease is only starting to be understood.[73]

Fight the Anger Urge Anger usually results when we feel we have lost control of a situation or are frustrated by events we can do little about. Major sources of anger include (1) perceived *threats* to self or others we care about; (2) *reactions to injustice*; (3) *fear*; (4) *faulty emotional reasoning* or misinterpretation of normal events; (5) *low frustration tolerance*, often fueled by stress, drugs, or lack of sleep; (6) *unreasonable expectations* for ourselves and others; and (7) *people rating*, or applying derogatory ratings to others.

To deal with anger, you can express, suppress, or calm it. Surprisingly, expressing anger is probably the healthiest option, if you do so assertively rather than aggressively. Several strategies can help redirect aggression into assertion:[74]

- **Recognize anger patterns and learn to de-escalate them.** Note what angers you. What thoughts or feelings led up to your boiling point? Try changing your self-talk or interrupting anger patterns by counting to ten or taking deep breaths.
- **Verbally de-escalate.** When conflict arises, be respectful and state your needs or feelings rather than shooting zingers. Avoid "you always" or "you never" and instead say, "I feel___ when you_____" or "I would really appreciate it if you could___."
- **Plan ahead.** Explore ways to minimize your exposure to anger triggers, such as traffic jams.
- **Vent to your friends.** Find a few close friends you trust and who can be honest with you about your situation. Allow them to listen to provide perspective. Don't wear down supporters with continual rants.
- **Develop realistic expectations.** Anger is often the result of unmet expectations, frustrations, resentments, and impatience. Are your expectations of yourself and others realistic?
- **Turn complaints into requests.** Try reworking a problem into a request. Instead of screaming because your neighbors' music woke you up at 2 A.M., talk with them. Try to reach an agreement.
- **Leave past anger in the past.** Learn to resolve issues that have caused pain, frustration, or stress. If necessary, seek professional counsel.

Invest in Loved Ones Too often, we don't make time for the people most important to us: friends and family. Cultivate and nurture relationships built on trust, mutual acceptance and understanding, honesty, and caring. Treating others empathically provides them with a measure of emotional security and reduces *their* anxiety.

Cultivate Your Spiritual Side Spiritual health and spiritual practice can link you to a community and offer perspective on the things that truly matter.

Spending time communicating and socializing can be an important part of building a support network and reducing your stress level.

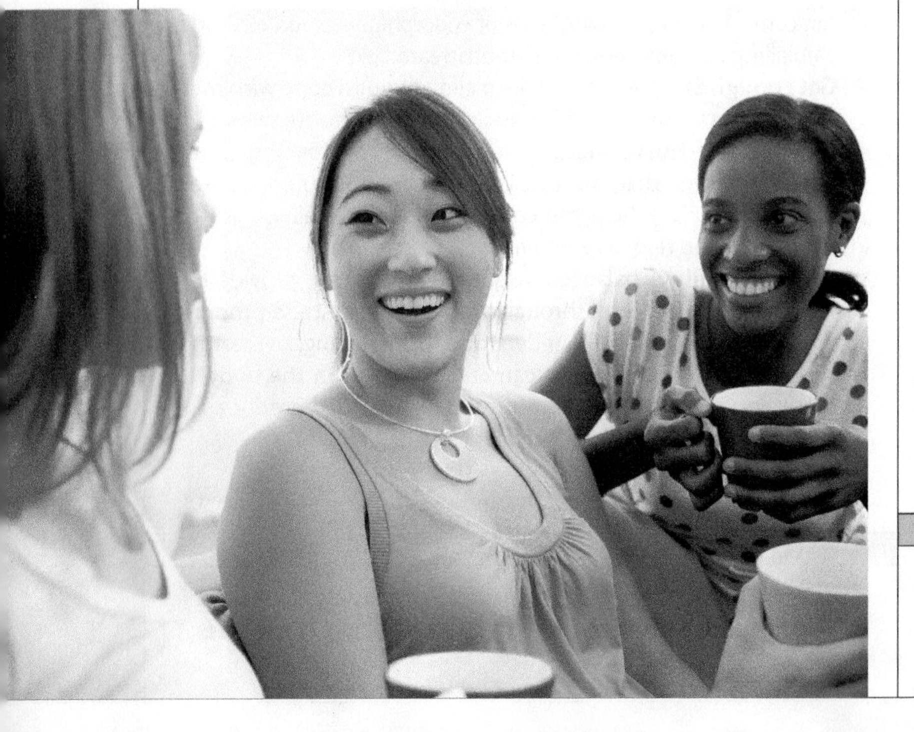

check yourself

- **How can emotions affect your stress levels?**
- **List three strategies to express anger assertively rather than aggressively.**

Stress Management Techniques: Managing Your Time and Your Finances

learning outcome

4.10 Describe strategies for managing your time and your finances.

Managing Your Time

Ever put off writing a paper until the night before it was due? We all **procrastinate**—voluntarily delay doing some task despite expecting to be worse off for it. Procrastination results in academic difficulties, financial problems, relationship problems, and stress-related ailments.

According to psychologist Peter Gollwitzer and colleagues, one key to beating procrastination is to set clear "implementation intentions."[75] Having a plan that includes specific deadlines (and rewards for meeting deadlines) can help you stay on task. Start with a simple plan and be flexible.

What else can you do to make better use of your time? Try logging your activities for 2 days—everything from going to class to doing laundry to texting friends—and the amount of time you spend doing each. Assess your results and make changes accordingly. Use these time-management tips to help you:

- **Do one thing at a time.** Don't try to watch television, wash clothes, and write your term paper all at once.
- **Clear your desk.** Toss unnecessary papers; file those you'll need later. Read your mail, recycle what you don't need, and file the rest for later action.
- **Prioritize tasks.** Make a daily "to do" list and stick to it. Categorize things you must do today, things you must do but not immediately, and "nice to dos" that you can take on if you finish the others or if they include something fun.
- **Find a clean, comfortable place to work, and avoid interruptions.** For a project that requires concentration, schedule uninterrupted time. Close your door and turn off your phone—or go to a quiet room in the library or student union.
- **Reward yourself.** Did you finish a task? Do something nice for yourself. Breaks give you time to recharge.
- **Work when you're at your best.** If you're a morning person, study in the morning. Take breaks when you start to slow down.

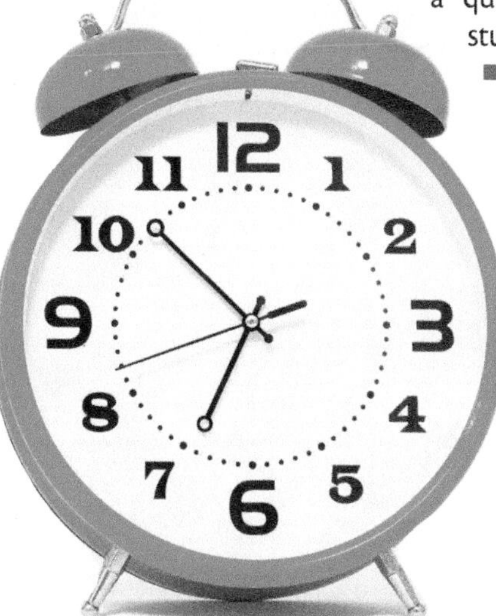

- **Learn to say no.** Avoid overcommitment by scheduling your time wisely. Don't give in to guilt or pressure when others request your time. Avoid spontaneous "yes" responses to new projects.

Managing Your Finances

Higher education can impose a huge financial burden on parents and students—and consequently become a major stressor. Over one-third of college students queried in a recent survey said finances have been "traumatic or very difficult to handle" in the past year.[76] These helpful tips can create a less stressful financial situation:

- **Create a budget.** Set a goal to avoid debt as much as possible. Track expenses such as tuition, books, rent, food, and entertainment. List your income to see if what you're spending is equitable to what you're earning or if it's putting you on the debt track.
- **Use credit cards wisely.** Resist credit card offers; racking up debt in school can affect your finances for years to come. Reserve credit cards you do have for less frequent, big-ticket buying, and carry cash whenever possible.
- **Complete a financial inventory.** How much money will you need to do the things you want to do in the future? Will you live alone or share costs with roommates? Do you need to buy a car, or can you rely on public transportation? Consider options for saving money; you need to prepare for emergencies and for future plans.

Consider Downshifting Many people, questioning whether "having it all" is worth it, are taking a step back and simplifying their lives. This trend has been labeled **downshifting**, or **voluntary simplicity**. Moving from a large urban area to a smaller town or leaving a high-stress job for one that makes you happy are examples of downshifting.

Downshifting involves a fundamental alteration in values and honest introspection about what is important in life. It means cutting down on shopping habits, buying only what you need to get by, and living within modest means. When you contemplate any form of downshift, move slowly by planning attainable goals to simplify your life.

check yourself

- **What are some time management strategies that could help reduce your stress levels?**
- **What are some strategies to improve your financial situation?**

4.11 Relaxation Techniques for Stress Management

learning outcome

4.11 Discuss relaxation techniques that can reduce stress.

Relaxation techniques to reduce stress have been practiced for centuries, and there is a wide array of practices from which to choose. Common techniques include yoga, qigong, tai chi, deep breathing, meditation, visualization, progressive muscle relaxation, massage therapy, biofeedback, and hypnosis.

Yoga Yoga is an ancient practice that combines meditation, stretching, and breathing exercises designed to relax, refresh, and rejuvenate. It began about 5,000 years ago in India and has been evolving ever since. In the United States today, some 20 million adults practice many versions of yoga.[77]

Classical yoga is the ancestor of nearly all modern forms of yoga. Breathing, poses, and verbal mantras are often part of classical yoga. Of the many branches of classical yoga, *Hatha yoga* is the most well known because it is the most body focused. This style of yoga involves the practice of breath control and *asanas*—held postures and choreographed movements that enhance strength and flexibility. Research shows increased evidence of benefits of Hatha yoga in reducing inflammation, boosting mood, increasing relaxation, and reducing stress among those who practice regularly.[78]

Qigong *Qigong* (pronounced "chee-kong"), one of the fastest-growing and most widely accepted forms of mind-body health exercises, is used by some of the country's largest health care organizations, particularly for people suffering from chronic pain or stress. Qigong is an ancient Chinese practice that involves becoming aware of and learning to control *qi* (or *chi*, pronounced "chee"), or vital energy in your body. According to Chinese medicine, a complex system of internal pathways called *meridians* carry *qi* throughout your body. If your *qi* becomes stagnant or blocked, you'll feel sluggish or powerless. Qigong incorporates a series of flowing movements, breath techniques, mental visualization exercises, and vocalizations of healing sounds designed to restore balance and integrate and refresh the mind and body.

Tai Chi *Tai chi* (pronounced "ty-chee") is sometimes described as "meditation in motion." Originally developed in China as a form of self-defense, this graceful form of exercise has existed for about 2,000 years. Tai chi is noncompetitive and self-paced. To do tai chi, you perform a defined series of postures or movements in a slow, graceful manner. Each movement or posture flows into the next without pause. Tai chi has been widely practiced in China for centuries and is becoming increasingly popular around the world, both as a basic exercise program and as a complement to other health

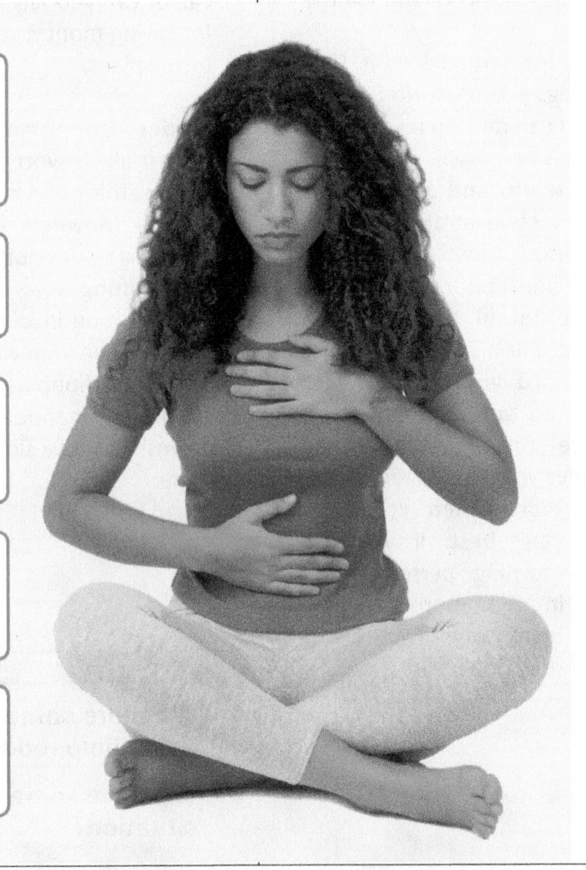

1. Assume a natural, comfortable position either sitting up straight with your head, neck, and shoulders relaxed, or lying on your back with your knees bent and your head supported. Close your eyes and loosen binding clothes.
2. In order to feel your abdomen moving as you breathe, place one hand on your upper chest and the other just below your rib cage.
3. Breathe in slowly and deeply through your nose. Feel your stomach expanding into your hand. The hand on your chest should move as little as possible.
4. Exhale slowly through your mouth. Feel the fall of your stomach away from your hand. Again, the hand on your chest should move as little as possible.
5. Concentrate on the act of breathing. Shut out external noise. Focus on inhaling and exhaling, the route the air is following, and the rise and fall of your stomach.

Figure 4.5 Diaphragmatic Breathing
This exercise will help you learn to breathe deeply as a way to relieve stress. Practice this for 5 to 10 minutes several times a day and soon diaphragmatic breathing will become natural for you.

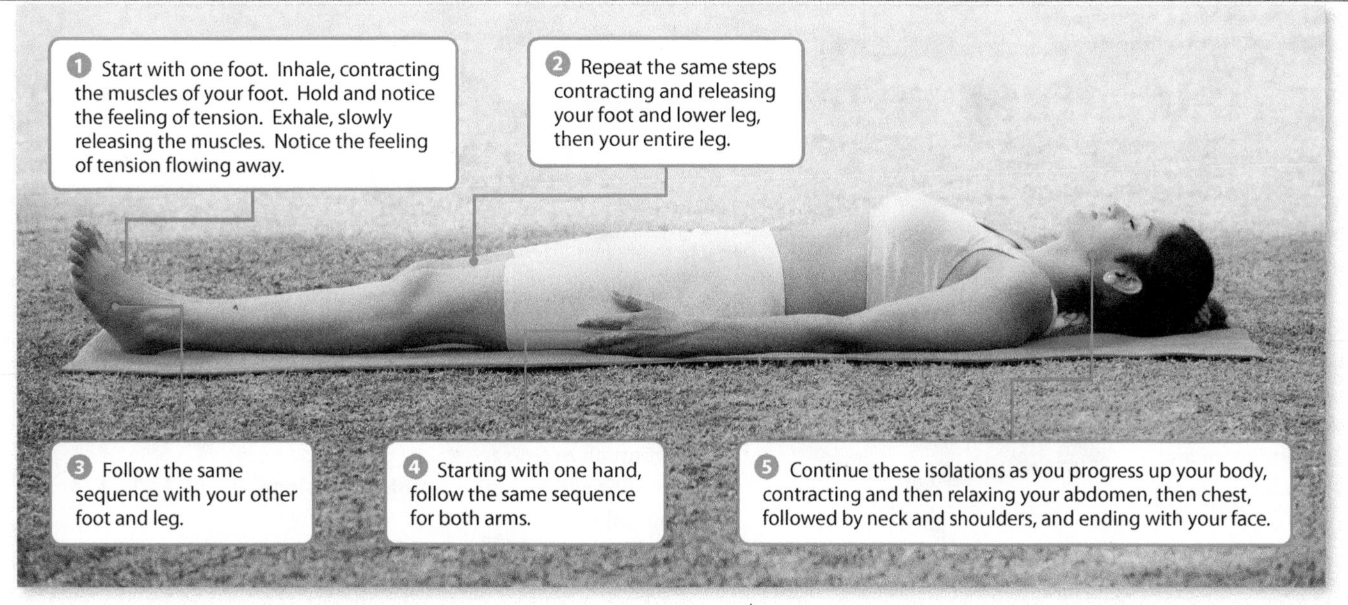

Figure 4.6 Progressive Muscle Relaxation
Sit or lie down in a comfortable position and follow the steps described to increase your awareness of tension in your body.

care methods. Health benefits include stress reduction, improved balance, and increased flexibility.

Diaphragmatic or Deep Breathing Typically, we breathe using only the upper chest and thoracic region rather than involving the abdominal region. Simply stated, diaphragmatic breathing is deep breathing that maximally fills the lungs by involving the movement of the diaphragm and lower abdomen. This technique is commonly used in yoga exercises and in other meditative practices. Try the diaphragmatic breathing exercise in Figure 4.5 right now and see if you feel more relaxed!

Meditation There are many different forms of **meditation**. Most involve sitting quietly for 15 minutes or longer, focusing on a particular word or symbol or observing one's thoughts, and controlling breathing. Practiced by Eastern religions for centuries, meditation is seen as an important form of introspection and personal renewal. Recent research found that one form of meditation, *transcendental meditation*, results in adults reducing their blood pressure as well as need for blood pressure medications.[79]

Visualization Often it is our own thoughts and imagination that provoke distress by conjuring up worst-case scenarios. Our imagination, however, can also be tapped to reduce stress. In **visualization**, you create mental scenes using your imagination. The choice of mental images is unlimited, but natural settings such as ocean beaches and mountain lakes are often used to represent stress-free environments. Recalling specific physical senses of sight, sound, smell, taste, and touch can replace stressful stimuli with peaceful or pleasurable thoughts.

Progressive Muscle Relaxation Progressive muscle relaxation involves systematically contracting and relaxing different muscle groups in your body. The standard pattern is to begin with the feet and work your way up your body, contracting and releasing as you go (Figure 4.6). The process is designed to teach awareness of the different feelings of muscle tension and muscle release. With practice, you can quickly identify tension in your body when you are facing stressful situations, then consciously release that tension to calm yourself.

Massage Therapy If you have ever had someone massage your stiff neck or aching feet, you know that massage is an excellent way to relax. Techniques vary from deep-tissue massage to gentler acupressure.

Biofeedback **Biofeedback** is a technique in which a person learns to use the mind to consciously control body functions like heart rate, body temperature, and breathing rate. Using machines from those as simple as stress dots that change color with body temperature variation to sophisticated electrical sensors, individuals learn to listen to their bodies and make necessary adjustments, such as relaxing certain muscles, changing breathing, or concentrating to slow heart rate and relax. Eventually, you develop the ability to recognize and lower stress responses without the help of the machine.

Hypnosis **Hypnosis** requires a person to focus on one thought, object, or voice, thereby freeing the right hemisphere of the brain to become more active. The person then becomes unusually responsive to suggestion. Whether self-induced or induced by someone else, hypnosis can reduce certain types of stress.

check yourself

- **What are three potential benefits to learning a variety of relaxation techniques?**
- **Which relaxation technique is the most effective for you? Why?**

4.12

What's Your Stress Level?

An interactive version of this assessment is available online in MasteringHealth.

Let's face it: Some periods in life, including your college years, can be especially stressful! Learning to "chill" starts with an honest examination of your life experiences and your reactions to stressful situations. Respond to each section, assigning points as directed. Total the points from each section, then add them and compare to the life-stressor scale.

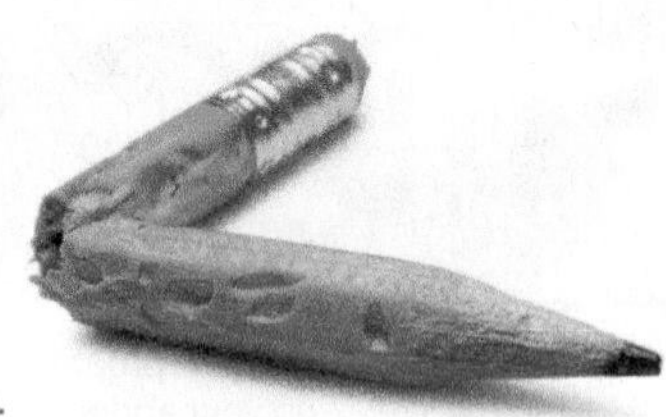

1 Recent History

In the last year, how many of the following major life events have you experienced? (Give yourself five points for each event you experienced; if you experienced an event more than once, give yourself ten points, etc.)

1. Death of a close family member or friend ____
2. Ending a relationship (whether by choice or not) ____
3. Major financial upset jeopardizing your ability to stay in college ____
4. Major move, leaving friends, family, and/or your past life behind ____
5. Serious illness (you) ____
6. Serious illness (of someone you're close with) ____
7. Marriage or entering a new relationship ____
8. Loss of a beloved pet ____
9. Involved in a legal dispute or issue ____
10. Involved in a hostile, violent, or threatening relationship ____

Total ____

2 Self-Reflection

For each of the following, indicate where you are on the scale of 0 to 5.

Strongly Disagree — Strongly Agree

1. I have a lot of worries at home and at school. 0 1 2 3 4 5
2. My friends and/or family put too much pressure on me. 0 1 2 3 4 5
3. I am often distracted and have trouble focusing on schoolwork. 0 1 2 3 4 5
4. I am highly disorganized and tend to do my schoolwork at the last minute. 0 1 2 3 4 5
5. My life seems to have far too many crisis situations. 0 1 2 3 4 5
6. Most of my time is spent sitting; I don't get much exercise. 0 1 2 3 4 5
7. I don't have enough control in decisions that affect my life. 0 1 2 3 4 5
8. I wake up most days feeling tired/like I need a lot more sleep. 0 1 2 3 4 5
9. I often have feelings that I am alone and that I don't fit in very well. 0 1 2 3 4 5
10. I don't have many friends or people I can share my feelings or thoughts with. 0 1 2 3 4 5
11. I am uncomfortable in my body, and I wish I could change how I look. 0 1 2 3 4 5
12. I am very anxious about my major and whether I will get a good job after I graduate. 0 1 2 3 4 5
13. If I have to wait in a restaurant or in lines, I quickly become irritated and upset. 0 1 2 3 4 5
14. I have to win or be the best in activities or in classes or I get upset with myself. 0 1 2 3 4 5
15. I am bothered by world events and am cynical and angry about how people behave. 0 1 2 3 4 5
16. I have too much to do, and there are never enough hours in the day. 0 1 2 3 4 5
17. I feel uneasy when I am caught up on my work and am relaxing or doing nothing. 0 1 2 3 4 5
18. I sleep with my cell phone near my bed and often check messages/tweets/texts during the night. 0 1 2 3 4 5
19. I enjoy time alone but find that I seldom get enough alone time each day. 0 1 2 3 4 5
20. I worry about whether or not others like me. 0 1 2 3 4 5
21. I am struggling in my classes and worry about failing. 0 1 2 3 4 5
22. My relationship with my family is not very loving and supportive. 0 1 2 3 4 5
23. When I watch people, I tend to be critical and think negatively about them. 0 1 2 3 4 5
24. I believe that people are inherently selfish and untrustworthy, and I am careful around them. 0 1 2 3 4 5
25. Life is basically unfair, and most of the time there is little I can do to change it. 0 1 2 3 4 5

	Strongly Disagree					Strongly Agree
26. I give more than I get in relationships with people.	0	1	2	3	4	5
27. I tend to believe that what I do is often not good enough or that I should do better.	0	1	2	3	4	5
28. My friends would describe me as highly stressed and quick to react with anger and/or frustration.	0	1	2	3	4	5
29. My friends are always telling me I "need a vacation to relax."	0	1	2	3	4	5
30. Overall, the quality of my life right now isn't all that great.	0	1	2	3	4	5
Total						______

Scoring: Total your points from Sections 1 and 2. ______

Although the following scores are not meant to be diagnostic, they do serve as an indicator of potential problem areas. If your scores are:

0–50, your stress levels are low, but it is worth examining areas where you did score points and taking action to reduce your stress levels.

51–100, you may need to reduce certain stresses in your life. Long-term stress and pressure from your stresses can be counterproductive. Consider what you can do to change your perceptions of things, your behaviors, or your environment.

100–150, you are probably pretty stressed. Examine what your major stressors are and come up with a plan for reducing your stress levels right now. Don't delay or blow this off because it could lead to significant stress-related problems, affecting your grades, your social life, and your future!

151–200, you are carrying high stress, and if you don't make changes, you could be heading for some serious difficulties. Find a counselor on campus to talk with about some of the major issues you identified above as causing stress. Try to get more sleep and exercise, and find time to relax. Surround yourself with people who are supportive of you and make you feel safe and competent.Figure Figure

Your Plan for Change

The Assess Yourself activity gave you the chance to look at your sources of chronic stress, identify major stressors in your life, and see how you typically respond to stress. Now that you are aware of these patterns, you can change behaviors that lead to increased stress.

Today, you can:

○ Practice one new stress-management technique. For example, you could spend 10 minutes doing a deep-breathing exercise or find a good spot on campus to meditate.

○ In a journal, write down stressful events or symptoms of stress that you experience.

Within the next 2 weeks, you can:

○ Attend a class or workshop in yoga, tai chi, qigong, meditation, or some other stress-relieving activity. Look for beginner classes offered on campus or in your community.

○ Make a list of the papers, projects, and tests that you have over the coming semester and create a schedule for them. Break projects and term papers into small, manageable tasks, and try to be realistic about how much time you'll need to get these tasks done.

By the end of the semester, you can:

○ Keep track of the money you spend and where it goes. Establish a budget and follow it for at least a month.

○ Find some form of exercise you can do regularly. You may consider joining a gym or just arranging regular "walk dates" or pickup basketball games with your friends. Try to exercise at least 30 minutes every day.

Summary

To hear an MP3 Tutor session, scan here or visit the Study Area in **MasteringHealth.**

LO 4.1 Stress is an inevitable part of our lives. *Eustress* refers to stress associated with positive events; *distress* refers to negative events.

LO 4.2 The alarm, resistance, and exhaustion phases of the general adaptation syndrome (GAS) involve physiological responses to both real and imagined stressors and cause complex hormonal reactions.

LO 4.3 Undue stress for extended periods of time can compromise the immune system. Stress has been linked to cardiovascular disease (CVD), weight gain, hair loss, diabetes, digestive problems, and increased susceptibility to infectious diseases. Psychoneuroimmunology is the science that analyzes the relationship between the mind's reaction to stress and immune function.

LO 4.3 Stress can affect intellectual and psychological health and contribute to depression and anxiety.

LO 4.4 The most common types of headaches are tension and migraine. Relaxation techniques can ease headaches triggered by stress.

LO 4.5 Sleep conserves body energy and restores physical and mental functioning.

LO 4.6 Psychosocial factors contributing to stress include change, hassles, relationships, pressure, conflict, overload, and environmental stressors. Persons subjected to discrimination or bias may face unusually high levels of stress.

LO 4.7 Some sources of stress are internal and related to appraisal, self-esteem, self-efficacy, personality, and psychological hardiness and resilience.

LO 4.8–4.11 College can be stressful. Recognizing the signs of stress is the first step toward better health. To manage stress, find coping skills that work for you—probably some combination of managing emotional responses, taking mental or physical action, downshifting, time management, managing finances, and relaxation techniques.

Pop Quiz

Visit MasteringHealth to personalize your study plan with Chapter Review Quizzes and Dynamic Study Modules.

LO 4.1 1. Even though Andre experienced stress when he graduated from college and moved to a new city, he viewed these changes as an opportunity for growth. What is Andre's stress called?
a. Strain
b. Distress
c. Eustress
d. Adaptive response

LO 4.1 2. Which of the following is an example of a chronic stressor?
a. Giving a talk in public
b. Meeting a deadline for a big project
c. Dealing with a permanent disability
d. Preparing for a job interview

LO 4.2 3. During what phase of the general adaptation syndrome has the physical and psychological energy used to fight the stressor been depleted?
a. Alarm phase
b. Resistance phase
c. Endurance phase
d. Exhaustion phase

LO 4.2 4. In which stage of the general adaptation syndrome does the fight-or-flight response occur?
a. Exhaustion stage
b. Alarm stage
c. Resistance stage
d. Response stage

LO 4.2 5. The branch of the autonomic nervous system that is responsible for energizing the body for either fight-or-flight and for triggering many other stress responses is the
a. central nervous system.
b. parasympathetic nervous system.
c. sympathetic nervous system.
d. endocrine system.

LO 4.6 6. A state of physical and mental exhaustion caused by excessive stress is called
a. conflict.
b. overload.
c. hassles.
d. burnout.

LO 4.6 7. Losing your keys is an example of what psychosocial source of stress?
a. Pressure
b. Inconsistent behaviors
c. Hassles
d. Conflict

LO 4.7 8. Which of the following test-taking techniques is not recommended to reduce test-taking stress?
a. Plan ahead and study over a period of time for the test.
b. Eat a balanced meal before the exam.
c. Do all your studying the night before the exam so it is fresh in your mind.
d. Remind yourself of three reasons you will pass the exam.

LO 4.10 9. After 5 years of 70-hour workweeks, Tom decided to leave his high-paying, high-stress law firm and lead a simpler lifestyle. What is this trend called?
a. Adaptation
b. Conflict resolution
c. Burnout reduction
d. Downshifting

LO 4.10 10. Which of the following is not an example of a time-management technique?
a. Doing one thing at a time
b. Rewarding yourself for finishing a task
c. Practicing procrastination in completing homework assignments
d. Breaking tasks into smaller pieces

Answers to these questions can be found on page A-1. If you answered a question incorrectly, review the module identified by the Learning Outcome. For even more study tools, visit MasteringHealth.

CVD, Cancer, and Diabetes

5

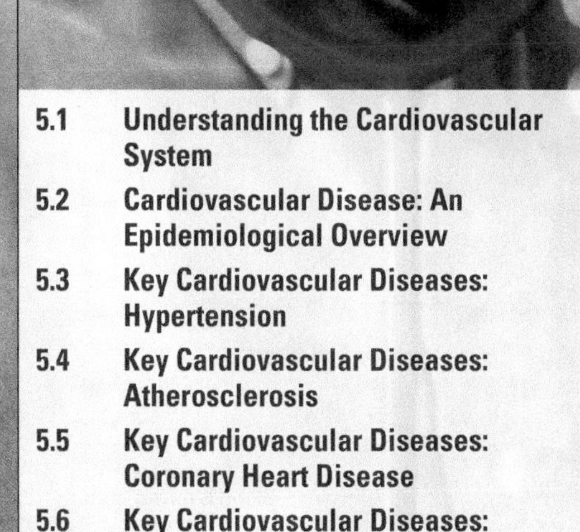

An overwhelming percentage of deaths in the United States are due to three major causes: cardiovascular disease, diabetes, and cancer. Nearly 84 million Americans—1 of every 3 adults—suffer from one or more types of **cardiovascular disease (CVD)**, diseases of the heart and blood vessels.[1] CVD has been the leading killer of U.S. adults every year since 1900, with the exception of the flu pandemic of 1918. Growing rates of obesity, hypertension, and diabetes contribute to CVD in the United States and worldwide.

Diabetes is one of the fastest growing health threats in the world today, with over 382 million people classified as diabetic in 2013.[2] Diabetes is the primary cause of death each year for over 71,000 Americans and a contributing factor to over 231,000 deaths from cardiovascular disease, kidney disease, and other diseases.[3]

As recently as 50 years ago, a cancer diagnosis was typically a death sentence. Cancer remains the second leading cause of death in the United States.[4] Although there were nearly 1.7 million *new* cancer diagnoses and over 585,000 deaths in 2014, the good news is that cancer death rates have been declining by over 2 percent per year in the last decades. Early detection and better treatments have dramatically improved the prognosis for many people, particularly for those diagnosed early.[5]

5.1 Understanding the Cardiovascular System

learning outcome

5.1 Identify the elements and functions of the cardiovascular system.

The cardiovascular system is the network of organs and vessels through which blood flows as it carries oxygen and nutrients to all parts of the body. It includes the heart, arteries, arterioles (small arteries), veins, venules (small veins), and capillaries (minute blood vessels).

The Heart: A Mighty Machine

The heart is a muscular, four-chambered pump, roughly the size of your fist. It is a highly efficient, extremely flexible organ that contracts 100,000 times each day and pumps the equivalent of 2,000 gallons of blood to all areas of the body. In a 70-year lifetime, an average human heart beats 2.5 billion times.

The human body contains approximately 6 quarts of blood, which transports nutrients, oxygen, waste products, hormones, and enzymes throughout the body. Blood aids in regulating body temperature, cellular water levels, and acidity levels of body components and helps defend the body against toxins and harmful microorganisms. Adequate blood supply is essential to health.

The heart's four chambers work together to circulate blood constantly throughout the body. The two large upper chambers, **atria**, receive blood from the rest of the body; the two lower chambers, **ventricles**, pump the blood out again. Small valves regulate steady, rhythmic flow of blood and prevent leakage or backflow between chambers.

Flow of Blood through the Heart and Blood Vessels

Heart activity depends on a complex interaction of biochemical, physical, and neurological signals. To understand blood flow through the heart, follow the steps in Figure 5.1, from deoxygenated blood entering the heart to oxygenated blood being pumped into the blood vessels. Different types of blood vessels are required for different parts of this process. **Arteries** carry blood away from the heart. All arteries carry oxygenated blood, *except* for the pulmonary arteries, which carry deoxygenated blood to the lungs, where the blood picks up oxygen and gives up carbon dioxide. The arteries branch off from the heart, then divide into smaller vessels called **arterioles**, then into even smaller **capillaries**. Capillaries have thin walls that permit the exchange of oxygen, carbon dioxide, nutrients, and waste products with body cells. Carbon dioxide and other waste products are transported to the lungs and kidneys through **veins** and **venules** (small veins).

Your heartbeat is governed by an electrical impulse that directs the heart muscle to move, resulting in sequential contraction of the chambers. This signal starts in a small bundle of highly specialized cells in the right atrium, called the **sinoatrial node (SA node)**, that serves as a natural pacemaker. The average adult heart at rest beats 70 to 80 times per minute.

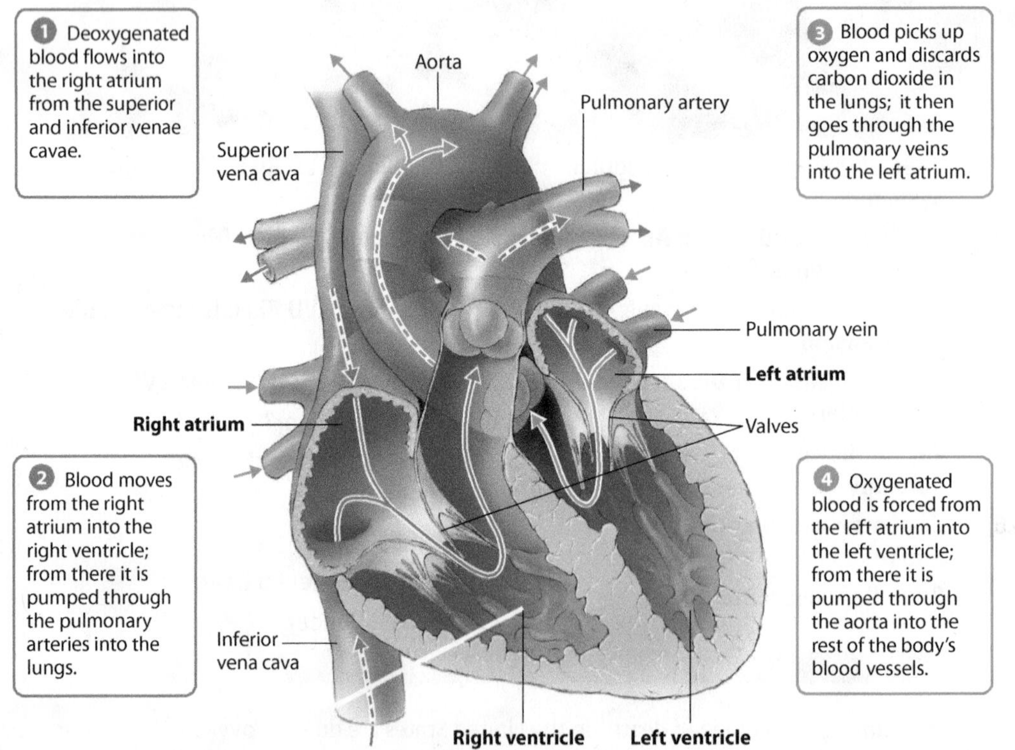

Figure 5.1 Blood Flow within the Heart

check yourself

- **Describe the pathway that blood follows as it circulates through the heart.**

5.2 Cardiovascular Disease: An Epidemiological Overview

learning outcome

5.2 Describe patterns in the prevalence of cardiovascular disease relative to gender and ethnicity.

Cardiovascular disease claims more lives each year than the next three leading causes of death combined (cancer, chronic lower respiratory diseases, and accidents), accounting for nearly 33 percent of all deaths in the United States.[6] Consider the following:

- Many CVD-related fatalities are sudden cardiac deaths, an abrupt, profound loss of heart function (cardiac arrest) that causes death either instantly or shortly after symptoms occur. Fifty percent of men and 64 percent of women who die suddenly have had no previous symptoms.[7]
- CVD has claimed the lives of more women than men every year since 1984. Only among people aged 20 to 39 is CVD significantly more prevalent among men than among women (Figure 5.2).[8] Women also have a higher lifetime prevalence of stroke.[9]
- Among women, African Americans and Asian/Pacific Islanders (particularly South Asians) have the highest percentages of CVD deaths, at 34 and 33 percent, respectively.[10]
- Among men, Asian/Pacific Islanders and African Americans have the highest percentages of CVD deaths, at 32.8 percent and 31.7 percent, respectively.[11]
- American Indian and Alaska Natives have the lowest percentages of deaths from CVD.[12]
- Among those aged 20 to 39, 20.3 percent have metabolic syndrome (MetS), a dangerous grouping of key risk factors for CVD. Among those aged 40 to 59, rates jump to 40.8 percent, and for those 60 and over, rates are nearly 52 percent.[13]

Although millions of Americans are living longer with CVD problems, many lack adequate health insurance and fail to obtain screenings and treatments early enough. Large numbers of CVD survivors suffer from physical and emotional disability in the form of fear, depression, and/or inability to perform activities of daily living. While actual death rates have declined, soaring costs for medicines, home health care, rehabilitation services and hospital care, and outpatient tests make recovery challenging. In spite of major improvements in medication, surgery, and other health care procedures, 25 percent of men and 38 percent of women will die within 1 year of having an initial heart attack.[14] The older the age at first heart attack, the greater the risk of dying.[15]

The economic burden of cardiovascular disease on our society is huge—more than $315 billion in direct and indirect costs.[16] Of this amount, nearly $194 billion is direct costs, including physicians and other professionals, hospital services, prescribed medication, and home health care.[17] Indirect costs, attributed to projected losses in future productivity, make up the remainder of the roughly $122 billion in costs.[18] Based on current trends, projections indicate total direct and indirect costs of CVD will surpass $918 billion by 2030.[19]

While economic concerns are huge, the effects of CVD on patients, families, communities, and society may be even greater.

With an international trend toward obesity, more and more countries face epidemic CVD rates. The World Health Organization (WHO) estimates CVD accounts for 30 percent of all deaths globally.[20] Unfortunately, over 80 percent of the world's deaths from CVD occur in low- and middle-income countries, places where people have more risks and fewer options for prevention and treatment.[21]

Although death rates are relatively easy to calculate, the short- and long-term psychological problems that occur after a person has a heart attack are harder to measure. Imagine the anxiety caused by wondering if your heart will fail each time you exercise, or fearing that sexual activity might cause another heart attack. Knowing more about your specific CVD risks, your limitations, and what you can do about them is key to taking healthy action.

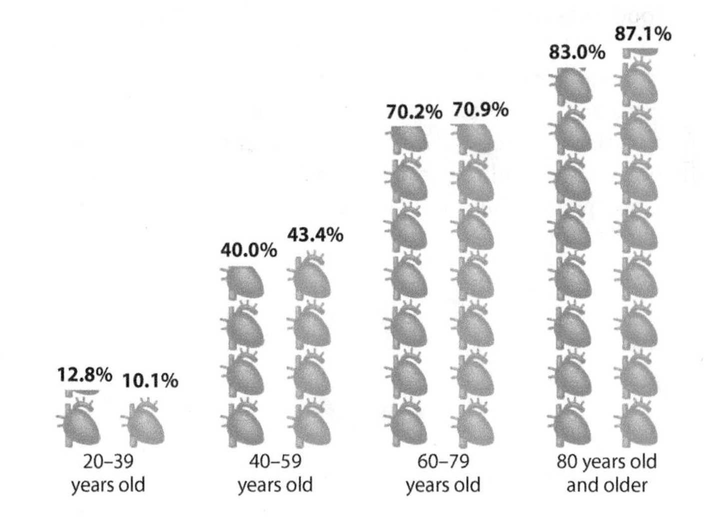

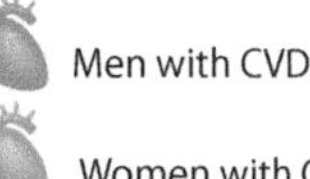

Figure 5.2 Prevalence of Cardiovascular Disease (CVD) in U.S. Adults Aged 20 and Older by Age and Sex

Source: Data from A. S. Go et al., "Heart Disease and Stroke Statistics—2014 Update: A Report from the American Heart Association," *Circulation* 129 (2014): e28-e292.

check yourself

- **What are some patterns in cardiovascular disease relative to gender and ethnicity?**

5.3 Key Cardiovascular Diseases: Hypertension

learning **outcome**

5.3 Define hypertension and explain how it is measured.

The major cardiovascular diseases include hypertension, atherosclerosis, coronary heart disease, and stroke. Each of these cardiovascular diseases causes deaths and disabilities; their causes and treatments are discussed in the following modules.

Hypertension refers to sustained high blood pressure. In general, the higher your blood pressure, the greater your risk for CVD. Hypertension is known as the silent killer—it often has few overt symptoms, and people often don't know they have it.

The prevalence of hypertension in the United States continues to increase in spite of significant efforts aimed at treatment and control; today more than 1 in 3 U.S. adults has high blood pressure. At nearly 47 percent, African Americans have the highest rate of high blood pressure in the United States.[22] Rates are also much higher among the elderly, men, and those who don't have a high school education.[23]

Blood pressure is measured by two numbers—for example, 110/80 mm HG, stated as "110 over 80 millimeters of mercury." The top number refers to **systolic pressure**, the pressure applied to the walls of the arteries when the heart contracts, pumping blood to the rest of the body. The bottom number is **diastolic pressure**, the pressure applied to the walls of the arteries during the heart's relaxation phase, when blood reenters the chambers of the heart in preparation for the next heartbeat.

2,150

Americans die every day of CVD.

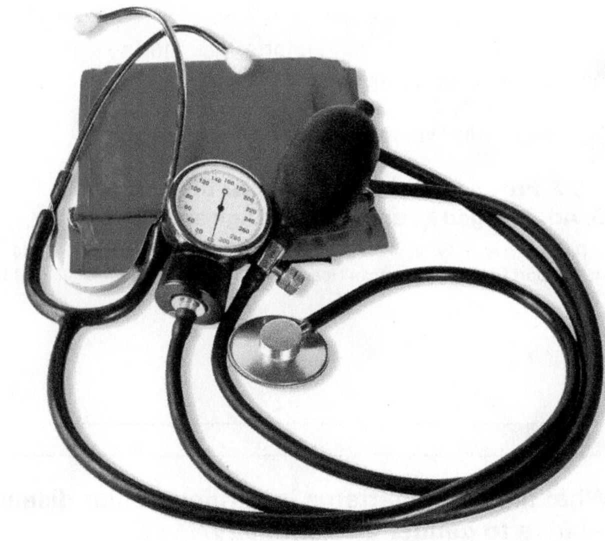

TABLE 5.1 **Blood Pressure Classifications**

Classification	Systolic Reading (mm Hg)		Diastolic Reading (mm Hg)
Normal	Less than 120	And	Less than 80
Prehypertension	120–139	Or	80–89
Hypertension			
Stage 1	140–159	Or	90–99
Stage 2	Greater than or equal to 160	Or	Greater than or equal to 100

Note: If systolic and diastolic readings fall into different categories, treatment is determined by the highest category. Readings are based on the average of two or more properly measured, seated readings on each of two or more health care provider visits.

Source: National Heart, Lung, and Blood Institute, *The Seventh Report of the Joint National Committee on Prevention, Detection, Evaluation, and Treatment of High Blood Pressure*, NIH Publication no. 03-5233, (Bethesda, MD: National Institutes of Health, 2003).

Normal blood pressure varies depending on weight, age, and physical condition. High blood pressure is usually diagnosed when systolic pressure is 140 or above. When only systolic pressure is high, the condition is known as *isolated systolic hypertension (ISH)*, the most common form of high blood pressure in older Americans. See Table 5.1 for a summary of blood pressure guidelines.

Systolic blood pressure tends to increase with age, whereas diastolic blood pressure increases until age 55 and then declines. Men under the age of 45 are at nearly twice the risk of becoming hypertensive as their female counterparts; however women tend to have higher rates of hypertension after age 65.[24] Over 30 percent of the population are considered to be **prehypertensive**, meaning that their blood pressure is above normal, but not yet in the hypertensive range. These individuals have a significantly greater risk of becoming hypertensive.[25]

Treatment of hypertension can involve dietary changes (reducing sodium and calorie intake), weight loss (when appropriate), use of diuretics and other medications (when prescribed by a physician), regular exercise, treatment of sleep disorders such as sleep apnea, and the practice of relaxation techniques and effective coping and communication skills.

check yourself

- **What is hypertension, and what are its causes and treatments?**

5.4 Key Cardiovascular Diseases: Atherosclerosis

learning outcome

5.4 List the major factors contributing to atherosclerosis.

Atherosclerosis comes from the Greek words *athero* (meaning gruel or paste) and *sclerosis* (hardness). In this condition, fatty substances, cholesterol, cellular waste products, calcium, and fibrin (a clotting material in the blood) build up in the inner lining of an artery. *Hyperlipidemia* (an abnormally high blood lipid level) is a key factor in this process, and the resulting buildup is called **plaque**.

As plaque accumulates, vessel walls become narrow and may eventually block blood flow or cause vessels to rupture (Figure 5.3). The pressure buildup is similar to that achieved when putting your thumb over the end of a hose while water is on. Pressure builds within arteries just as pressure builds in the hose. If vessels are weakened and pressure persists, the vessels may burst or the plaque itself may break away from the walls of the vessels and obstruct blood flow. In addition, fluctuation in the blood pressure levels within arteries can damage internal arterial walls, making it even more likely that plaque will stick to injured wall surfaces and accumulate.

Atherosclerosis is often called **coronary artery disease (CAD)** because of the damage to the body's main coronary arteries on the outer surface of the heart. These are the arteries that provide blood supply to the heart muscle itself. Most heart attacks result from blockage of these arteries. Atherosclerosis and other circulatory impairments also often reduce blood flow and limit the heart's blood and oxygen supply, a condition known as **ischemia**.

When atherosclerosis occurs in the lower extremities, such as in the feet, calves, or legs, or in the arms, it is called **peripheral artery disease (PAD)**. Over 8.5 million people—particularly those over 65, non-Hispanic blacks, and women in the United States—have PAD, and many are not receiving treatment because they are asymptomatic or don't recognize subtle symptoms.[26] Most often characterized by pain and aching in the legs, calves, or feet upon walking or exercise (known as *intermittent claudication*), PAD is a leading cause of disability in people over the age of 50. While it strikes both men and women, men, smokers, and diabetics tend to develop it more frequently.[27] In recent years, increased attention has been drawn to PAD's role in subsequent blood clots and resultant heart attacks, particularly among people who sit in cramped airplanes for long distances without getting up and moving. Sometimes PAD in the arms can be caused by trauma, certain diseases, radiation therapy, surgery, repetitive motion syndrome, or a combination of factors. Damage to vessels and threats to health can be severe, with a two- to three-times greater risk of stroke and heart attack among those who have PAD.[28]

Atherosclerosis treatment focuses on lifestyle changes, drugs that reduce the risk of plaque, medical procedures to open vessels, or surgery to open clogged vessels. Millions of Americans take drugs designed to reduce triglycerides and LDL (bad cholesterol) and increase HDL (good cholesterol). Statins are the most commonly prescribed; however they are not without risk. The most common risk is muscle pain that ranges from mild to severe. Other potential side effects include digestive issues, liver damage, increased risk of diabetes, and memory loss. People considering statins should discuss the risks versus the benefits with their doctors.

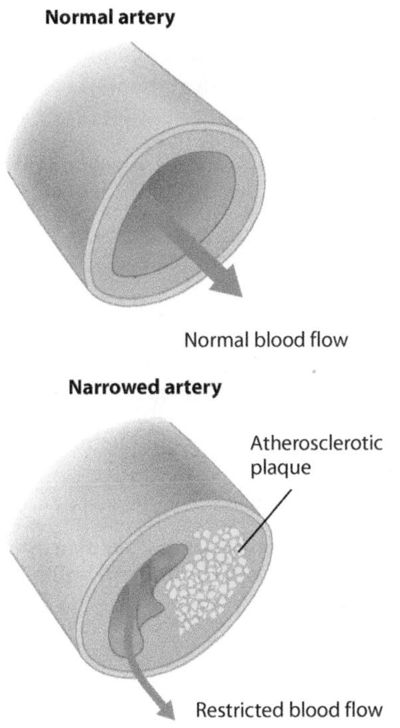

Normal artery

Normal blood flow

Narrowed artery

Atherosclerotic plaque

Restricted blood flow

Figure 5.3 Atherosclerosis and Coronary Artery Disease

In atherosclerosis, arteries become clogged by a buildup of plaque. When atherosclerosis occurs in coronary arteries, blood flow to the heart muscle is restricted and a heart attack may occur.

Sources: Adapted from Joan Salge Blake, *Nutrition and You*, 2nd ed. © 2012. Reprinted by permission of Pearson Education, Inc., Upper Saddle River, New Jersey.

VIDEO TUTOR
Atherosclerosis and Coronary Artery Disease

check yourself

- **What is atherosclerosis, and what are its causes?**
- **What are the symptoms of peripheral artery disease (PAD)? Who is most at risk?**

5.5 Key Cardiovascular Diseases: Coronary Heart Disease

learning outcome

5.5 List the major factors contributing to a heart attack and the signs of a heart attack.

Of all the major cardiovascular diseases, **coronary heart disease (CHD)** is the greatest killer, accounting for about 1 in 6 deaths in the United States. Nearly 1 million new and recurrent heart attacks occur in the United States each year.[29]

A **myocardial infarction (MI)**, or **heart attack**, involves an area of the heart that suffers permanent damage because its normal blood supply has been blocked. This condition is often brought on by a **coronary thrombosis** (clot) or an atherosclerotic narrowing that blocks a coronary artery (an artery supplying the heart muscle with blood). When a clot, or **thrombus**, becomes dislodged and moves through the circulatory system, it is called an **embolus.** Whenever blood does not flow readily, there is a corresponding decrease in oxygen flow to tissue below the blockage.

If the blockage is extremely minor, an otherwise healthy heart will adapt over time by enlarging existing blood vessels and growing new ones to reroute needed blood through other areas. This system, called **collateral circulation**, is a form of self-preservation that allows an affected heart muscle to cope with damage.

When a heart blockage is more severe, however, the body is unable to adapt on its own, and outside life-saving support is critical. The hour following a heart attack is the most crucial period.

It is important to know and recognize the symptoms of a heart attack so that help can be obtained immediately (Table 5.2). Ignoring symptoms or delays in seeking treatment can have fatal consequences. Be sure to be familiar with heart attack symptoms and know how to summon emergency help at home, work, and school.

Skills for Behavior Change

WHAT TO DO WHEN A HEART ATTACK HITS

People often miss the signs of a heart attack, or they wait too long to seek help, which can have deadly consequences. Knowing what to do in an emergency could save your life or somebody else's.

- **Keep a list of emergency rescue service numbers next to your telephone and in your pocket, wallet, or purse. Be aware of whether your local area has a 9-1-1 emergency service.**
- **Expect the person to deny the possibility of anything as serious as a heart attack, particularly if that person is young and appears to be in good health. If you're with someone who appears to be having a heart attack, don't take no for an answer; insist on taking prompt action.**
- **If you are with someone who suddenly collapses, perform cardiopulmonary resuscitation (CPR). See www.heart.org for information on the new chest-compression-only techniques recommended by the American Heart Association. If you're trained and willing, use conventional CPR methods.**

Sources: Adapted from American Heart Association, "Warning Signs of Heart Attack, Stroke, and Cardiac Arrest," 2012, www.heart.org.

TABLE 5.2 **Common Heart Attack Symptoms and Signs**

Sign or Symptom	Gender Who Most Commonly Experiences It
Crushing or squeezing chest pain	More common in men
Pain radiating down arm, neck, or jaw	More common in men
Chest discomfort or pressure with shortness of breath, nausea/vomiting, or lightheadedness	Women more likely to feel pressure than pain. Shortness of breath, nausea, and lightheadedness common in both women and men
Shortness of breath without chest pain, discomfort in back, neck, or jaw or in one or both arms	More common in women
Unusual weakness	More common in women
Unusual fatigue	More common in women
Sleep disturbances	More common in women
Indigestion, flulike symptoms	More common in women

Sources: American Heart Association, "Symptoms of Heart Attack in Women," 2012, www.heart.org.

check yourself

- **What is a heart attack, and what are its causes?**
- **What should you do if someone shows signs of a heart attack?**

Key Cardiovascular Diseases: Stroke

learning outcome

5.6 List the major factors contributing to stroke and the signs of a stroke.

A **stroke** (or *cerebrovascular accident*) occurs when blood supply to the brain is interrupted, killing brain cells, which have little capacity to heal or regenerate.

Strokes may be *ischemic* (caused by plaque or a clot that reduces blood flow) or *hemorrhagic* (due to bulging or rupture of a weakened blood vessel). Figure 5.4 illustrates blood vessel disorders that can lead to a stroke. An **aneurysm** is the most life-threatening hemorrhagic stroke.

Mild strokes cause temporary dizziness, weakness, or numbness. More serious interruptions in blood flow may impair speech, memory, or motor control. Others affect heart and lung function regulation, killing within minutes. Nearly 7 million Americans suffer a stroke every year, and almost 129,000 die as a result.[30] Strokes account for 1 in 19 deaths each year.[31] Even scarier, it is thought that more young people are having strokes than ever before, possibly due to increased obesity and hypertension.[32]

See It! Videos

See how two young women have regained their lives after experiencing a stroke. Watch **Stroke in Young Adults** in the Study Area of MasteringHealth.

Many major strokes are preceded days, weeks, or months earlier by **transient ischemic attacks (TIAs)**, brief interruptions of the brain's blood supply that cause temporary impairment.[33] Symptoms of TIAs include dizziness (particularly on rising), weakness, temporary paralysis or numbness in the face or other regions, temporary memory loss, blurred vision, nausea, headache, and difficulty speaking. Some people experience unexpected falls or have blackouts; others have no obvious symptoms.

The earlier a stroke is recognized and treatment started, the more effective the treatment. One of the great medical successes in recent years is the decline in the death rate from strokes, which in the United States has dropped by one-third since the 1980s.[34] Greater awareness of stroke symptoms, improvements in emergency medicine protocols and medicines, and a greater emphasis on fast rehabilitation and therapy after a stroke have helped many survive.

Despite improved treatments, stroke survivors do not always make a full recovery; often, problems with speech, memory, swallowing, and activities of daily living persist. Depression is also an issue for many survivors.

Skills for Behavior Change

A SIMPLE TEST FOR STROKE

People often ignore, minimize, or misunderstand stroke symptoms. Starting treatment within just a few hours is crucial for the best recovery outcomes. So if you suspect someone is having a stroke, use the tool many emergency teams do to assess what is happening: think FAST.

1. Facial Droop: Ask the person to smile. It is normal for both sides of the face to move equally, and it is abnormal if one side moves less easily.
2. Arm Weakness: Ask the person to raise both arms. It is normal if both arms move equally (or not at all). It is abnormal if one arm drifts or cannot be raised as high as the other.
3. Speech Difficulty: Have the patient restate a sentence such as, "You can't teach an old dog new tricks." It is normal if they can say the sentence correctly, and it is abnormal if they use inappropriate words, slur, or cannot speak.
4. Time to ACT and call 9-1-1. Don't delay if you note 1 to 3 above. Time is of the essence.

Source: Cincinnati Prehospital Stroke Scale, adapted from the Uniform Document for Georgia EMS Providers, Department of Public Health, State of Georgia. Available at http://ems.ga.gov.

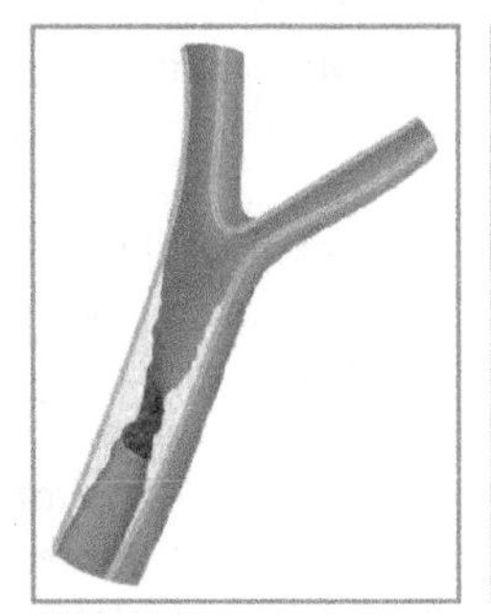

(a) A **thrombus** is a blood clot that forms inside a blood vessel and blocks the flow of blood at its origin.

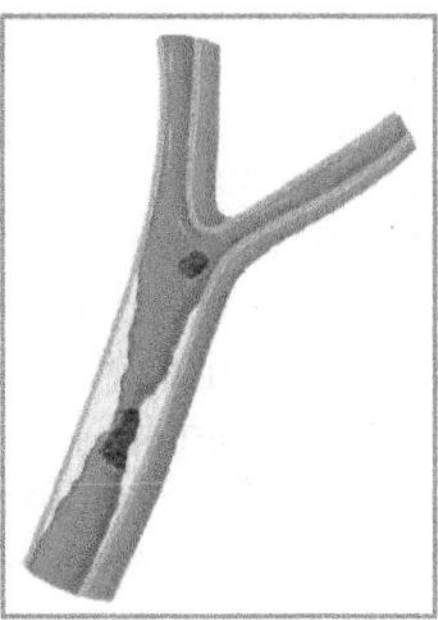

(b) An **embolus** is a blood clot that breaks off from its point of formation and travels in the bloodstream until it lodges in a narrowed vessel and blocks blood flow.

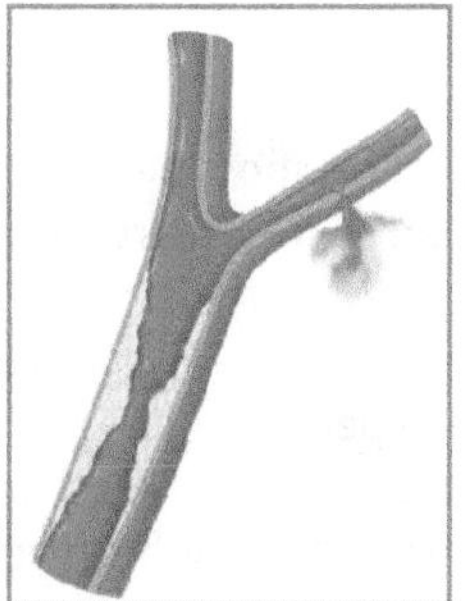

(c) A **hemorrhage** occurs when a blood vessel bursts allowing blood to flow into the surrounding tissue or between tissues.

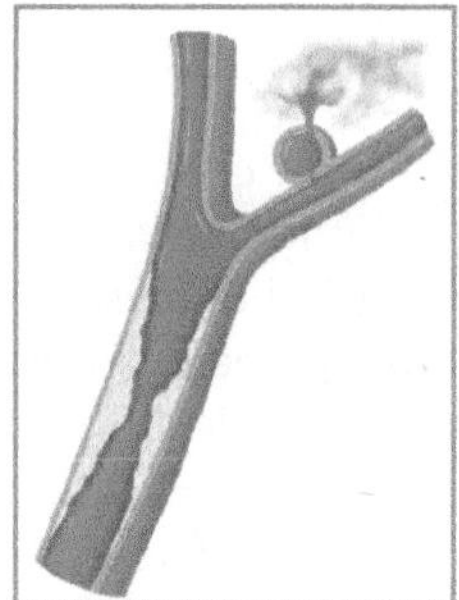

(d) An **aneurysm** is the bulging of a weakened blood vessel wall.

Figure 5.4 Blood Vessel Disorders That Can Lead to Stroke

check yourself

- **What is stroke, and what are its causes?**
- **What should you do if someone shows signs of a stroke?**

5.7 Other Cardiovascular Diseases

learning outcome

5.7 Know the signs and symptoms of angina pectoris, arrhythmias, congestive heart failure, and childhood cardiovascular defects.

Other cardiovascular diseases of concern include angina pectoris, arrhythmias, congestive heart failure, and childhood cardiovascular defects.

Angina Pectoris

Angina pectoris occurs when there is not enough oxygen to supply the heart muscle, resulting in chest pain or pressure. Nearly 8 million people in the U.S. suffer from mild-to-severe symptoms of angina—from indigestion or heartburn-like sensations to chest crushing pain.[35] Generally, the more serious the oxygen deprivation, the more severe the pain. Although angina pectoris is not a heart attack, it does indicate underlying heart disease.

Mild angina cases are treated with rest. Treatments for more severe cases involve drugs that affect either supply of blood to the heart muscle or the heart's demand for oxygen. Pain and discomfort are often relieved with *nitroglycerin*, a drug used to relax (dilate) veins, reducing the amount of blood returning to the heart and so lessening its workload. Patients with angina caused by spasms of the coronary arteries are often given *calcium channel blockers*, which prevent calcium atoms from passing through the arteries and causing the contractions. *Beta blockers* control potential overactivity of the heart muscle.

Arrhythmias

Over the course of a lifetime, most people experience some type of **arrhythmia**, an irregularity in heart rhythm that occurs when the electrical impulses in your heart that coordinate heartbeat don't work properly. A person with a racing heart in the absence of exercise or anxiety may be experiencing *tachycardia*, the medical term for abnormally fast heartbeat. On the other end of the continuum is *bradycardia*, or abnormally slow heartbeat. When a heart goes into **fibrillation**, it beats in a sporadic pattern that causes extreme inefficiency in moving blood through the cardiovascular system. If untreated, fibrillation may be fatal.

Not all arrhythmias are life-threatening. In many instances, excessive caffeine or nicotine consumption can trigger an arrhythmia episode. However, severe cases may require drug therapy or external electrical stimulus to prevent serious complications. When in doubt, it is always best to check with your doctor.

Congestive Heart Failure

When the heart muscle is damaged and can't pump enough blood to supply body tissues, fluids may begin to accumulate in various parts of the body, most notably the lungs, feet, ankles, and legs. Acute shortness of breath and fatigue are often key symptoms of **heart failure (HF)** or **congestive heart failure (CHF)**. Nearly 6.6 million adults age 20 and over in the United States have HF, with cases estimated to rise to nearly 10 million by 2030.[36] Underlying causes of HF may include heart injury that results in damage to heart muscle (**cardiomyopathy**), affects heart valves, or causes problems with heart rhythms. Infectious diseases, such as rheumatic fever, can damage heart valves. Bacteria and viruses can inflame blood vessels, increasing atherosclerotic plaque formation. Uncontrolled high blood pressure, coronary artery disease, diabetes, and other chronic conditions can all lead to heart failure. Certain prescription drugs such as NSAIDS and diabetes medications also increase risks, as do chronic drug and alcohol abuse. In some cases, damage is due to cancer radiation or chemotherapy treatments.

Untreated, HF can be fatal. However, most cases respond well to treatment, which includes *diuretics* (water pills) to relieve fluid accumulation; drugs such as *digitalis* that increase the heart's pumping action; and *vasodilators*, drugs that expand blood vessels and decrease resistance, making the heart's work easier.

Congenital and Rheumatic Heart Disease

Approximately 32,000 children are born in the United States each year with some form of **congenital cardiovascular defect** (*congenital* means the problem is present at birth).[37] These may be relatively minor, such as slight *murmurs* (low-pitched sounds caused by turbulent blood flow through the heart) caused by valve irregularities, which many children outgrow. About 25 percent of those born with congenital heart defects must undergo invasive procedures to correct problems within the first year of life.[38] Underlying causes are unknown but may be related to hereditary factors; maternal diseases, such as rubella, that occurred during fetal development; or a mother's chemical intake (particularly alcohol or methamphetamine) during pregnancy. With advances in pediatric cardiology, the prognosis for children with congenital heart defects is better than ever before.

Rheumatic heart disease is attributed to rheumatic fever, an inflammatory disease caused by an unresolved *streptococcal infection* of the throat (strep throat). Over time, the strep infection can affect connective tissues of the heart, joints, brain, or skin. In some cases, the infection can lead to an immune response in which antibodies attack the heart as well as the bacteria. Many operations on heart valves are related to rheumatic heart disease.

check yourself

- **Name and describe several common cardiovascular diseases.**

5.8 Reducing CVD Risk: Metabolic Syndrome

learning outcome

5.8 List the cluster of factors composing metabolic syndrome.

A large cluster of factors are related to increased risk for cardiovascular disease. Recently, the U.S. Burden of Disease Collaborators determined that the greatest contributor to overall CVD burden was suboptimal diet, followed by tobacco smoking, high body mass index, high blood pressure, high fasting plasma glucose, and physical inactivity.[39] A growing body of research has implicated selected CVD risks and conditions such as obesity and hypertension with an increased risk for impaired cognitive function and an increased risk for Alzheimer's disease.[40] **Cardiometabolic risks** are the combined risks, which indicate physical and biochemical changes that can lead to diseases. Some risks result from choices and behaviors and are modifiable, whereas others are inherited or are intrinsic (such as age and gender) and cannot be changed.

Over the past decade, health professionals have attempted to establish diagnostic cutoff points for a cluster of combined cardiometabolic risks, variably labeled *syndrome X*, *insulin resistance syndrome*, and most recently, **metabolic syndrome (MetS)**. Historically, MetS is believed to increase risk for atherosclerotic heart disease by as much as three times normal rates. Twenty percent of people age 20 to 39, 41 percent of people age 40 to 59, and nearly 52 percent of those over the age of 60 meet its criteria.[41] Although different professional organizations have slightly different criteria for MetS, that of the National Cholesterol Education Program's Adult Treatment Panel (NCEP/ATPIII) is most commonly used. According to these criteria, for a diagnosis of metabolic syndrome a person would have three or more of the following risks (Figure 5.5):[42]

- Abdominal obesity (waist measurement of more than 40 inches in men or 35 inches in women)
- Elevated blood fat (triglycerides greater than 150 mg/dL)
- Low levels of high-density lipoprotein (HDL; "good" cholesterol) (less than 40 mg/dL in men and less than 50 mg/dL in women)
- Blood pressure greater than 130/85 mm Hg
- Fasting glucose greater than 100 mg/dL (a sign of insulin resistance or glucose intolerance)

The use of the metabolic syndrome classification and other, similar terms has been important in highlighting the relationship between the number of risks a person possesses and that person's likelihood of developing CVD and diabetes. Groups such as the AHA and others are giving increased attention to multiple risks and emphasizing cardiovascular health in lifestyle interventions.

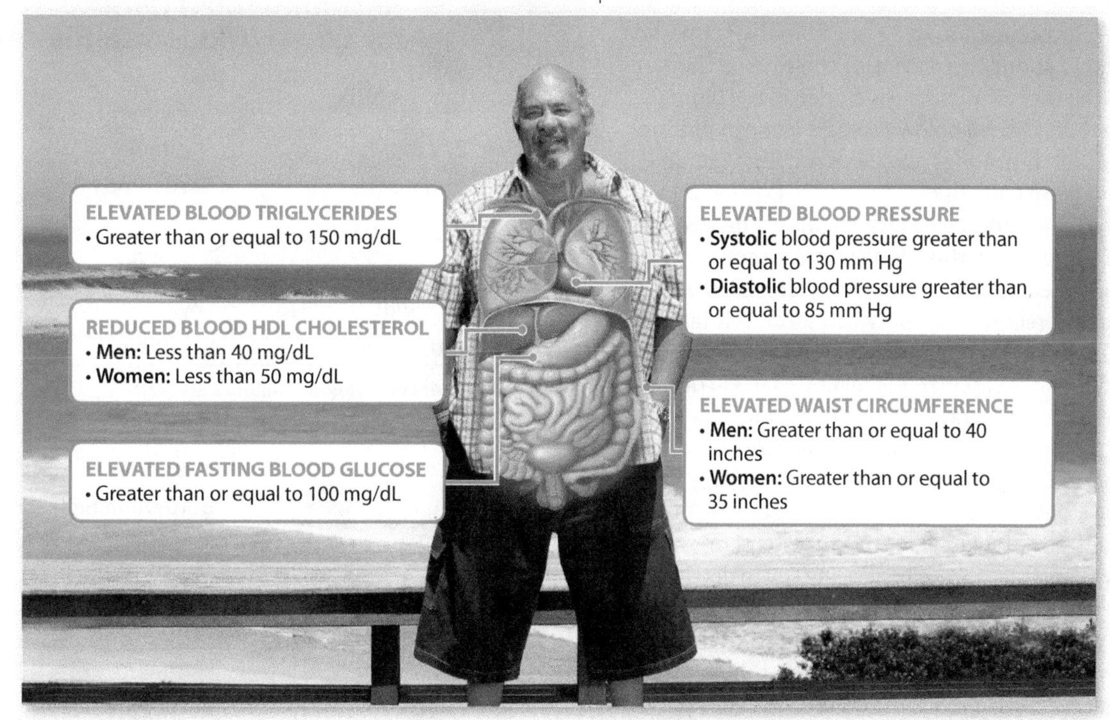

Figure 5.5 Risk Factors Associated with Metabolic Syndrome

check yourself

- **How does metabolic syndrome contribute to the risk of heart disease?**

5.9 Reducing CVD Risk: Modifiable Risks

learning outcome

5.9 Describe modifiable factors affecting CVD risk.

From the first moments of your life, you begin to accumulate risks for CVD. Your past and current lifestyle choices may haunt you as you enter your middle and later years. Behaviors you choose today and over the coming decades can actively reduce or promote your risk for CVD.

Avoid Tobacco Smoke

Cigarette smokers are 2 to 4 times more likely to develop coronary heart disease[43] and more than 10 times as likely to develop peripheral vascular diseases[44] than are nonsmokers. Smoking also doubles a person's risk of stroke.[45] Nonsmokers regularly exposed to secondhand smoke have a 25 to 30 percent increased risk of heart disease, with over 35,000 deaths per year.[46]

The good news is that if you stop smoking, your heart can mend itself. After 1 year, the former smoker's risk of heart disease drops by 50 percent. Between 5 and 15 years after quitting, the risk of stroke and CHD becomes similar to that of nonsmokers. Quitting by age 30 reduces chances of dying prematurely from tobacco-related diseases by more than 90 percent.[47]

Cut Back on Saturated Fat and Cholesterol

Cholesterol is a fat-like substance found in your bloodstream and cells. Your body products about 75 percent of cholesterol; the rest comes from foods in your diet. Cholesterol is carried in the blood by LDL and HDL lipoproteins (defined below); it plays a role in production of cell membranes and hormones and helps process vitamin D. However, high levels increase CVD risk.

Diets high in saturated fat and *trans* fats are widely believed to raise cholesterol levels and make the blood more viscous, which increases risk of heart attack, stroke, and atherosclerosis. However, researchers looking at the relationship between saturated fat and increased risk of CVD recently concluded that current evidence doesn't clearly support cardiovascular guidelines that encourage high consumption of polyunsaturated fatty acids and low consumption of total saturated fats.[48] Still, multiple factors play a role in CVD risk, and experts continue to recommend reducing saturated fats, maintaining a balanced diet, and exercising.

Historically, clinicians have looked at total cholesterol, triglycerides, and high and low-density lipoproteins as being key to determining CVD risks. **Low-density lipoprotein (LDL)**, or "bad" cholesterol, is believed to build up on artery walls; **high-density lipoprotein (HDL)**, or "good" cholesterol, appears to remove such buildup. In theory, if LDL levels get too high or HDL levels too low, cholesterol will accumulate inside arteries and lead to cardiovascular problems. However, new research indicates that raising HDL to prevent negative CVD outcomes may not be as beneficial as once thought.[49]

Other blood lipid factors may increase CVD risk. *Lipoprotein-associated phospholipase A2 (Lp-PLA2)* is an enzyme that circulates in the blood and attaches to LDL; it plays an important role in plaque accumulation and increased risk for stroke and coronary events, particularly in men.[50] *Apolipoprotein B (apo B)* is a primary component of LDL essential for cholesterol delivery to cells. Some researchers believe apo B levels may be more important to heart disease risk than total cholesterol or LDL levels.[51]

When you consume calories, the body converts any extra to **triglycerides**, which are stored in fat cells to provide energy. High counts of blood triglycerides are often found in people who are obese or overweight or who have high cholesterol levels, heart problems, or diabetes. A baseline cholesterol test (lipid panel or lipid profile) measures triglyceride, HDL, LDL, and total cholesterol. It should be taken at age 20, with follow-ups every 5 years, then annually for men over 35 and women over 45. (See Table 5.3 for recommended levels of cholesterol and triglycerides.)

See It! Videos

What habits can you change now to improve your heart health? Watch **Importance of Heart Health** in the Study Area of MasteringHealth.

TABLE 5.3 **Recommended Cholesterol Levels for Lower/Moderate-Risk Adults**

Total Cholesterol Level (lower numbers are better)	
Less than 200 mg/dL	Desirable
200 to 239 mg/dL	Borderline high
240 mg/dL and above	High
HDL Cholesterol Level (higher numbers are better)	
Less than 40 mg/dL (for men)	Low
60 mg/dL and above	Desirable
LDL Cholesterol Level (lower numbers are better)	
Less than 100 mg/dL	Optimal
100 to 129 mg/dL	Near or above optimal
130 to 159 mg/dL	Borderline high
160 to 189 mg/dL	High
190 mg/dL and above	Very high
Triglyceride Level (lower numbers are better)	
Less than 150 mg/dL	Normal
150–199 mg/dL	Borderline high
200–499 mg/dL	High
500 mg/dL and above	Very high

Source: Adapted from ATP III Guidelines At-a-Glance Quick Desk Reference, National Heart, Lung, and Blood Institute, National Institutes of Health. Update on Cholesterol Guidelines, 2004.

How can I improve my cholesterol level?

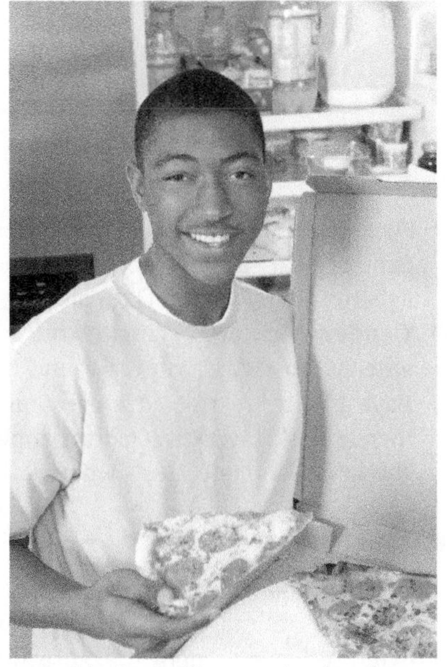

You get cholesterol from two primary sources: from your body (which involves genetic predisposition) and from food. The good news is that the 25 percent of the cholesterol you get from foods is the part where you can make real improvements in overall cholesterol profiles, even if you have a high genetic risk. Controlling your intake of saturated fats and *trans* fats will help you keep your cholesterol level in check.

In spite of all of the education on the dangers of high cholesterol, Americans continue to have higher-than-recommended levels and millions are on cholesterol-lowering drugs. Nearly 44 percent of adults age 20 and over have cholesterol levels at or above 200 mg/dL, and another 14 percent have levels in excess of 240 mg/dL.[52]

Modify Other Dietary Habits

Research continues into dietary modifications that may affect heart health. An overall approach, such as the DASH eating plan from the National Heart, Lung, and Blood Institute, has strong evidence to back up its claims of reducing CVD risk:

- Consume 5 to 10 milligrams per day of soluble fiber from sources such as oat bran, fruits, vegetables, legumes, and psyllium seeds.
- Consume about 2 grams per day of **plant sterols**, which are present in many fruits, vegetables, nuts, seeds, cereals, legumes, vegetable oils, and other plant sources.
- Eat less sodium. Excess sodium has been linked to high blood pressure, which can affect CVD risk.

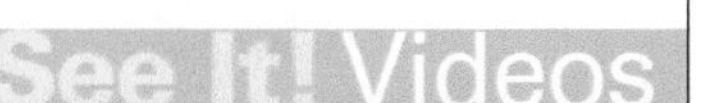

Can a way of eating reduce your risk of heart disease? Watch **Mediterranean Diet Could Help Reduce Heart Disease** in the Study Area of MasteringHealth.

Several foods, including fish high in omega-3 fatty acids, olive oil, whole grains, nuts, green tea, and dark chocolate, have been shown to reduce the chances that cholesterol will be absorbed in the cells, reduce levels of LDL cholesterol, or enhance the protective effects of HDL cholesterol.[53]

Maintain a Healthy Weight

Overweight people are more likely to develop heart disease and stroke even if they have no other risk factors. If you're heavy, losing even 5 to 10 pounds can make a significant difference.[54] This is especially true if you're an "apple" (thicker around upper body and waist) rather than a "pear" (thicker around hips and thighs).

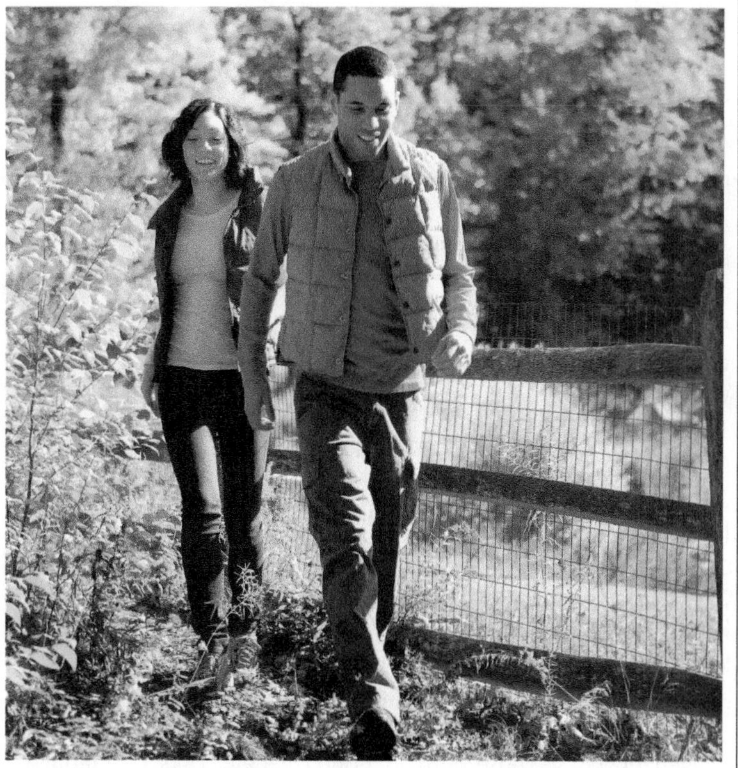

Even low-intensity activity can reduce your risk of CVD. Exercise can increase HDL, lower triglycerides, and reduce coronary risks in several ways.

Exercise Regularly

Inactivity is a definite risk factor for CVD.[55] Even light activity—walking, gardening, housework, dancing—is beneficial if done regularly and over the long term.

Control Diabetes and Blood Pressure

Heart disease death rates among adults with diabetes are two to four times higher than the rates for adults without diabetes. At least 68 percent of people with diabetes die of some form of heart disease or stroke.[56]

Although blood pressure typically creeps up with age, lifestyle changes can dramatically lower CVD risk. Among the most beneficial are losing extra pounds, cutting back on sodium, exercising more, reducing alcohol and caffeine intake, and quitting smoking.

Manage Stress Levels

Stress may trigger cardiac events or even sudden cardiac death, and it increases the risks of hypertension, stroke, and elevated cholesterol levels. Research indicates that everyday, chronic stressors can lead to increased risk of coronary events, HBP, strokes, and sudden cardiac death in much the same way as acute natural disasters do.[57]

check yourself

- **Of the risk factors described, which are of the most concern to you? What kind of changes could you make to improve in these areas?**

5.10 Reducing CVD Risk: Nonmodifiable Risks

learning outcome

5.10 Identify nonmodifiable factors affecting CVD risk.

Some risk factors for CVD cannot be prevented or controlled. Among these factors are the following:

- **Race and Ethnicity.** African Americans tend to have the highest overall rates of CVD and hypertension and the lowest rates of physical activity. The rate of high blood pressure in African Americans is among the highest in the world. Mexican Americans have the highest percentage of adults with cholesterol levels exceeding 200 mg/dL and the highest rates of obesity and overweight.[58] Figure 5.6 summarizes deaths from heart disease and stroke by ethnicity.
- **Heredity.** Family history of heart disease appears to increase CVD risk significantly. Amount of cholesterol produced, tendencies to form plaque, and a host of other factors seem to have genetic links. Those with identified genetic risks can reduce future risks through diet, exercise, or medication.

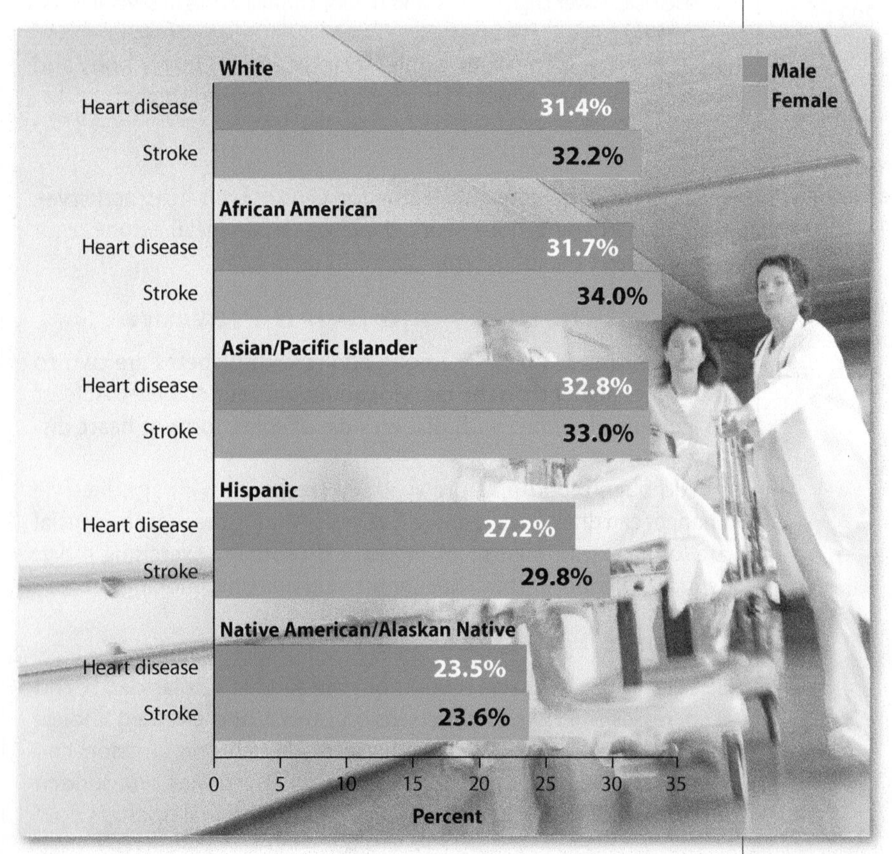

Figure 5.6 Deaths from Heart Disease and Stroke in the United States by Ethnicity

Sources: American Heart Association, "Statistics At a Glance—2014," Population Fact Sheets; A. S. Go et al., "Heart Disease and Stroke Statistics—2014 Update: A Report from the American Heart Association," *Circulation* 129 (2014):: e28–e292, Statistics, 2014, chart 13.8.

- **Age.** Although cardiovascular disease can affect all ages, 82 percent of heart attacks occur in people over age 65.[59] Increasing age ups the risk for CVD for all.
- **Gender.** Men are at greater risk for CVD until about age 60, when women catch up and then surpass them. Women under 35 have a fairly low risk, although oral contraceptives and smoking increase risk. Hormonal factors appear to reduce risk for women, though after menopause, women's LDL levels tend to rise.[60]

Inflammation and C-Reactive Protein

Inflammation—which occurs when tissues are injured, for example by bacteria, trauma, toxins, or heat—may play a major role in atherosclerosis development, because injured vessel walls are more prone to plaque formation. Cigarette smoke, high blood pressure, high LDL cholesterol, diabetes mellitus, certain forms of arthritis, and exposure to toxins have been linked to increased risk of inflammation. However, the greatest risk appears to be from infectious disease pathogens, most notably *Chlamydia pneumoniae* (a common cause of respiratory infections); *Helicobacter pylori* (a bacterium that causes ulcers); herpes simplex virus; and *cytomegalovirus* (another herpes virus infecting most Americans before age 40).

During an inflammatory reaction, C-reactive proteins (CRPs) tend to be present in blood at high levels. A recent meta-analysis shows a strong association between C-reactive proteins in the blood and increased risks for atherosclerosis and CVD.[61] Doctors can test patients using an assay called hs-CRP; if levels are high, action could be taken to prevent progression to reduce inflammation.

Homocysteine

Homocysteine, an amino acid normally present in blood, was thought to be a prelude to coronary heart disease, peripheral artery disease, and increased risk of stroke. Scientists hypothesized that homocysteine inflamed the inner lining of the arterial walls and promoted fat deposits and the development of blood clots.[62] Early studies indicated that folic acid and other B vitamins may help break down homocysteine in the body. However, professional groups such as the American Heart Association do not currently recommend taking folic acid supplements to lower homocysteine levels and prevent CVD; instead they recommend following a healthy diet.[63]

check yourself

- **Of the risk factors described, which is of the most concern to you and why?**

5.11

Diagnosing and Treating CVD

learning outcome

5.11 Describe techniques for diagnosing and treating CVD.

There are many diagnostic, treatment, prevention, and rehabilitation options for cardiovascular disease. Medications can strengthen heartbeat, control arrhythmias, remove fluids, reduce blood pressure, and improve heart function.

CVD Diagnostic Techniques

An **electrocardiogram (ECG)** is a record of the heart's electrical activity. Patients may undergo a *stress test*—exercise on a stationary bike or treadmill with an electrocardiogram—or a *nuclear stress test,* which involves injecting a radioactive dye and taking images of the heart to reveal blood flow problems. In **angiography** (*cardiac catheterization*), a thin tube called a *catheter* is threaded through heart arteries, a dye is injected, and an X-ray is taken to identify blocked areas. A **positron emission tomography (PET) scan** produces three-dimensional images of the heart as blood flows through it. In *magnetic resonance imaging (MRI)*, powerful magnets look inside the body to help identify damage, congenital defects, and disease. *Ultrafast computed tomography (CT)*, an especially fast heart X-ray, is used to evaluate bypass grafts, diagnose ventricular function, and identify irregularities. *Coronary calcium score* is derived from another type of ultrafast CT used to diagnose calcium levels in heart vessels; high levels increase risk.

Surgical Options

Coronary bypass surgery has helped many patients survive coronary blockages or heart attacks. In a coronary artery bypass graft (CABG, referred to as a "cabbage"), a blood vessel is taken from another site in the patient's body (usually the saphenous vein in the leg or the internal thoracic artery [ITA] in the chest) and implanted to "bypass" blocked coronary arteries and transport blood to heart tissue.

With an **angioplasty** (sometimes called a *balloon angioplasty*), a catheter is threaded through blocked heart arteries. The catheter has a balloon at the tip, which is inflated to flatten fatty deposits against arterial walls, allowing blood to flow more freely. New forms of laser angioplasty and *atherectomy*, a procedure that removes plaque, are done in several clinics.

Many people with heart blockage undergo angioplasty and receive a **stent**, a steel mesh tube inserted to prop open the artery. Although stents are highly effective, inflammation and tissue growth in the area may actually increase after the procedure, and in about 30 percent of patients, the treated arteries become clogged again within 6 months.[64] Newer stents are usually medicated to reduce this risk.

Drug Therapies

Although aspirin has been touted as possibly reducing risks for future heart attacks, the benefits of an aspirin regimen for otherwise healthy adults remains in question. New research indicates an increased risk of gastrointestinal bleeding and stroke in those who take it daily.[65] Furthermore, once a patient has taken aspirin regularly for possible protection against CHD, stopping this regimen may, in fact, increase his or her risk.[66]

Clot-busting therapy with **thrombolysis** can be performed within the first 1 to 3 hours after an attack. Thrombolysis involves injecting an agent such as *tissue plasminogen activator* (*tPA*) to dissolve the clot and restore some blood flow, thereby reducing the amount of tissue that dies from ischemia.[67]

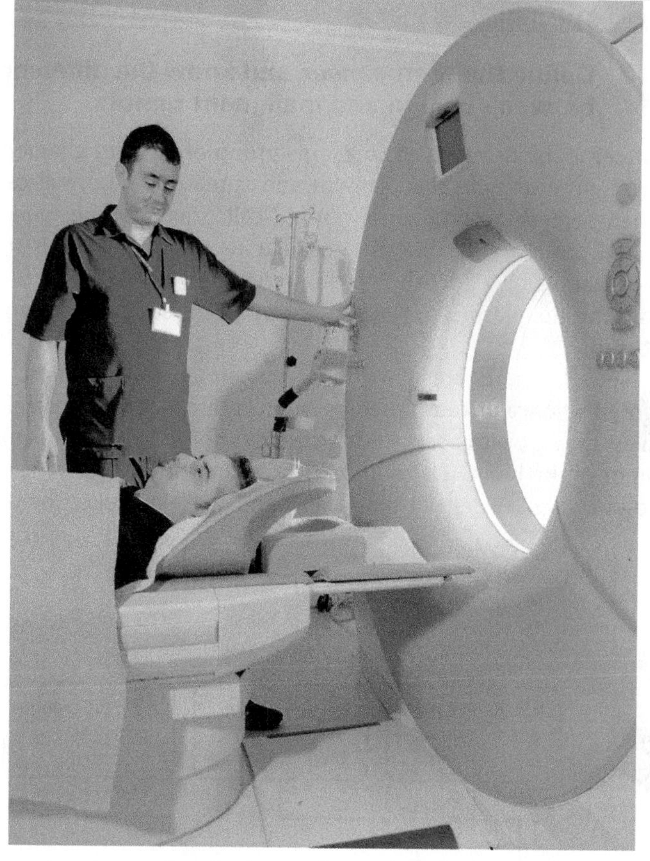

Magnetic resonance imaging is one of several methods used to detect heart damage, abnormalities, or defects.

Cardiac Rehabilitation and Recovery

Every year, more than 1 million Americans survive heart attacks. Millions more have a number of medical interventions to help them survive and thrive. Strategies for rehabilitation may include exercise training and classes on nutrition and CVD risk management. Not all patients choose to participate, due to lack of insurance, fear of another attack due to exercise, or other barriers. However, the benefits of rehabilitation far outweigh the risks.

check yourself

- **How is CVD commonly diagnosed and treated?**

5.12

What Is Cancer?

learning outcome

5.12 Define the term *cancer,* and know the difference between benign and malignant tumors.

Cancer is the name given to a large group of diseases characterized by the uncontrolled growth and spread of abnormal cells. When something interrupts normal cell programming, uncontrolled growth and abnormal cellular development result in a **neoplasm**, a new growth of tissue serving no physiological function. This neoplasmic mass often forms a clump of cells known as a **tumor**.

Not all tumors are **malignant** (cancerous); in fact, most are **benign** (noncancerous). Benign tumors are generally harmless unless they grow to obstruct or crowd out normal tissues. A benign tumor of the brain, for instance, may become life threatening if it grows enough to restrict blood flow and cause a stroke. The only way to determine whether a tumor is malignant is through **biopsy**, or microscopic examination of cell development.

Benign tumors generally consist of ordinary-looking cells enclosed in a fibrous shell or capsule that prevents their spreading to other body areas. In contrast, malignant tumors are usually not enclosed in a protective capsule and can therefore spread to other organs (Figure 5.7). This process, known as **metastasis**, makes some forms of cancer particularly aggressive in their ability to overwhelm bodily defenses. Malignant tumors frequently metastasize throughout the body, making treatment extremely difficult. Unlike benign tumors, which merely expand to take over a given space, malignant cells invade surrounding tissue, emitting clawlike protrusions that disturb the RNA and DNA within normal cells. Disrupting these substances, which control cellular metabolism and reproduction, produces **mutant cells** that differ in form, quality, and function from normal cells.

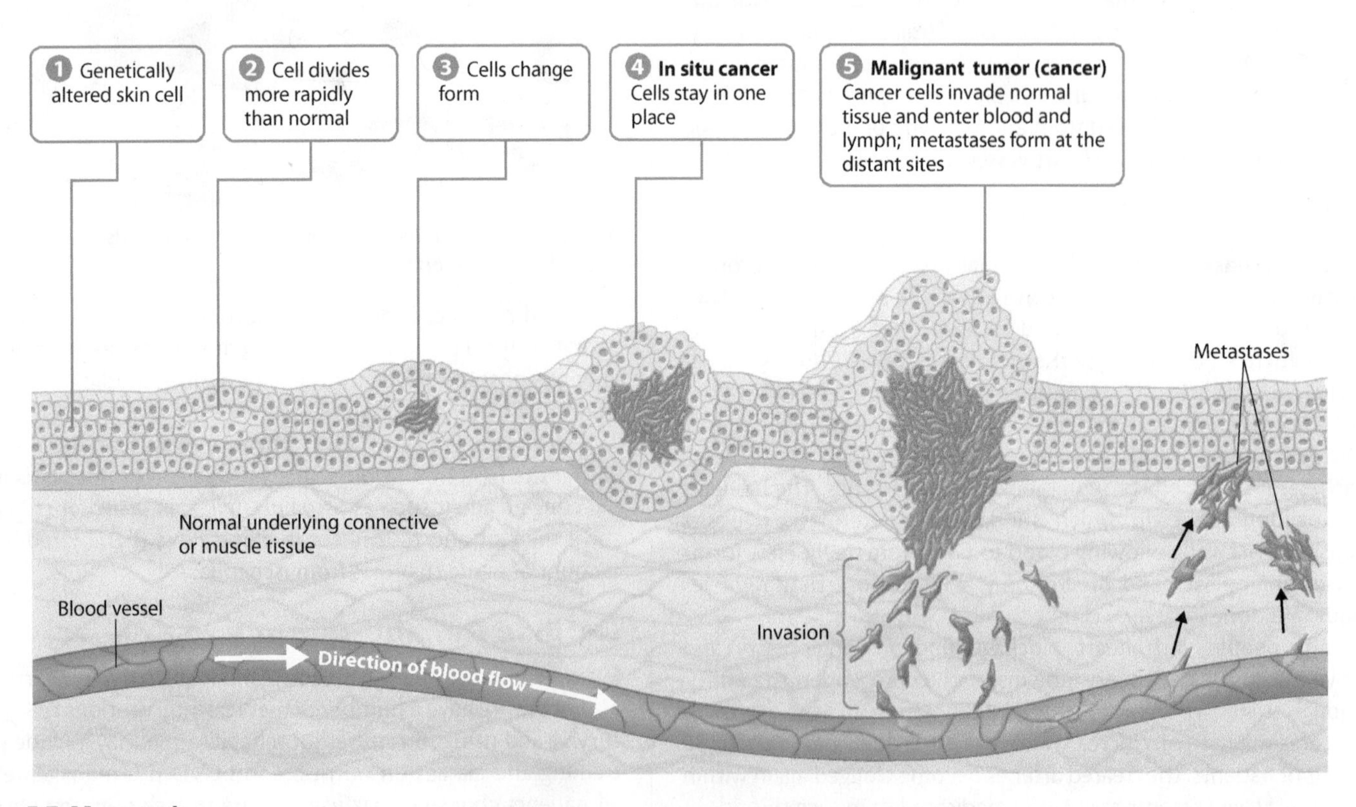

Figure 5.7 Metastasis
A mutation to the genetic material of a skin cell triggers abnormal cell division and changes cell formation, resulting in a cancerous tumor. If the tumor remains localized, it is considered in situ cancer. If the tumor spreads, it is considered a malignant cancer.

VIDEO TUTOR
Metastasis

check yourself

- **What is cancer?**
- **What is the difference between benign and malignant tumors?**

5.13 Types and Sites of Cancer

learning outcome

5.13 List the major types and most common sites of cancer.

The word *cancer* refers not to a single disease, but to hundreds of different diseases. They are grouped into four broad categories based on the type of tissue from which the cancer arises:

- **Carcinomas.** Epithelial tissues (tissues covering body surfaces and lining most body cavities) are the most common sites for cancers; cancers occurring in epithelial tissue are called *carcinomas*. These cancers affect the outer layer of the skin and mouth as well as the mucous membranes. They metastasize initially through the circulatory or lymphatic system and form solid tumors.
- **Sarcomas.** Sarcomas occur in the mesodermal, or middle, layers of tissue—for example, in bones, muscles, and general connective tissue. In the early stages of disease, they metastasize primarily via the blood. These cancers are less common but generally more virulent than carcinomas. They also form solid tumors.
- **Lymphomas.** Lymphomas develop in the lymphatic system—the infection-fighting regions of the body—and metastasize through the lymphatic system. Hodgkin's disease is an example. Lymphomas also form solid tumors.
- **Leukemias.** Cancer of the blood-forming parts of the body, particularly the bone marrow and spleen, is called leukemia. A nonsolid tumor, leukemia is characterized by an abnormal increase in the number of white blood cells that the body produces.

Figure 5.8 shows the most common sites of cancer and the estimated number of new cases and deaths from each type in 2011.

Estimated New Cases of Cancer*		Estimated Deaths from Cancer*	
Female	**Male**	**Female**	**Male**
Breast 232,670 (29%)	Prostate 232,670 (29%)	Lung & bronchus 72,330 (26%)	Lung & bronchus 86,930 (28%)
Lung & bronchus 108,210 (13%)	Lung & bronchus 108,210 (13%)	Breast 40,000 (15%)	Prostate 29,480 (10%)
Colon & rectum 65,000 (8%)	Colon & rectum 71,830 (9%)	Colon & rectum 24,040 (9%)	Colon & rectum 26,270 (8%)
Uterine corpus 52,630 (6%)	Urinary bladder 56,390 (7%)	Pancreas 19,420 (7%)	Pancreas 20,170 (7%)
Thyroid 47,790 (6%)	Melanoma of the skin 43,890 (5%)	Ovary 14,270 (5%)	Liver & intrahepatic bile duct 15,870 (5%)
Non-Hodgkin lymphoma 32,530 (4%)	Kidney & renal pelvis 39,140 (5%)	Leukemia 10,050 (4%)	Leukemia 14,040 (5%)
Melanoma of the skin 32,210 (4%)	Non-Hodgkin lymphoma 38,270 (4%)	Uterine corpus 8,590 (3%)	Esophagus 12,450 (4%)
Kidney & renal pelvis 24,780 (3%)	Oral cavity & pharynx 30,220 (4%)	Non-Hodgkin lymphoma 8,520 (3%)	Urinary bladder 11,170 (4%)
Pancreas 22,890 (3%)	Leukemia 30,100 (4%)	Liver & intrahepatic bile duct 7,130 (3%)	Non-Hodgkin lymphoma 10,470 (3%)
Leukemia 22,280 (3%)	Pancreas 22,289 (3%)	Brain & other nervous system 6,230 (2%)	Kidney & renal pelvis 8,900 (3%)
All Sites 810,320 (100%)	All Sites 855,220 (100%)	All Sites 275,370 (100%)	All Sites 310,010 (100%)

*Excludes basal and squamous cell skin cancers and in situ carcinoma except urinary bladder. Percentages may not total 100% due to rounding.

Figure 5.8 Leading Sites of New Cancer Cases and Deaths, 2014 Estimates

Source: Data from Table on page 4, American Cancer Society, *Cancer Facts & Figures 2014* (Atlanta, GA: American Cancer Society, Inc.). Note that percentages do not add up to 100 due to omissions of certain rare cancers as well as rounding of statistics.

check yourself

- **What are the major types of cancer?**
- **What sites are the most common sites of cancer?**

5.14 Risk Factors for Cancer

learning outcome

5.14 List lifestyle, genetic, environmental, and medical risk factors for cancer.

Specific risk factors for cancer fall into two major classes: hereditary risk and acquired (environmental) risk. Hereditary factors cannot be modified, whereas environmental factors are potentially modifiable.

Lifestyle Risks for Cancer

Anyone can develop cancer; however, nearly 77 percent of cancers are diagnosed at age 55 and above.[68] *Lifetime risk* refers to the probability that an individual, over the course of a lifetime, will develop cancer or die from it. In the United States, men have a lifetime risk of about 1 in 2 and women 1 in 3.[69]

Relative risk is a measure of the strength of the relationship between risk factors and a particular cancer. For example, a male smoker's relative risk of getting lung cancer is about twice that of a male nonsmoker.[70]

Tobacco Use Of all the risk factors for cancer, smoking is among the greatest. In the United States, tobacco is responsible for nearly 1 in 5 deaths annually, or about 443,000 premature deaths each year.[71] Smoking is associated with increased risk of at least 15 different cancers, including causal relationships between smoking and liver cancer, colorectal polyps, and colorectal cancer.[72] Smoking accounts for 30 percent of all cancer deaths and 87 percent of all lung cancer deaths in the United States.[73] Chances of developing cancer are 23 times higher among male smokers and 13 times higher among female smokers, compared to nonsmokers.[74]

Of the several lifestyle risk factors for cancer, tobacco use is perhaps the most significant and the most preventable.

Alcohol and Cancer Risk Countless studies have implicated alcohol as a risk factor for cancer. Light to moderate alcohol intake (more than one drink per day) appears to increase risk of breast cancer among women.[75] Moderate alcohol intake (above one drink per day) in women also appears to increase the risk of cancers of the oral cavity and pharynx, esophagus, and larynx, and binge drinking may increase gastric and pancreatic cancer risk.[76] For men, regular heavy consumption of alcohol appears to increase the risk of esophageal and liver cancers more than sevenfold. The risk of colon, stomach, and prostate cancers in men was about 80 percent higher among heavy drinkers, while lung cancer risk rose by almost 60 percent compared to nondrinkers.[77]

Poor Nutrition, Physical Inactivity, and Obesity About one-third of U.S. cancer deaths may be due to lifestyle factors such as overweight or obesity, physical inactivity, and nutrition.[78] Dietary choices and physical activity are the most important modifiable determinants of cancer risk (besides not smoking). Several studies indicate a relationship between high body mass index (BMI) and death rates for cancers of the esophagus, colon, rectum, liver, stomach, kidney, and pancreas, and others.[79] Women who gain 55 pounds or more after age 18 have almost a 50 percent greater risk of breast cancer compared to those who maintain their weight.[80] The relative risk of colon cancer in men is 40 percent higher for obese men than for nonobese men. Numerous other studies support the link between cancer and obesity.[81]

Stress and Psychosocial Risks People who are under chronic, severe stress or who suffer from depression or other persistent emotional problems show higher rates of cancer than their healthy counterparts. Sleep disturbances or an unhealthy diet may weaken the body's immune system, increasing susceptibility to cancer. Another possible contributor to cancer development is poverty and the health disparities associated with low socioeconomic status.

Genetic and Physiological Risks

Scientists believe that about 5 percent of all cancers are strongly hereditary; some people may be more predisposed to the malfunctioning of genes that ultimately cause cancer.[82]

Suspected cancer-causing genes are called **oncogenes**. Though these genes are typically dormant, certain conditions such as age; stress; and exposure to carcinogens, viruses, and radiation may activate them, causing cells to grow and reproduce uncontrollably. Scientists are uncertain whether only people who develop cancer have oncogenes or whether we all have genes that can become oncogenes under certain conditions.

Certain cancers, particularly those of the breast, stomach, colon, prostate, uterus, ovaries, and lungs, appear to run in families. Hodgkin's disease and certain leukemias show similar familial patterns. Can we attribute these patterns to genetic susceptibility or to the fact that people in the same families experience similar environmental risks? The complex interaction of hereditary predisposition, lifestyle, and environment makes it a challenge to determine a single cause. Even among those predisposed to mutations, avoiding risks may decrease chances of cancer development.

Reproductive and Hormonal Factors Increased numbers of fertile years (early menarche, late menopause), not having children or having them later in life, recent use of birth control pills or hormone replacement therapy, and opting not to breast-feed all appear to increase risks of breast cancer.[83] However, although these factors appear to play a significant role in increased risk for non-Hispanic white women, they do not appear to have as strong an influence on Hispanic women.[84] Although earlier studies suggested that hormone therapy may slightly increase the risk of lung cancer, newer research has shown no significant increases due to hormone therapy.[85]

Inflammation Risks

Inflammatory processes in the body are thought to play a significant role in the development of cancer—from initiation and promoting cancer cells to paving the way for them to invade, spread, and weaken the immune response.[86] According to some researchers, 90 percent of cancers are caused by cellular mutations and environmental factors that occur as a result of inflammation. These researchers believe that up to 20 percent of cancers are the result of chronic infections, 30 percent are the result of tobacco smoking and inhaled particulates such as asbestos, and 35 percent are due to dietary factors.[87]

Occupational and Environmental Risks

Though workplace hazards account for only a small percentage of all cancers, several substances are known to cause cancer when exposure levels are high or prolonged. Asbestos, nickel, chromate, benzene, arsenic, and vinyl chloride are **carcinogens** (cancer-causing agents), as are certain dyes and radioactive substances, coal tars, inhalants, and possibly some herbicides and pesticides.

Radiation Ionizing radiation (IR)—radiation from X-rays, radon, cosmic rays, and ultraviolet radiation (primarily UVB radiation)—is the only form of radiation proven to cause human cancer. Virtually any part of the body can be affected by IR, but bone marrow and the thyroid are particularly susceptible. Radon exposure in homes can increase lung cancer risk, especially in cigarette smokers. To reduce the risk of harmful effects, diagnostic medical and dental X-rays are set at the lowest dose levels possible.

Nonionizing radiation produced by radio waves, cell phones, microwaves, computer screens, televisions, electric blankets, and other products has been a topic of great concern in recent years, though research has not proven excess risk to date.

Chemicals in Foods Much of the concern about chemicals in food centers on possible harm from pesticide and herbicide residue. Continued research regarding pesticide and herbicide use is essential, and scientists and consumer groups stress the importance of a balance between chemical use and the production of high-quality food products.

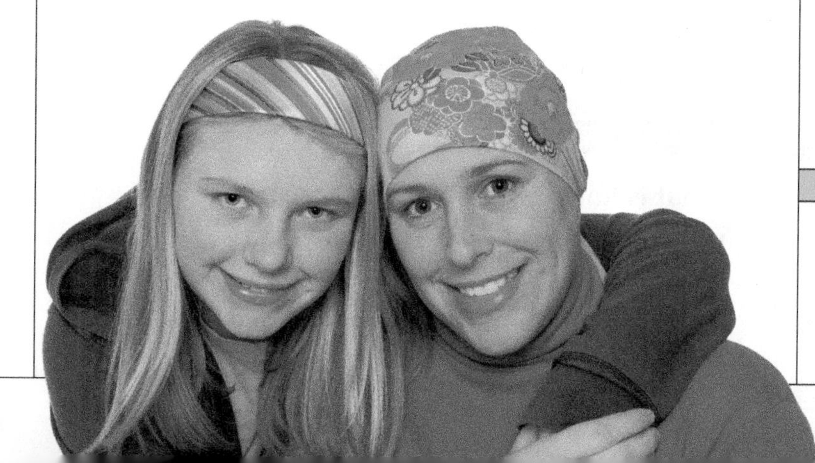

Some forms of cancer have strong genetic bases; daughters of women with breast cancer have an increased risk of developing the disease.

Infectious Disease Risks

Over 10 percent of all cancers in the United States are caused by infectious agents such as viruses, bacteria, or parasites.[88] Worldwide, approximately 15–20 percent of human cancers have been traced to infectious agents.[89] Infections are thought to influence cancer development in several ways, most commonly through chronic inflammation, suppression of the immune system, or chronic stimulation.

Hepatitis B, Hepatitis C, and Liver Cancer Viruses such as the ones that cause chronic forms of hepatitis B (HBV) and C (HCV) chronically inflame liver tissue, which may make it more hospitable for cancer development.

Human Papillomavirus and Cervical Cancer Between 70 and 100 percent of women with cervical cancer have evidence of human papillomavirus (HPV) infection, which is also believed to be a cause of vaginal and vulvar cancers in women and penile cancers in men. A vaccine is available to help protect men and women from becoming infected with HPV. The vaccine seems to be effective in reducing risks of cervical and penile cancer.[90]

***Helicobacter pylori* and Stomach Cancer** *Helicobacter pylori* is a bacterium found in the stomach lining of approximately 30 to 40 percent of Americans. It causes irritation, scarring, and ulcers, damaging the lining of the stomach and leading to cellular changes that may lead to cancer. More than half of all cases of stomach cancer may be linked to *H. pylori* infection, even though most infected people don't develop cancer.[91] Treatment with antibiotics often cures the ulcers, which appears to reduce risk of new stomach cancer.[92]

Medical Factors

Some medical treatments can increase a person's risk for cancer. The use of estrogen for relieving women's menopausal symptoms is now recognized to have contributed to multiple cancer risks; hence prescriptions for estrogen therapy have declined dramatically. Some chemotherapy drugs have been shown to increase risks for other cancers; weighing the benefits versus harms of these treatments is always necessary.

check yourself

- **What are some major lifestyle, genetic, environmental, and medical risk factors for cancer?**
- **What are your risks for cancer? What lifestyle changes can you make to mitigate these risks?**

5.15 Lung Cancer

learning outcome

5.15 Identify the major factors contributing to lung cancer.

Lung cancer is the leading cause of cancer deaths for both men and women in the United States. It killed an estimated 160,000 Americans in 2014, accounting for nearly 27 percent of all cancer deaths.[93] The lifetime risks for males and females getting lung cancer is 1 in 13 and 1 in 16, respectively. Risks begin to rise around age 40 and continue to climb through all age groups thereafter.[94]

Since 1987, more women have died each year from lung cancer than from breast cancer, which over the previous 40 years was the major cause of cancer deaths in women. Although lower smoking rates have boded well for cancer statistics, there is growing concern about the number of young people, particularly women and persons of low income and low educational levels, who continue to pick up the habit.

There is also concern about increase in lung cancers among *never smokers*—people who have never smoked, but nevertheless have as many as 15 percent of all lung cancers. Never smokers' lung cancer is believed to be related to exposure to secondhand smoke, radon gas, asbestos, indoor wood-burning stoves, and aerosolized oils caused by cooking with oil and deep fat frying.[95] Unfortunately, because doctors often don't think of lung cancer when a never smoker presents with a cough, patients are often put on antibiotics or cough suppressants as therapy. By the time they recognize that it's really lung cancer, their cancer is likely to be more advanced and treatment more challenging.

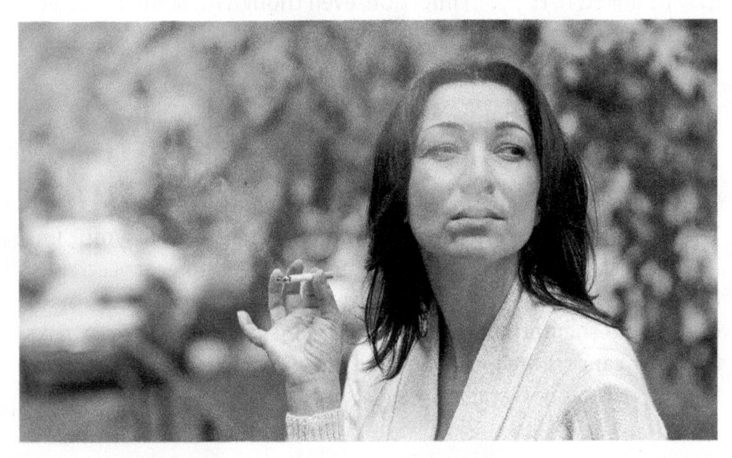

If my mom quits smoking now, will it reduce her risk of cancer, or is it too late?

It's never too late to quit. Stopping smoking at any time will reduce your risk of lung cancer, in addition to the numerous other health benefits that are gained. Studies of women have shown that within 5 years of quitting, their risk of death from lung cancer had decreased by 21 percent, when compared with people who had continued smoking.

90%

of all lung cancers could be avoided if people did not smoke.

Detection, Symptoms, and Treatment

Symptoms of lung cancer include a persistent cough, blood-streaked sputum, voice change, chest pain or back pain, and recurrent attacks of pneumonia or bronchitis. Newer computerized tomography (CT) scans, molecular markers in saliva, and newer biopsy techniques have improved screening accuracy for lung cancer but have a long way to go.

Treatment depends on type and stage of cancer. Surgery, radiation therapy, chemotherapy, and targeted biological therapies are all options. If the cancer is localized, surgery is usually the treatment of choice. If it has spread, surgery is combined with radiation, chemotherapy and other targeted drug treatments. Fewer than 15 percent of lung cancer cases are diagnosed at the early, localized stages. Early stage cancers have a 54 percent 1-year survival rate, falling to 6–18 percent at 5 years after diagnosis.[96]

Risk Factors and Prevention

Risks for cancer increase dramatically based on the quantity of cigarettes smoked and the number of years smoked, often referred to as *pack years*. The greater the number of pack years smoked, the greater the risk of developing cancer. Quitting smoking does reduce the risk of developing lung cancer.[97] Exposure to industrial substances or radiation also highly increases the risk for lung cancer.

check yourself

- **What is lung cancer, and what are its causes?**
- **What can you do to protect yourself against lung cancer?**
- **What are the symptoms and treatment of lung cancer?**

Colon and Rectal Cancers

learning outcome

5.16 Identify the major factors contributing to colorectal cancer.

Colorectal cancers (cancers of the colon and rectum) continue to be the third most commonly diagnosed cancer in both men and women and the third leading cause of cancer deaths, even though death rates are declining.[98] In 2014, there were 96,830 cases of colon cancer and 40,000 cases of rectal cancer diagnosed in the United States, as well as 50,310 deaths.[99] Ninety percent of colorectal cancers occur in individuals who are over the age of 50. From birth to age 49, men have a 1 in 305 risk of developing it, while women have a 1 in 334 chance.[100]

Detection, Symptoms, and Treatment

Because colorectal cancer tends to spread slowly, the prognosis is quite good if it is caught in the early stages. In fact, when caught at an early, localized stage, 5-year survival rates are over 90 percent.[101] But in its early stages, colorectal cancer typically has no symptoms. As the disease progresses, bleeding from the rectum, blood in the stool, and changes in bowel habits are the major warning signals.

An excellent way to catch such cancers early is through testing. Colonoscopies and other screening tests should begin at age 50 for most people. Virtual colonoscopies and fecal DNA testing are newer diagnostic techniques that have shown promise. However, only 10 percent of all Americans over age 50 have had the most basic screening test—the at-home *fecal occult blood* test (FBOT)—in the past year, and slightly over 50 percent have had an endoscopy test.[102] Only 59 percent of those over age 50 who should be screened actually get screened, and Hispanics and non-English-speaking individuals have even lower rates of screening.[103]

Treatment often consists of radiation or surgery. Chemotherapy, although not used extensively in the past, is today a possibility.

Risk Factors and Prevention

Anyone can get colorectal cancer, but people who are older than age 50, who are obese, who have a family history of colon and rectal cancer, who have a personal or family history of polyps (benign growths) in the colon or rectum, or who have inflammatory bowel problems such as colitis run an increased risk. A history of diabetes also seems to increase risk. Other possible risk factors include diets high in fat or low in fiber, high consumption of red and processed meats, smoking, sedentary lifestyle, high alcohol consumption, and low intake of fruits and vegetables. New research shows an alarming increase in colorectal cancer among young adults. If these trends continue, we may see a 90% increase in incidence among those 20–34 years old between 2010 and 2030.[104]

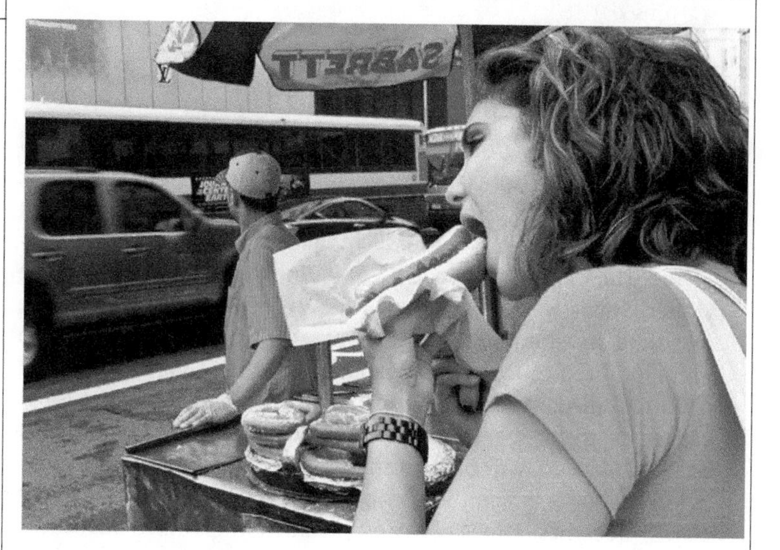

The consumption of red meat and processed meats is a risk factor for colorectal cancer, as is obesity. Food additives, particularly sodium nitrate, are used to preserve and give color to red meat and to protect against pathogens, particularly *Clostridium botulinum*, the bacterium that causes botulism. Concern about the carcinogenic properties of nitrates, which are often used in hot dogs, hams, and luncheon meats, has led to the introduction of meats that are nitrate-free or contain reduced levels of the substance.

Regular exercise, a diet with lots of fruits and other plant foods, a healthy weight, and moderation in alcohol consumption appear to be among the most promising prevention strategies. Consumption of milk and calcium also appears to decrease risks. New research suggests that nonsteroidal anti-inflammatory drugs (NSAIDs) such as aspirin, postmenopausal hormones, folic acid, calcium supplements, selenium, and vitamin E may also help.[105]

check yourself

- **What is colorectal cancer, and what are its causes?**
- **What can you do to protect against colorectal cancer?**

5.17 Breast Cancer

learning outcome

5.17 Identify the major factors contributing to breast cancer.

Breast cancer is a group of diseases that cause uncontrolled cell growth in breast tissue, particularly in the glands that produce milk and the ducts that connect those glands to the nipple. Cancers can also form in the connective and lymphatic tissues of the breast.

In 2014, approximately 232,679 women and 2,360 men in the United States were diagnosed with invasive breast cancer for the first time. In addition, 63,570 new cases of in situ breast cancer, a more localized cancer, were diagnosed. About 40,430 women (and 430 men) died, making breast cancer the second leading cause of cancer death for women.[106] Women have a 1 in 8 lifetime risk of being diagnosed with breast cancer. From birth to age 49, the risk is 1 in 53, but between the ages of 50 and 59, the chance for breast cancer becomes 1 in 43.[107] Most health groups have advocated screening for breast cancer more thoroughly after age 40.

Detection

The earliest signs of breast cancer are usually observable on mammograms, often before lumps can be felt. However, mammograms are not foolproof, and there is debate regarding the optimal age at which women should start regularly receiving them. Hence, regular breast self-examination (BSE) is also important (see below for information on BSE). Although not recommended as a screening tool per se, a newer form of magnetic resonance imaging (MRI) appears to be even more accurate, particularly in women with genetic risks for tumors or those who have suspicious areas of the breast or surrounding tissue that warrant a clearer image. If you are referred for a breast MRI, be sure to go to a facility where they can perform a breast biopsy if there are any areas that need further investigation.[108]

Symptoms

If breast cancer grows large enough, it can produce the following symptoms: a lump in the breast or surrounding lymph nodes, thickening, dimpling, skin irritation, distortion, retraction or scaliness of the nipple, nipple discharge, or tenderness.

Breast Awareness and Self-Exam

Breast self-exam has been recommended by major health organizations as a form of early breast cancer screening for the last two decades (Figure 5.9). However, a 2009 "study of studies" done by the U.S. Preventive Services Task Force determined that breast self-exams did not decrease suffering and death and, in fact, often lead to unnecessary worry, unnecessary tests, and increased health care costs. As a result of this research, several groups have downgraded the recommendation about BSE from "do them and do them regularly" to "learn how to do them, and if you desire, do them to know your body and be able to recognize changes."

To do a breast self-exam, begin by standing in front of a mirror to inspect the breasts, looking for their usual symmetry. Some breasts are not symmetrical, and if this is not a change, it is okay. Raise and lower both arms while checking that the breasts move evenly and freely. Next, inspect the skin, looking for areas of redness, thickening, or dimpling, which might have the appearance of an orange peel. Look for any scaling on the nipple.

To feel for lumps, raise one arm above your head while either standing or lying. This will flatten out the breast, making it easier to feel the tissue. Using the index, middle, and fourth fingers of your opposite hand, gently push down on the breast tissue and move the fingers in small circular motions, varying pressure from light to more firm. Start at

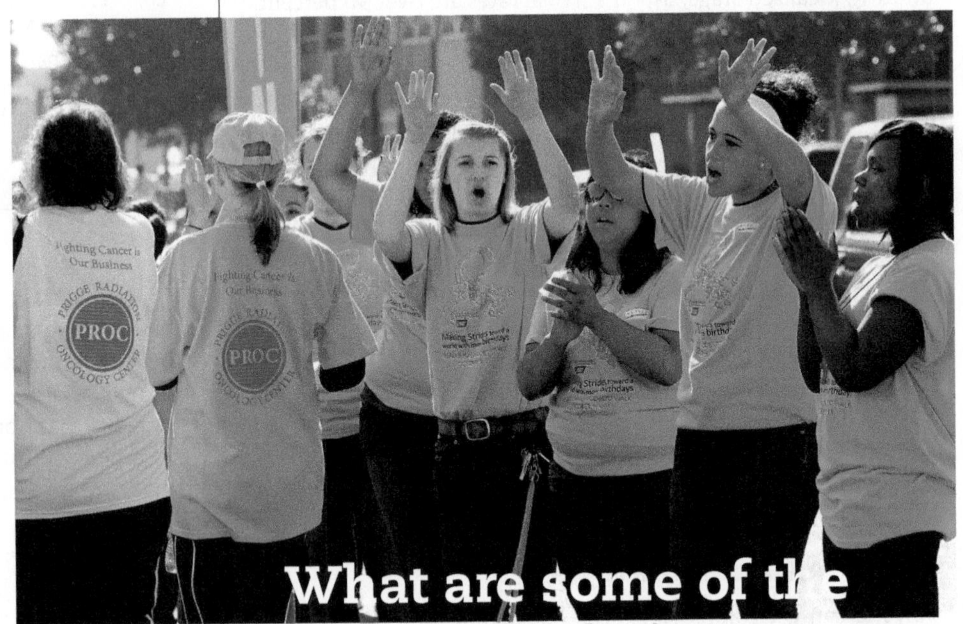

What are some of the challenges facing cancer survivors?

The journey through cancer survivorship is not always smooth. Even after the 5-year benchmark is reached, living a full, positive life in cancer's wake can be a major challenge. There may be physical, emotional, and financial issues to cope with for years after diagnosis and treatment. Survivors may find themselves struggling with access to health insurance and life insurance, financial strains, difficulties with employment, and the toll on personal relationships. Survivors also have to live with the possibility of a recurrence. However, cancer survivors can and do live active, productive lives despite these challenges.

one edge of the breast and move upward and then downward, working your way across the breast until all of the breast tissue has been covered. Often, breast tissue will feel dense and irregular, and this is usually normal. It helps to do regular self-exams to become familiar with what your breast tissue feels like; then, if there is a change, you will notice. Cancers usually feel like a dense or firm little rock and are very different from the normal breast tissue.

Next, lower the arm and reach into the top of the underarm and pull downward with gentle pressure feeling for any enlarged lymph nodes. To complete the exam, squeeze the tissue around the nipple. If you notice discharge from the nipple and you have not recently been breastfeeding, consult your doctor. Likewise, if you notice any asymmetry, skin changes, scaling on the nipple, or new lumps in the breast, you should see your doctor for evaluation.

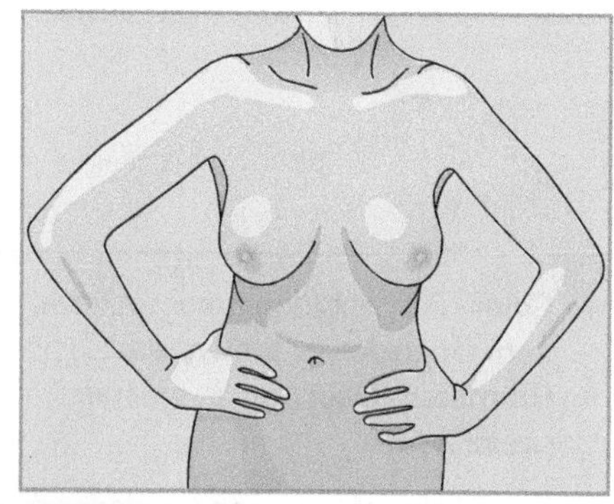

1 Face a mirror and check for changes in symmetry.

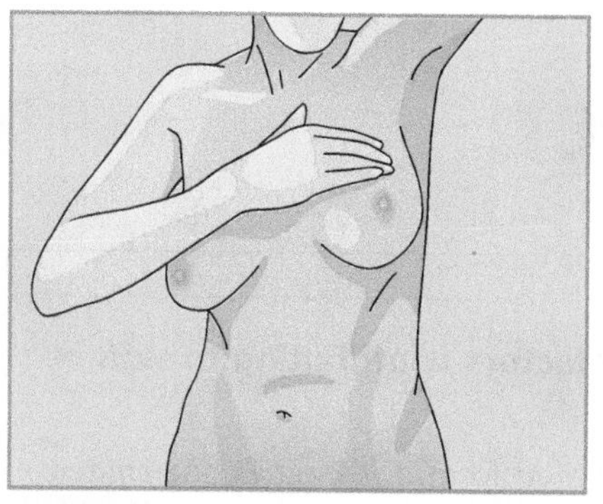

2 Either standing or lying down, use the pads of the three middle fingers to check for lumps. Follow an up and down pattern on the breast to ensure all tissue gets inspected.

Figure 5.9 Breast Self-Examination

Treatment

Treatments range from a lumpectomy to radical mastectomy to various combinations of radiation or chemotherapy. Among nonsurgical options, promising results have been noted among women using *selective estrogen-receptor modulators* (*SERMs*) such as tamoxifen and raloxifene, particularly among women whose cancers appear to grow in response to estrogen. These drugs, as well as new *aromatase inhibitors*, work by blocking estrogen. The 5-year survival rate for people with localized breast cancer has risen from 80 percent in the 1950s to 99 percent today.[109] However, these statistics vary dramatically, based on the stage of the cancer when it is first detected and whether it has spread. If the cancer has spread to the lymph nodes or other organs, the 5-year survival rate drops to as low as 24 percent.[110]

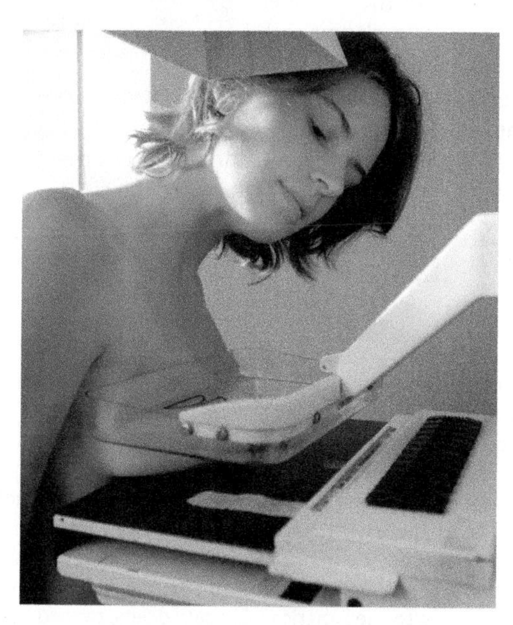

Early detection through mammography and other techniques greatly increase a woman's chance of surviving breast cancer.

Risk Factors and Prevention

The incidence of breast cancer increases with age. Although there are many possible risk factors, those well supported by research include family history of breast cancer, menstrual periods that started early and ended late in life, weight gain after the age of 18, obesity after menopause, recent use of oral contraceptives or postmenopausal hormone therapy, never bearing children or bearing a first child after age 30, consuming two or more drinks of alcohol per day, and physical inactivity. In addition, there is new evidence that heavy smoking, particularly among women who started smoking before their first pregnancy, increases risk. Other factors that increase risk include having dense breasts, type 2 diabetes, high bone mineral density, and exposure to high-dose radiation.[111] Although the *BRCA1* and *BRCA2* gene mutations are rare and occur in less than 1 percent of the population, they account for approximately 5 to 10 percent of all cases of breast cancer.[112] Women who possess these genes have up to an 80 percent risk of developing breast cancer in their lives and tend to develop breast cancer at earlier ages. Because these genes are rare, routine screening for them is not recommended unless there is a strong family history (particularly among younger primary relatives) of breast cancer.[113]

See It! Videos

Could you have inherited breast cancer from a female relative? Watch **Breast Cancer Patients Getting Younger** in the Study Area of MasteringHealth.

International differences in breast cancer incidence correlate with variations in diet, especially fat intake, although a causal role for these dietary factors has not been firmly established. Sudden weight gain has also been implicated. Research also shows that regular exercise can reduce risk.[114] Research indicates if you eat more fiber, breast cancer rates seem to go down, and if you eat less, rates seem to increase.[115]

check yourself

- **What is breast cancer, and what are its causes?**
- **What can you do to protect against breast cancer?**

5.18 Skin Cancer

learning outcome

5.18 Identify the major factors contributing to skin cancer.

Skin cancer is the most common form of cancer in the United States today, with over 3.5 million diagnosed cases in 2014.[116] Millions more remain undiagnosed and untreated, and 1 in 5 people in the United States will be diagnosed in their lifetime. In 2014, an estimated 12,980 deaths from skin cancer will occur, 9,710 from melanoma and 3,370 from other skin cancers.[117]

The two most common types of skin cancer—basal cell and squamous cell carcinomas—are highly curable. **Malignant melanoma**, the third most common form of skin cancer, is the most deadly. The majority of these deaths are in white men over the age of 50, with only rare cases among African Americans. Between 65 and 90 percent of melanomas are caused by exposure to ultraviolet (UV) light or sunlight.[118]

Detection, Symptoms, and Treatment

Basal and squamous cell carcinomas show up most commonly on the face, ears, neck, arms, hands, and legs as warty bumps, colored spots, or scaly patches. Bleeding, itchiness, pain, or oozing are other symptoms that warrant attention. Although surgery may be necessary to remove these, they are seldom life threatening.

In striking contrast is melanoma, an invasive killer that may appear as a skin lesion. Typically, the lesion's size, shape, or color changes and it spreads to regional organs and throughout the body. Malignant melanomas account for over 75 percent of all skin cancer deaths. Figure 5.10 shows melanoma compared to basal cell and squamous cell carcinomas. The *ABCD* rule can help you remember the warning signs of melanoma:

- **Asymmetry.** One half of the mole or lesion does not match the other half.
- **Border irregularity.** The edges are uneven, notched, or scalloped.
- **Color.** Pigmentation is not uniform. Melanomas may vary in color from tan to deeper brown, reddish black, black, or deep bluish black.
- **Diameter.** Diameter is greater than 6 millimeters (about the size of a pea).

Treatment of skin cancer depends on the type of cancer, its stage, and its location. Surgery, laser treatments, topical chemical agents, *electrodessication* (tissue destruction by heat), and *cryosurgery* (tissue destruction by freezing) are common treatments. For melanoma, treatment may involve surgical removal of the regional lymph nodes, radiation, or chemotherapy.

Risk Factors and Prevention

Anyone who overexposes himself or herself to ultraviolet (UV) radiation without adequate protection is at risk for skin cancer. The risk is greatest for people who:

- Have fair skin; blonde, red, or light brown hair; blue, green, or gray eyes
- Always burn before tanning, or burn easily and peel readily
- Don't tan easily but spend lots of time outdoors
- Use no or low-SPF (sun protection factor) sunscreens or expired suntan lotions
- Have had skin cancer or have a family history of skin cancer
- Experienced severe sunburns during childhood

Preventing skin cancer is a matter of limiting exposure to harmful UV rays. Upon exposure, the skin responds by increasing its thickness and the number of pigment cells (melanocytes), which produce the "tan" look. Ultraviolet light damages the skin's immune cells, lowering the normal immune protection of skin and priming it for cancer. Photodamage also causes wrinkling by impairing collagens that keep skin soft and pliable.

See It! Videos

Is there such a thing as a "safe" tan? Watch **Extreme Tanning** in the Study Area of MasteringHealth.

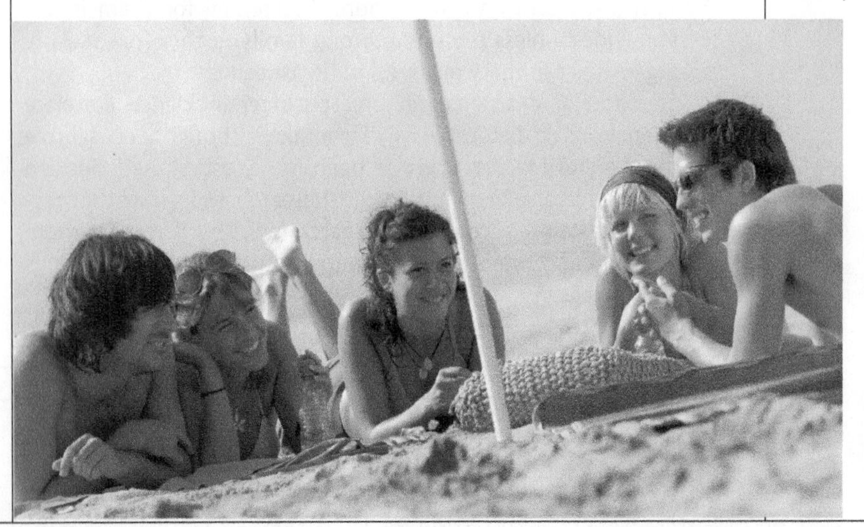

Is there any safe way to get a tan?

Unfortunately, no. There is no such thing as a "safe" tan, because a tan is visible evidence of UV-induced skin damage. The injury accumulated through years of tanning contributes to premature aging, as well as increasing your risk for disfiguring forms of skin cancer, eye problems, and possible death from melanoma. Whether the UV rays causing your tan came from the sun or from a tanning bed, the damage—and the cancer risk—is the same. Nor is an existing "base tan" protective against further damage. According to the American Cancer Society, tanned skin can provide only about the equivalent of sun protection factor (SPF) 4 sunscreen—much too weak to be considered protective.

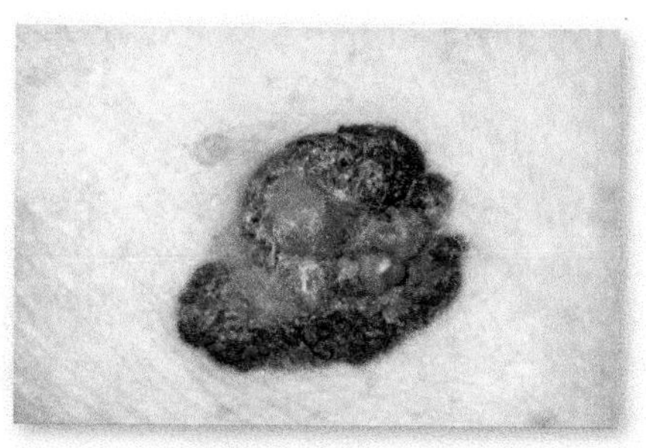

ⓐ Malignant melanoma

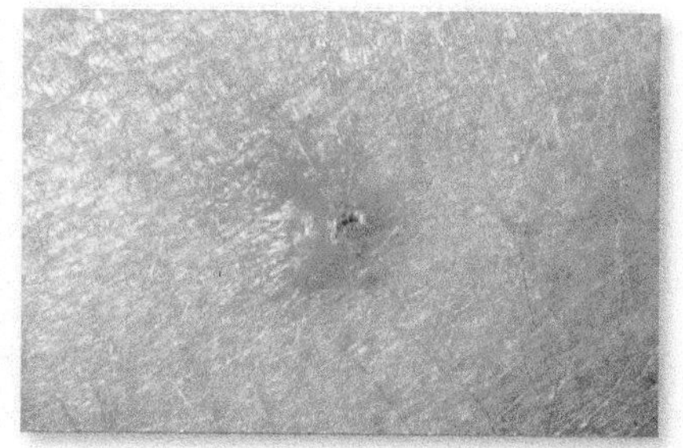

ⓑ Basal cell carcinoma

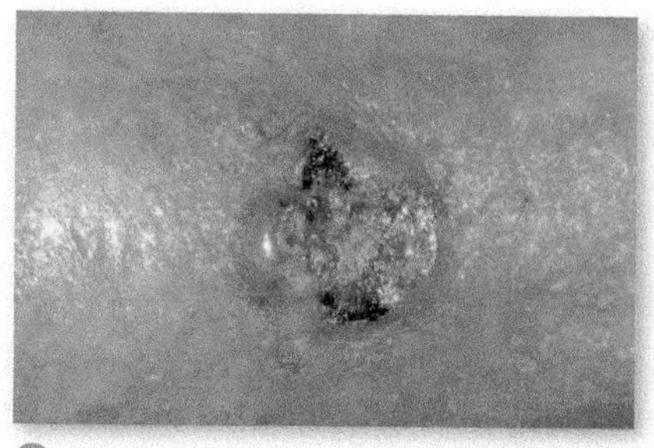

ⓒ Squamous cell carcinoma

Figure 5.10 Types of Skin Cancers

Preventing skin cancer includes keeping a careful watch for any new, pigmented growths and for changes to any moles. The ABCD warning signs of melanoma (a) include *asymmetrical* shapes, irregular *borders*, *color* variation, and an increase in *diameter*. Basal cell carcinoma (b) and squamous cell carcinoma (c) should be brought to your physician's attention but are not as deadly as melanoma.

Artificial Tans: Sacrificing Health for Beauty

In spite of the risks, many Americans strive for a tan each year, prompting some psychologists to speculate that there might be a form of compulsion to tan termed "*tanorexia*." Tanning is thought to be addictive due to some form of brain response to UVR light, prompting physiological or psychological responses. Recent studies of young adults exposed to indoor tanning suggests a possible link to tanning dependence and activation of the reward system.[119] However, critics argue that this research is preliminary and that large-scale clinical trials are necessary to confirm an association.

In our culture, being tan is equated with being healthy, chic, and attractive. Indoor tanning is a multi-billion-dollar industry. Teens and 20-somethings are the most likely to be users of indoor tanning overall, but users should know that their "glow" comes with a greatly increased cancer risk.

Many people believe—incorrectly—that tanning booths are safer than sitting in the sun. But all tanning lamps emit UVA rays, and most emit UVB rays as well. Both types of light rays cause long-term skin damage and can contribute to cancer. Consider the following:[120]

- There is a 59 percent increased risk of melanoma in those exposed to regular UV radiation from tanning beds. Tanning devices have been listed as carcinogenic for humans.
- People who use tanning beds are 2.5 times more likely to develop squamous cell carcinoma and 1.5 times more likely to develop basal cell carcinoma.
- High-pressure sunlamps used in some salons emit doses of UV radiation that can be as much as 12 times that of the sun.
- Up to 90 percent of visible skin changes commonly blamed on aging are caused by the sun.
- Some tanning facilities don't calibrate the UV output of their tanning bulbs, which can lead to more or less exposure than is paid for.
- Tanning booths and beds pose significant hygiene risks. Don't assume that those little colored water sprayers used to "clean" the inside of the beds are sufficient to kill organisms. The busier the facility, the more likely you'll come into contact with germs that could make you ill.

Skills for Behavior Change

TIPS FOR PROTECTING YOUR SKIN IN THE SUN

Avoid the sun or seek shade from 10 A.M. to 4 P.M., when the sun's rays are strongest. Even on a cloudy day, up to 80 percent of the sun's rays can get through.

- **Apply an SPF 15 or higher sunscreen evenly to all uncovered skin before going outside. Look for a "broad-spectrum" sunscreen that protects against both UVA and UVB radiation. If the label does not specify, apply the sunscreen 15 minutes before going outside.**
- **Know your SPFs. An SPF 15 product typically blocks about 94 percent of UVB rays, while an SPF 30 may block 97 percent. If you pay more for a 70–100 SPF product , you are probably just paying extra for no greater benefit.**
- **Check the expiration date on your sunscreen. Sunscreens lose effectiveness over time.**
- **Remember to apply sunscreen to your eyelids, lips, nose, ears, neck, hands, and feet. If you don't have much hair, apply sunscreen to the top of your head, too.**
- **Reapply sunscreen often. The label will tell you how often you need to do this. If it isn't waterproof, reapply it after swimming, or when sweating a lot.**
- **Wear loose-fitting, light-colored clothing. You can now purchase in most sporting goods stores clothing that has SPF protection. Wear a wide-brimmed, light-colored hat to protect your head and face.**
- **Use sunglasses with 99 to 100 percent UV protection to protect your eyes. Look for polarization in your shades.**
- **Check your skin for cancer, keeping an eye out for changes in birthmarks, moles, or sunspots.**

Source: Based on U.S. Food and Drug Administration, "FDA Sheds Light on Sunscreens," 2013, www.fda.gov.

check yourself

- **What is skin cancer, and what are its causes?**
- **What can you do to protect against skin cancer?**

5.19 Prostate and Testicular Cancer

learning outcome

5.19 Identify the major factors contributing to prostate and testicular cancer.

Prostate Cancer

Prostate cancer is the most frequently diagnosed cancer in American males today, after skin cancer, and it is the second leading cause of cancer deaths in men after lung cancer. In 2014, about 233,000 new cases of prostate cancer were diagnosed in the United States. About 1 in 6 men will be diagnosed with prostate cancer during his lifetime. However, with improved screening and early diagnosis, 5-year survival rates are nearly 100 percent for all but the most advanced cases. Men who are obese and smoke have an increased risk of dying from prostate cancer.[121]

Detection, Symptoms, and Treatment The prostate is a muscular, walnut-sized gland that surrounds part of a man's urethra, the tube that transports urine and sperm out of the body. A part of the reproductive system, its primary function is to produce seminal fluid. Symptoms of prostate cancer may include weak or interrupted urine flow; difficulty starting or stopping urination; feeling the urge to urinate frequently; pain on urination; blood in the urine; or pain in the low back, pelvis, or thighs. Many men have no symptoms in the early stages.

Men over age 40 should have an annual digital rectal prostate examination. Another screening method for prostate cancer is the **prostate-specific antigen (PSA)** test, a blood test that screens for an indicator of prostate cancer. However, the United States Preventive Services Task Force recommends that otherwise asymptomatic men no longer receive the routine PSA test because, overall, it does not save lives and may lead to unnecessary treatments.

Risk Factors and Prevention Increasing age is one of the biggest risks for prostate cancer, as is African ancestry or a family history of prostate cancer. Over 97 percent of all cases occur in men over the age of 50.[122] African American men and Jamaican men of African descent have the highest documented prostate cancer incidence rates in the world and are more likely to be diagnosed at more advanced stages than other racial groups.[123] Having a father or brother with prostate cancer more than doubles a man's risk of getting prostate cancer. Men who have had several relatives with prostate cancer, especially those with relatives who developed prostate cancer at younger ages, are also at higher risk.[124]

Eating more fruits and vegetables, particularly those containing *lycopene*, a pigment found in tomatoes and other red fruits, may lower the risk of prostate cancer death.[125] Diets high in processed meats or dairy and obesity appear to increase risks.[126] The best advice is to follow recommendations for a balanced diet and to maintain a healthy weight.

Testicular Cancer

Testicular cancer is one of the most common types of solid tumors found in young adult men, affecting nearly 8,820 young men in 2014.[127] Over one-half of all cases occur between the ages of 20 and 34.[128] However, with a 95 percent 5-year survival rate, it is one of the most curable forms of cancer, particularly if caught in localized stages. Men with undescended testicles appear to be at greatest risk, and some studies indicate a genetic influence. Risk is also higher if you are white, if you have HIV or AIDS, or if a primary relative (father or brother, in particular) has had testicular cancer.[129]

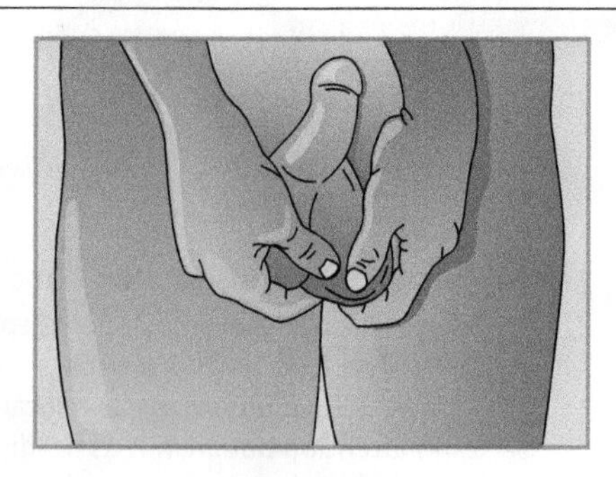

Figure 5.11 Testicular Self-Examination

Testicular Self-Exam

Testicular tumors first appear as an enlargement of the testis or thickening in testicular tissue. Some men report a heavy feeling, dull ache, or pain that extends to the lower abdomen or groin area. Testicular self-exams have long been recommended for teen boys and young men to perform monthly as a means of detecting testicular cancer (Figure 5.11). However, recent studies discovered that findings from monthly self-exams result in testing for noncancerous conditions and thus are not cost-effective. For this reason, the U.S. Preventive Services Task Force has dropped their recommendation for monthly testicular exams. Regardless, most cases of testicular cancer are discovered through self-exam, and there is currently no other screening test for the disease.

How To Examine Your Testicles

The testicular self-exam is best done after a hot shower, which will relax the scrotum and make the exam easier. Standing in front of a mirror, hold the testicle with one hand while gently rolling its surface between the thumb and fingers of your other hand. Feel underneath the scrotum for the tubes of the epididymis and blood vessels that sit close to the body. Repeat with the other testicle. Look for any lump, thickening, or pea-like nodules, paying attention to any areas that may be painful over the entire surface of the scrotum. When done, wash your hands with soap and water. Doing regular self-exams will help you to know what is normal for you and to note any irregularity. Consult a doctor if you note anything that is unusual.

check yourself

- **What are prostate and testicular cancer, and what are their causes?**

Other Cancers

learning outcome

5.20 Know the signs and symptoms of ovarian and uterine cancers, leukemia, and lymphoma.

Ovarian Cancer

Ovarian cancer is the fifth leading cause of cancer deaths for women, with about 22,000 women diagnosed in 2012 and 14,270 dying from it.[130] It causes more deaths than any other cancer of the reproductive system; women tend not to discover it until the cancer is at an advanced stage. If detected when localized, 5-year survival rates are 92 percent. If diagnosed at the regional level, rates drop to 72 percent, and if metastasis is diffuse and distant, survival rates drop to 27 percent.[131]

A woman may complain of feeling bloated, having pain in the pelvic area, feeling full quickly, or feeling the need to urinate more frequently. Some may experience persistent digestive disturbances; other symptoms include fatigue, pain during intercourse, unexplained weight loss, unexplained changes in bowel or bladder habits, and incontinence. If these vague symptoms persist for more than a week or two, prompt medical evaluation is a must.

Early-stage treatment typically includes surgery, chemotherapy, and occasionally radiation. Depending on the patient's age and desire to bear children, one or both ovaries, fallopian tubes, and the uterus may be removed.

Primary relatives (mother, daughter, sister) of a woman who has had ovarian cancer are at increased risk. A family or personal history of breast or colon cancer is also associated with increased risk. Women who have never been pregnant are more likely to develop ovarian cancer than those who have given birth to a child; the more children a woman has had, the less risk she faces. The use of estrogen postmenopausal therapy may increase a woman's risk, as will smoking and obesity.[132]

Using birth control pills, adhering to a low-fat diet, having multiple children, and breast-feeding can reduce risk of ovarian cancer.[133]

To protect yourself, get a complete pelvic examination. Women over 40 should have a cancer-related checkup every year. Uterine ultrasound or a blood test is recommended for those with risk factors or unexplained symptoms.

Cervical and Endometrial (Uterine) Cancer

Most uterine cancers develop in the body of the uterus, usually in the endometrium. The rest develop in the cervix, located at the base of the uterus. In 2014, an estimated 12,360 new cases of cervical cancer and 52,630 cases of endometrial cancer were diagnosed in the United States.[134] As more women have regular **Pap test** screenings—a procedure in which cells taken from the cervical region are examined for abnormal activity—rates should decline even further in the future. Pap tests are very effective for detecting early-stage cervical cancer, though less effective for detecting cancers of the uterine lining. Women have a lifetime risk of 1 in 151 for being diagnosed with cervical cancer and a 1 in 37 risk of being diagnosed with uterine corpus cancer.[135] Early warning signs of uterine cancer include bleeding outside the normal menstrual period or after menopause or persistent unusual vaginal discharge.

Risk factors for cervical cancer include early age at first intercourse, multiple sex partners, cigarette smoking, and certain sexually transmitted infections, including HPV (the cause of genital warts) and herpes. For endometrial cancer, age, estrogen, and obesity are strong risk factors. Risks are increased by treatment with tamoxifen for breast cancer, metabolic syndrome, late menopause, never bearing children, history of polyps in the uterus or ovaries, history of other cancers, and race (white women are at higher risk).[136]

See It! Videos

How can you prevent cervical cancer? Watch **Preventing Cervical Cancer** in the Study Area of MasteringHealth.

Leukemia and Lymphoma

Leukemia is a cancer of the blood-forming tissues that leads to proliferation of millions of immature white blood cells. These abnormal cells crowd out normal white blood cells (which fight infection), platelets (which control hemorrhaging), and red blood cells (which carry oxygen to body cells). This results in symptoms such as fatigue, paleness, weight loss, easy bruising, repeated infections, nosebleeds, and other forms of hemorrhaging occur.

Leukemia can be acute or chronic and can strike both sexes and all age groups. An estimated 52,380 new cases were diagnosed in the United States in 2014.[137] Chronic leukemia can develop over several months and have few symptoms. It is usually treated with radiation and chemotherapy. Other methods of treatment include bone marrow and stem cell transplants.

Lymphomas, a group of cancers of the lymphatic system that include Hodgkin's disease and non-Hodgkin lymphoma, are among the fastest growing cancers, with an estimated 79,990 new cases in 2014.[138] Much of this increase has occurred in women. The cause is unknown; however, a weakened immune system is suspected—particularly one exposed to viruses such as HIV, hepatitis C, and Epstein-Barr virus (EBV). Treatment varies by type and stage; chemotherapy and radiotherapy are commonly used.

check yourself

- **What are the signs and symptoms of ovarian and uterine cancers, leukemia, and lymphoma?**

5.21 Cancer Detection and Treatment

learning outcome

5.21 Describe several common cancer detection and treatment options.

Detecting Cancer

Magnetic resonance imaging (MRI) uses a huge electromagnet to detect tumors by mapping the vibrations of atoms in the body on a computer screen. The **computerized axial tomography (CAT) scan** uses X-rays to examine parts of the body. *Prostatic ultrasound* (a rectal probe using ultrasonic waves to produce an image of the prostate) is being investigated as a means to increase early detection of prostate cancer, combined with the PSA blood test. In 2011, the FDA approved the first 3D mammogram machines, which offer significant improvements in imaging and breast cancer detection but deliver nearly double the radiation risk of conventional mammograms. Table 5.4 shows screening recommendations for selected cancers.

Cancer Treatments

Treatments vary according to type and stage of cancer. Surgery to remove the tumor and surrounding tissue may be performed alone or with other treatments. The surgeon may operate using traditional surgical instruments or a laser, laparoscope, or other tools.

Stereotactic radiosurgery, also known as **gamma knife surgery**, uses a targeted dose of gamma radiation to zap tumors without any blood loss. **Radiotherapy** (use of radiation) and **chemotherapy** (use of drugs) that kill cancerous cells are also used. Radiation is most effective in treating localized cancer because it can be targeted to a particular area. Side effects include fatigue, changes to skin in the affected area, and slightly greater chances of developing another type of cancer.

Chemotherapy may be used to shrink a tumor before or after surgery or radiation therapy or on its own. Powerful drugs are administered, usually in cycles so the body can recover from their effects. Side effects, which may include nausea, hair loss, fatigue, increased chance of bleeding, bruising, infection, and anemia, fade after treatment. Other effects, such as loss of fertility, may be permanent. Long-term damage to the cardiovascular and other body systems from radiotherapy and chemotherapy can be significant.

Participation in clinical trials (people-based studies of new drugs or procedures) has provided hope for many. Deciding whether to participate in a clinical trial can be difficult. Despite the risks, which should be carefully considered, thousands of clinical trial participants have benefited from treatments otherwise unavailable to them. Before beginning any form of cancer therapy, be a vigilant and vocal consumer. Read and seek information from cancer support groups. Check the skills of your surgeon, radiation therapist, and doctor in terms of clinical experience and interpersonal interactions. Look at Oncovin and other websites supported by the National Cancer Institute and the American Cancer Society (ACS) to check out clinical trials, reports on treatment effectiveness, experimental therapies, etc. And although you may like and trust your family doctor, it is always a good idea to seek consultation or advice from larger cancer facilities.

77%

of cancers are diagnosed in adults age 55 or older.

New Cancer Treatments

Surgery, chemotherapy, and radiation therapy remain the most common cancer treatments. However, newer techniques may be more effective for certain cancers or certain patients:

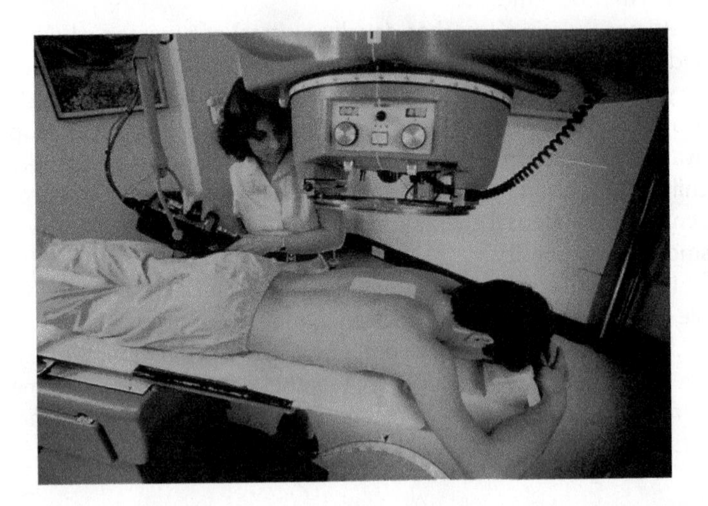

How does radiation therapy work?

Radiation therapy is often used to target and destroy cancerous tumors. The machine in this photograph emits gamma rays, which are typically used to treat localized secondary cancers and also provide pain relief for otherwise untreatable cancers. Gamma rays are less powerful than the X rays emitted from linear accelerators, another machine frequently used in radiation therapy.

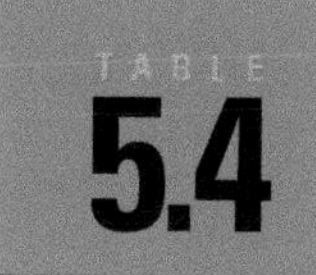

TABLE 5.4 Screening Guidelines for Early Cancer Detection in Average Risk and Asymptomatic People

Cancer Site	Screening Procedure	Age and Frequency of Test
Breast	Mammograms	The National Cancer Institute (NCI) recommends that women in their forties and older have mammograms every 1 to 2 years. Women who are at higher-than-average risk of breast cancer should talk with their health care provider about whether to have mammograms before age 40 and how often to have them.
Cervix	Pap test (Pap smear)	Women should begin having Pap tests 3 years after they begin having sexual intercourse or when they reach age 21 (whichever comes first). Most women should have a Pap test at least once every 3 years.
Colon and rectum	***Fecal occult blood test:*** Sometimes cancer or polyps bleed. This test can detect tiny amounts of blood in the stool. ***Sigmoidoscopy:*** Checks the rectum and lower part of the colon for polyps. ***Colonoscopy:*** Checks the rectum and entire colon for polyps and cancer.	People aged 50 and older should be screened. People who have a higher-than-average risk of cancer of the colon or rectum should talk with their doctor about whether to have screening tests before age 50 and how often to have them.
Prostate	Prostate-specific antigen (PSA) test	Some groups encourage yearly screening for men over age 50, and some advise men who are at a higher risk for prostate cancer to begin screening at age 40 or 45. Others caution against routine screening. Currently, Medicare provides coverage for an annual PSA test for all men age 50 and older.

Sources: National Cancer Institute, National Institutes of Health, "What You Need to Know About Cancer Screening," www.cancer.gov; National Cancer Institute, "Fact Sheet, Prostate-Specific Antigen (PSA) Test," www.cancer.gov.

- **Immunotherapy.** Immunotherapy is designed to enhance the body's disease-fighting systems. Biological response modifiers such as interferon and interleukin-2 are under study.
- **Biological therapies.** *Cancer-fighting vaccines* alert the body's immune defenses to cells gone bad. Rather than preventing disease as other vaccines do, they help people who are already ill.
- **Gene therapies.** Viruses may carry genetic information that makes the cells they infect (such as cancer cells) susceptible to an antiviral drug. Scientists are also looking at ways to transfer genes that increase immune response to the cancerous tumor or that confer drug resistance to bone marrow so higher doses of chemotherapeutic drugs can be given.
- **Angiogenesis inhibitors.** Some compounds may stop tumors from forming new blood vessels, a process called *angiogenesis*. Without adequate blood supply, tumors either die or grow very slowly.
- **Disruption of cancer pathways.** Steps in the *cancer pathway* include oncogene actions, hormone receptors, growth factors, metastasis, and angiogenesis. Preliminary studies are under way to design compounds that inhibit actions at each of these steps.
- **Smart drugs.** *Targeted smart-drug therapies* attack only the cancer cells and not the entire body.
- **Enzyme inhibitors.** An enzyme inhibitor, *TIMP2*, shows promise for slowing metastasis of tumor cells. A metastasis suppressor gene, *NM23*, has also been identified.
- **Neoadjuvant chemotherapy.** This method uses chemotherapy to shrink the tumor before surgically removing it.
- **Stem cell research.** Transplants of stem cells from donor bone marrow are used when a patient's bone marrow has been destroyed by disease, chemotherapy, or radiation.

check yourself

- **What are the screening recommendations for several common cancers?**
- **Have you been screened for any cancers for which you might be at risk? Why or why not?**
- **What are some traditional and new treatments for cancer?**

5.22 What Is Diabetes?

learning **outcome**

5.22 Explain the development of diabetes and distinguish between type 1 and type 2 diabetes.

Over 382 million people were classified as diabetic in 2013, and cases are expected to rise to 592 million by 2035.[139] While the number of people with diabetes has increased in virtually all countries of the world, 80 percent of those with diabetes live in low- and middle-income countries where access to prevention and treatment may be lacking. Globally, most people with diabetes are between 40 and 59 years of age.[140]

The United States isn't immune to epidemic rates of diabetes. Over the past 2 decades, diabetes rates have increased dramatically.[141] The Centers for Disease Control and Prevention (CDC) estimates that nearly 26 million people—almost 10 percent of the U.S. population—have diabetes.[142] Experts predict more than 1 in 3 Americans will have diabetes by 2050. Diabetes kills more Americans each year than breast cancer and AIDS, and millions suffer the physical and emotional burdens of dealing with this difficult disease.[143]

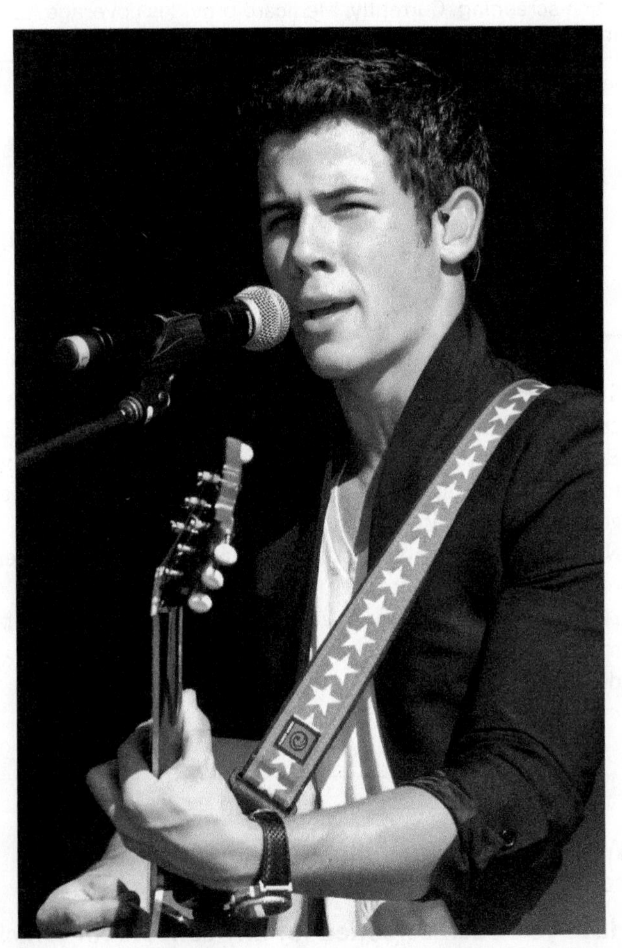

Singer and pop star Nick Jonas is one of the 5 to 10 percent of diabetics diagnosed with type 1.

Diabetes rates climb with age. While they aren't as high for college-age adults, overall rates have increased, even among the youngest populations. Among persons aged 18 to 44, approximately 2.4 percent have diabetes, compared to roughly 12.7 percent of those aged 45 to 65, and over 21 percent of those 65 to 74.[144] Diabetes is the primary cause of death each year for over 71,000 Americans.[145] All told, diabetes contributes to over 231,000 deaths, ravaging the immune system, contributing to CVD, kidney, respiratory, liver, and a host of other problems.[146] Additionally, the costs of diagnosing and treating diabetes are staggering. The younger a person is when he or she develops the disease, the greater the long-term costs.

Diabetes mellitus is actually a group of diseases, each with its own mechanism, but all characterized by a persistently high level of glucose, a type of sugar, in the blood. High blood glucose levels—or **hyperglycemia**—in diabetes can lead to serious health problems and premature death.

In a healthy person, carbohydrates from foods are broken down into a monosaccharide called *glucose*. Red blood cells use only glucose for fuel; brain and other nerve cells prefer glucose over other fuels. Excess glucose is stored as glycogen in the liver and muscles. The average adult has 5 to 6 grams of glucose in the blood at any given time, enough to provide energy for about 15 minutes of activity. Once circulating glucose is used, the body draws upon its glycogen reserves.

See It! Videos

Are diabetes patients getting even younger? Watch **Young Adults and Diabetes** in the Study Area of MasteringHealth.

1 in 3

people in the U.S. will have diabetes by 2050, based on current trends.

8 million people in the U.S. are undiagnosed diabetics.

Whenever a surge of glucose enters the bloodstream, the **pancreas**, an organ just beneath the stomach, secretes a hormone called **insulin**, stimulating cells to take up glucose from the bloodstream and carry it into cells. Conversion of glucose to glycogen for storage in the liver and muscles is also assisted by insulin.

Type 1 Diabetes

Type 1 diabetes (insulin-dependent diabetes) is an autoimmune disease in which the immune system attacks and destroys insulin-making cells in the pancreas, reducing or stopping insulin production. Without insulin, cells cannot take up glucose, and blood glucose levels become permanently elevated.

Type 1 diabetes used to be called *juvenile diabetes* because it most often appears during childhood or adolescence. Only about 5 percent of diabetic cases are type 1.[147] European ancestry, a genetic predisposition, and certain viral infections all increase the risk.[148] People with type 1 diabetes require daily insulin injections or infusions and must carefully monitor their diet and exercise levels.

Type 2 Diabetes

Type 2 diabetes (non-insulin-dependent diabetes) accounts for 90 to 95 percent of all cases.[149] In type 2, either the pancreas does not make sufficient insulin or the body cells become resistant to its effects and don't efficiently use available insulin (Figure 5.12), a condition referred to as **insulin resistance**.

Unlike type 1 diabetes, which can appear suddenly, type 2 usually develops slowly. In early stages, cells begin to resist the effects of insulin. One contributor to insulin resistance is an overabundance of free fatty acids in fat cells (common in obese individuals). These free fatty acids inhibit cells' glucose uptake and diminish the liver's ability to self-regulate conversion of glucose into glycogen.

As blood levels of glucose gradually rise, the pancreas attempts to compensate by producing more insulin. Over time, more and more pancreatic insulin-producing cells sustain damage and become nonfunctional. As insulin output declines, blood glucose levels rise enough to warrant diagnosis of type 2 diabetes.

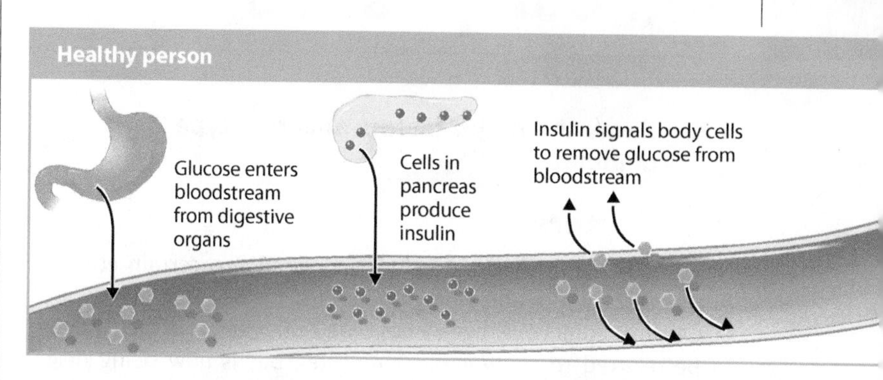

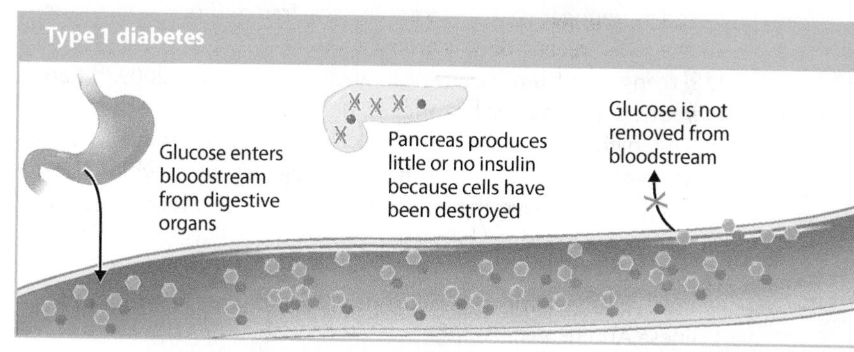

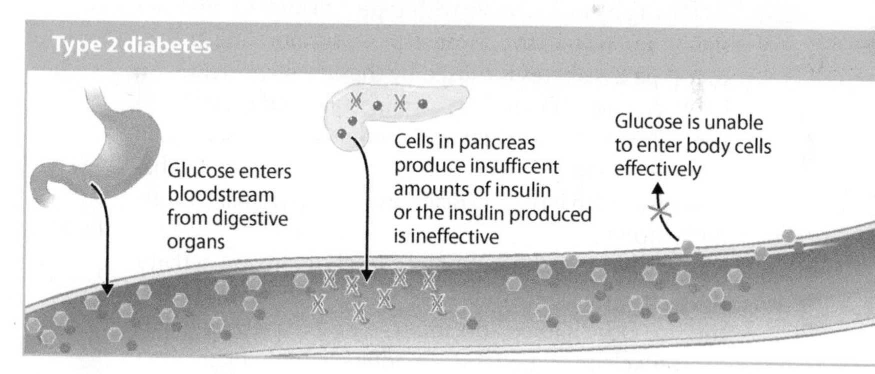

Figure 5.12 Diabetes: What It Is and How It Develops
In a healthy person, a sufficient amount of insulin is produced and released by the pancreas and used efficiently by the cells. In type 1 diabetes, the pancreas makes little or no insulin. In type 2 diabetes, either the pancreas does not make sufficient insulin or cells are resistant to insulin and thus are not able to use it efficiently.

VIDEO TUTOR How Diabetes Develops

check yourself

- **What is the role of glucose and insulin in diabetes?**
- **What is the difference between type 1 and type 2 diabetes?**
- **Why do you think diabetes rates have increased so dramatically in the United States?**

5.23 Diabetes: Risk Factors, Symptoms, and Complications

learning outcome

5.23 Know the major factors affecting type 2 diabetes.

Risk Factors

Nonmodifiable risk factors include increased age, certain ethnicities, genetic factors, and biological factors.

One in 4 adults over age 65 has type 2 diabetes.[150] In fact, it used to be referred to as *adult-onset diabetes*, but is now being diagnosed at younger ages, even among children and teens. According to the most recent data, type 2 diabetes rates are soaring among U.S. teens—up from 9 percent in 2000 to 23 percent 2009.[151] Rates of youth diabetes have historically increased with age, with females having higher rates than males.[152] Non-Hispanic whites, Native Americans, and black youth have the highest rates, while Asian/Pacific Islanders have the lowest rates.[153] However, recent research points to a surprising shift, with South Asians having significantly higher rates of diabetes (23%) than other ethnic groups (6% in whites, 18% in African Americans, 12.7% in Latinos, and 13% in Chinese Americans).[154]

Having a close relative with type 2 diabetes is another significant risk factor. Most experts support the theory that type 2 diabetes is caused by the complex interaction between environmental factors, lifestyle, and genetic susceptibility. Although numerous potential genes have been identified as likely culprits in increased risk, the mechanisms by which inherited diabetes develops remain poorly understood.[155]

Body weight, dietary choices, level of physical activity, sleep patterns, and stress level are all modifiable risk factors. In both children and adults, type 2 diabetes is linked to overweight and obesity. In adults, a body mass index (BMI) of 25 or greater increases the risk.[156] In particular, excess weight carried around the waistline—a condition called *central adiposity*—and measured by waist circumference is a significant risk factor for older women.[157]

Inadequate sleep may contribute to the development of both obesity and type 2 diabetes—possibly due to the fact that sleep-deprived people tend to engage in less physical activity.[158] There also seems to be a link between the body clock hormone *melatonin* and type 2 diabetes. Melatonin regulates the release of insulin, which adjusts blood sugar levels. Accordingly, body clock disruptions may lead to disruptions in insulin and issues with blood sugar control. People who have genetic defects in receptors for melatonin and have disrupted sleep may increase their risk of type 2 diabetes by six times.[159] Even pulling an "all-nighter" during exams may induce insulin resistance in young, healthy subjects.[160] People who routinely fail to get enough sleep have been shown to be at higher risk for a cluster of risk factors that include poor glucose metabolism.[161]

Recent data from large studies provide evidence of a link between diabetes and psychological or physical stress; however, a recent analysis of studies focused on the role of work-related stress on type 2 diabetes development has shown mixed results, with sleep being more important than stress. Shift workers, in particular, appear to have a greater risk of diabetes, even when BMI and other risks are consider.[162]

A study of young adults with impaired fasting glucose experiencing significant financial stressors showed that physical activity played a key role in reducing stress and blood sugar levels.[163] Research on the effect of chronic stress and lack of sleep on insulin production and diabetes development is in its infancy. To reduce your risks, the best rules to follow are to manage stress and to increase exercise and sleep.[164]

Prediabetes

An estimated 79 million Americans 20 or older—35 percent of the adult population—have a set of symptoms known as **prediabetes**, a condition in which blood glucose levels are higher than normal, but not high enough to be classified as diabetes.[165] If this condition

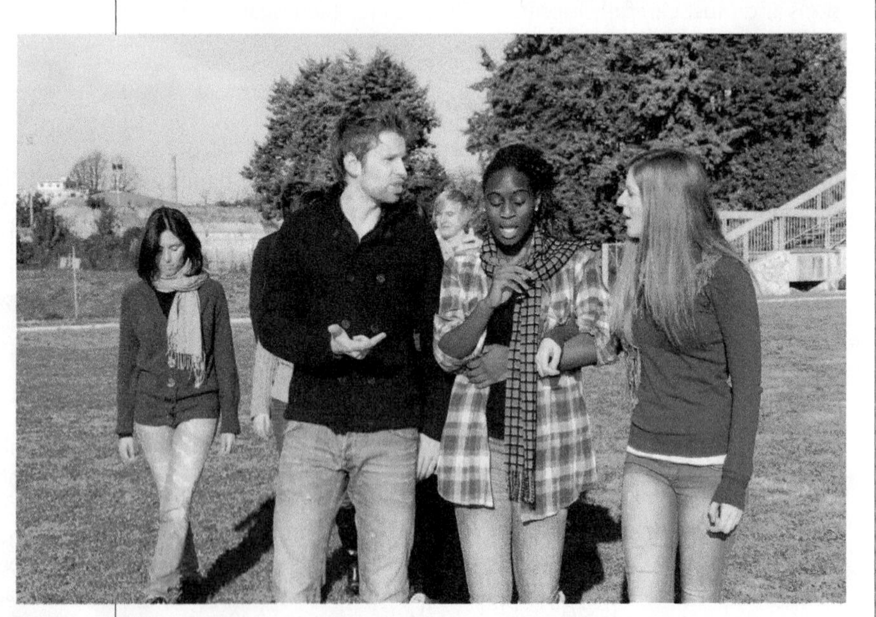

Do college students need to be concerned about diabetes?

Type 2 diabetes used to be almost nonexistent in young people, but in the past decade, cases of type 2 diabetes in people under the age of 20 have risen to the tens of thousands.

is not addressed, diabetes will eventually strike. Prediabetes is one of a cluster of six conditions linked to overweight and obesity that together constitute a dangerous health risk known as metabolic syndrome (MetS) (see Module 5.8). A person with MetS is five times more likely to develop type 2 diabetes than is a person without the syndrome.[166]

If you have already been diagnosed with prediabetes or type 2 diabetes, you can follow the tips in the Skills for Behavior Change box, "Key Steps to Begin Reducing Your Risk for Diabetes," to halt or slow the progression of your condition. Even if you've never had your blood glucose tested, these steps could reduce your risk.

Gestational Diabetes

A third type of diabetes, **gestational diabetes**, is a state of high blood glucose during pregnancy, thought to be associated with metabolic stresses that occur in response to changing hormonal levels. As many as 18 percent of pregnancies are affected by gestational diabetes, posing added risks for the mother and developing fetus.[167] Between 40 and 50 percent of women with gestational diabetes may progress to type 2 diabetes if they fail to make significant lifestyle changes.[168]

Symptoms of Diabetes

Common symptoms of diabetes are similar for type 1 and type 2:

- **Thirst and excessive urination.** Kidneys filter excessive glucose by diluting it with water. This can pull too much water from the body and result in dehydration and increased need to urinate.
- **Weight loss.** Because so many calories are lost in the glucose that passes into urine, a person with diabetes often feels hungry. Despite eating more, he or she typically loses weight.
- **Fatigue.** When glucose cannot enter cells, fatigue and weakness become inevitable.
- **Nerve damage.** High glucose levels damage the smallest blood vessels of the body, leading to numbness and tingling.
- **Blurred vision.** High blood glucose levels can dry out the cornea or damage microvessels in the eye.
- **Poor wound healing and increased infections.** High levels of glucose can affect ability to ward off infection and overall immune function.

Diabetes Complications

Poorly controlled diabetes can lead to a variety of complications:[169]

- **Diabetic coma.** In the absence of glucose, body cells break down stored fat for energy. This produces acidic molecules called *ketones*, excessive amounts of which dangerously elevate blood acid. The diabetic slips into a coma and, without prompt medical intervention, can die.
- **Cardiovascular disease.** More than 68 percent of diabetics have one or more forms of cardiovascular disease, including hypertension, increasing risk of heart attack and stroke significantly. Blood vessels become damaged as glucose-laden blood flows more sluggishly and nutrients and other substances are not transported as effectively.
- **Kidney disease.** Kidneys become scarred by their extraordinary workload and by high blood pressure in their vessels. More than 224,000 Americans are currently living with kidney failure due to diabetes.[170]
- **Amputations.** More than 60 percent of nontraumatic amputations of legs, feet, and toes are due to diabetes. Each year nearly 66,000 nontraumatic lower-limb amputations (180 per day) are performed on people with diabetes.[171]
- **Eye disease and blindness.** Nearly 7.7 million people over the age of 40 have *early-stage retinopathy*, which could lead to blindness without treatment.[172]
- **Infectious diseases.** Persons with diabetes have increased risk of poor wound healing and greater susceptibility to infectious diseases, particularly influenza and pneumonia.
- **Other complications.** Diabetics may have gum and tooth disease, foot neuropathy, and chronic pain that makes walking, driving, and simple tasks more difficult. In addition, persons with diabetes are more likely to suffer from depression, making intervention and treatment more difficult.

Skills for Behavior Change

KEY STEPS TO BEGIN REDUCING YOUR RISK FOR DIABETES

- Maintain a healthy weight, and lose weight if you need to.
- Eat smaller portions and choose foods with less fat, salt, and added sugars. Keep calories equal to energy expended. Eat more fruits, vegetables, and complex carbohydrates, and make sure you consume lean protein
- Get your body moving. Aim for at least 30 minutes of moderate activity 5 days a week.
- Quit smoking; in addition to cancer and heart disease, smoking increases blood glucose levels.
- Reduce or eliminate alcohol consumption. It's high in calories and can interfere with blood glucose regulation.
- Get enough sleep.
- Inoculate yourself against stress. Learn to take yourself less seriously, find time for fun, develop a strong support network, and use relaxation skills.
- If you have a family history, or several risk factors, get regular checkups.

Sources: Centers for Disease Control and Prevention, "National Diabetes Prevention Program," 2014, www.cdc.gov.

check yourself

- **Name three possible complications of poorly controlled diabetes.**
- **What factors put someone at greatest risk for type 2 diabetes?**
- **What are common symptoms of type 1 and type 2 diabetes?**

5.24 Diabetes: Diagnosis and Treatment

learning outcome

5.24 Explain how diabetes is diagnosed and treated.

Diagnosing and Monitoring Diabetes

Generally, a physician orders one of the following blood tests to diagnose prediabetes or diabetes:

- The *fasting plasma glucose (FPG) test* requires the patient to fast overnight; a small sample of blood is then tested for glucose concentration. An FPG level greater than or equal to 100 mg/dL indicates prediabetes, and a level greater than or equal to 126 mg/dL indicates diabetes (Figure 5.13).
- The *oral glucose tolerance test (OGTT)* requires the patient to drink a fluid containing concentrated glucose. Blood is drawn for testing 2 hours later. A reading greater than or equal to 140 mg/dL indicates prediabetes, whereas a reading greater than or equal to 200 mg/dL indicates diabetes.
- The *A1C* or *glycosylated hemoglobin test (HbA1C)* gives the average value of a patient's blood glucose over the past 2 to 3 months, instead of at one moment in time. In general, an A1C of 5.7 to 6.4 means that you are at high risk for diabetes or are prediabetic. If your A1C is 6.5 or higher, diabetes may be diagnosed.[173] *Estimated average glucose (eAG)* shows how AIC numbers correspond to the blood glucose numbers people are used to seeing. For example, someone with an A1C value of 6.1 would be able to look at a chart and see that their average blood glucose was around 128—a high level that should encourage healthy lifestyle modifications.

People with diabetes need to check their blood glucose level several times throughout each day to make sure they stay within their target range. To check blood glucose, diabetics must prick their finger to obtain a drop of blood. A handheld glucose meter is then used to evaluate the blood sample.

Treating Diabetes

Lifestyle changes can prevent or delay the development of type 2 diabetes by up to 58 percent.[174] For those with type 2 diabetes, such lifestyle changes can prevent or delay need for medication or insulin injections.

Weight loss significantly lowers risk of progressing from prediabetes to diabetes. A loss of as little as 5 to 7 percent of current body weight and regular physical activity significantly lowers the risk of progressing to diabetes.[175]

A low-fat, reduced-calorie diet aids weight loss. Researchers have also studied a variety of foods for their effect on blood glucose levels. A diet high in whole grains reduces risk of type 2 diabetes.[176] Eating high-fiber foods—fruits, vegetables, beans, nuts, and

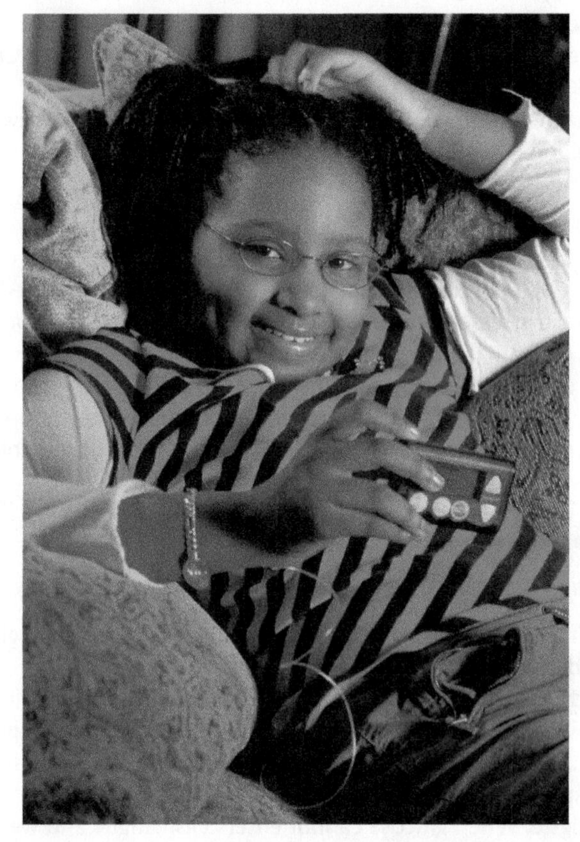

Some type 2 diabetics can control their condition with changes in diet and lifestyle habits or with oral medications. However, some type 2 diabetics and all type 1 diabetics require insulin injections or infusions.

seeds—may reduce diabetes risk.[177] Eating low-carbohydrate diets also appears to reduce overall CVD risks and may have a significant effect on preventing and controlling type 2 diabetes. In addition, consumption of fish high in omega-3 fatty acids is linked with decreased progression of insulin resistance.[178]

It is also important for people with diabetes to prevent surges in blood sugar after they eat. The **glycemic index (GI)** compares foods with the same amount of carbohydrates and determines how quickly and how much each raises blood glucose levels. Foods low on the GI have far less effect on blood glucose than those that are high on the GI. A food's **glycemic load (GL)** is defined as its GI (potential to raise blood glucose) multiplied by the grams of carbohydrates it provides, divided by 100. By learning to combine high- and low-GI foods to avoid surges in blood glucose, diabetics can help control their average blood glucose levels throughout the day. Eating smaller amounts, several times a day, from low GI sources is an important part of glucose control.

At least 30 minutes of physical activity 5 days a week reduces risk of type 2 diabetes.[179] The more muscle mass you have and the

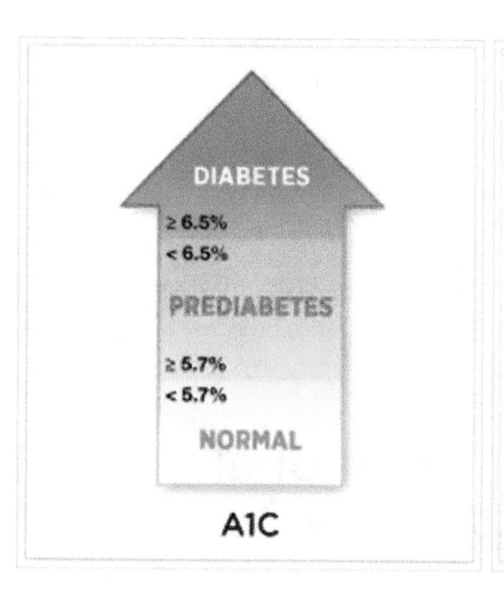

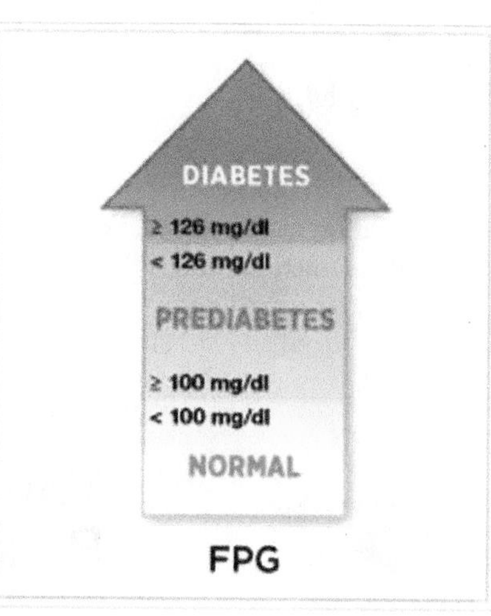

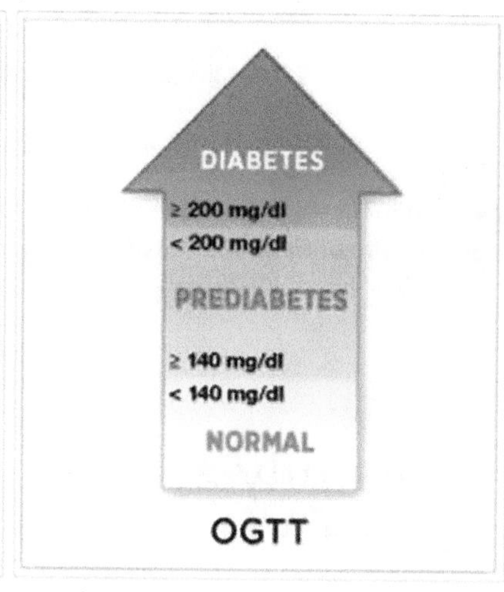

Figure 5.13 Blood Glucose Levels in Prediabetes and Untreated Diabetes
The fasting plasma glucose (FPG) test measures levels of blood glucose after a person fasts overnight. The oral glucose tolerance test (OGTT) measures levels of blood glucose after a person consumes a concentrated amount of glucose. The A1C or glycosylated hemoglobin test (HbA1C) gives the average value of a patient's blood glucose over the past 2 to 3 months.
Source: American Diabetes Association, "Diagnosing Diabetes and Learning about Prediabetes," March 2014, www.diabetes.org.

more you use your muscles, the more efficiently cells use glucose for fuel, meaning there will be less glucose circulating in the bloodstream. For most people, activity of moderate intensity can help keep blood glucose levels under control.

When lifestyle changes fail to control type 2 diabetes, one of several oral medications may be prescribed, each of which influences blood glucose in a different way—reducing the liver's glucose production, slowing absorption of carbohydrates from the small intestine, increasing pancreatic insulin production, or increasing cells' insulin sensitivity.

The newest class of diabetes drugs are known as SGLT2 inhibitors. These drugs cause the kidneys to actually excrete more glucose, which lowers the levels of glucose circulating in the body. All diabetic drugs have side effects and contraindications; however, each person must balance risks of medications with risks of elevated blood glucose.

When lifestyle changes prove challenging and risks are high and increasing, surgery is another option. People who undergo gastric/bariatric surgery for weight loss have shown remarkable reductions in blood glucose and diabetes symptoms for 2–3 years after surgery.[180] Those who combined gastric bypass or sleeve gastrectomy (a surgery where about 80% of the stomach is removed, leaving a small sleeve of stomach tissue connected to the intestines) with intensive medical therapy had similar outcomes.[181] In many cases, former diabetics can stop taking medications for some of their CVD risks and stop diabetes symptoms altogether. Many professional groups are pushing for wider use of these more drastic weight loss methods.[182] Gastric bypass surgeries are not without risks, however, and can include death and serious complications.

With type 1 diabetes, the pancreas cannot produce adequate insulin, making added insulin essential. People with type 2 diabetes whose blood glucose cannot be controlled with other treatments also require insulin. Insulin cannot be taken in pill form because it's a protein, and thus would be digested in the gastrointestinal tract. It must therefore be inserted into the fat layer under the skin, from which it is absorbed into the bloodstream.

Today, many diabetics use an *insulin infusion pump* rather than injections. The pump, small and easily hidden by clothes, delivers insulin in minute amounts throughout the day through a catheter inserted under the skin.

Losing 5%–7% of body weight can cause significant reductions in blood glucose levels and help prevent diabetes.

check yourself

- **What tests are commonly used to diagnose diabetes?**
- **What are some of the treatments for diabetes?**
- **How do people with diabetes monitor their blood glucose level?**

What's Your Personal CVD Risk?

An interactive version of this assessment is available online in MasteringHealth.

Each of us has a unique level of risk for various diseases, including cardiovascular disease. Answer each of the following questions and total your points in each section.

1 Your Family Risk for CVD

	Yes (1 point)	No (0 points)	Don't Know
1. Do any of your primary relatives (parents, grandparents, siblings) have a history of heart disease or stroke?	○	○	○
2. Do any of your primary relatives have diabetes?	○	○	○
3. Do any of your primary relatives have high blood pressure?	○	○	○
4. Do any of your primary relatives have a history of high cholesterol?	○	○	○
5. Would you say that your family consumed a high-fat diet (lots of red meat, whole dairy, butter/margarine) during your time spent at home?	○	○	○

Total points:__________

2 Your Lifestyle Risk for CVD

	Yes (1 point)	No (0 points)	Don't Know
1. Is your total cholesterol level higher than it should be?	○	○	○
2. Do you have high blood pressure?	○	○	○
3. Have you been diagnosed as prediabetic or diabetic?	○	○	○
4. Do you smoke?	○	○	○
5. Would you describe your life as being highly stressful?	○	○	○

Total points:__________

3 Your Additional Risks for CVD

1. **How would you best describe your current weight?**
   a. Lower than it should be for my height (0 points)
   b. About what it should be for my height (0 points)
   c. Higher than it should be for my height (1 point)
2. **How would you describe the level of exercise that you get each day?**
   a. Less than I should be exercising each day (1 point)
   b. About how much I should be exercising each day (0 points)
   c. More than I should be exercising each day (0 points)
3. **How would you describe your dietary behaviors?**
   a. Eating only the recommended number of calories each day (0 points)
   b. Eating less than the recommended number of calories each day (0 points)
   c. Eating more than the recommended number of calories each day (1 point)
4. **Which of the following statements best describes your typical dietary behavior?**
   a. I eat from the major food groups, especially trying to get the recommended fruits and vegetables. (0 points)
   b. I eat too much red meat and consume too much saturated and *trans* fats from meat, dairy products, and processed foods each day. (1 point)
   c. Whenever possible, I try to substitute olive oil or canola oil for other forms of dietary fat. (0 points)

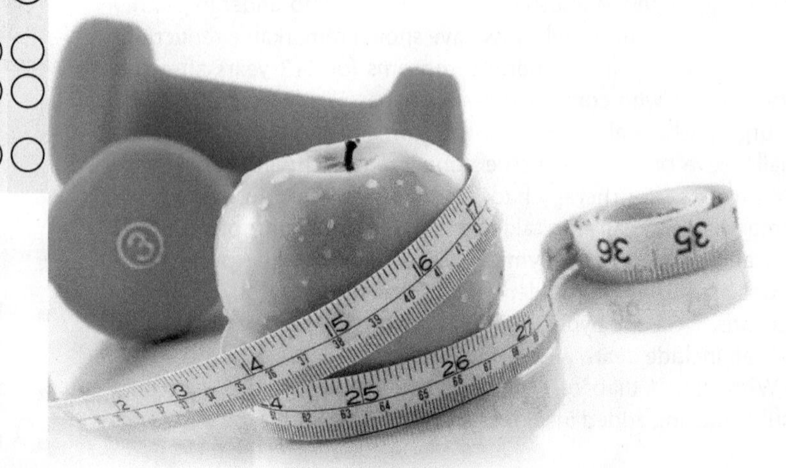

5. Which of the following (if any) describes you?
   a. I watch my sodium intake and try to reduce stress in my life. (0 points)
   b. I have a history of chlamydia infection. (1 point)
   c. I try to eat 5 to 10 milligrams of soluble fiber each day and to substitute a soy product for an animal product in my diet at least once each week. (0 points)

Total points: __________

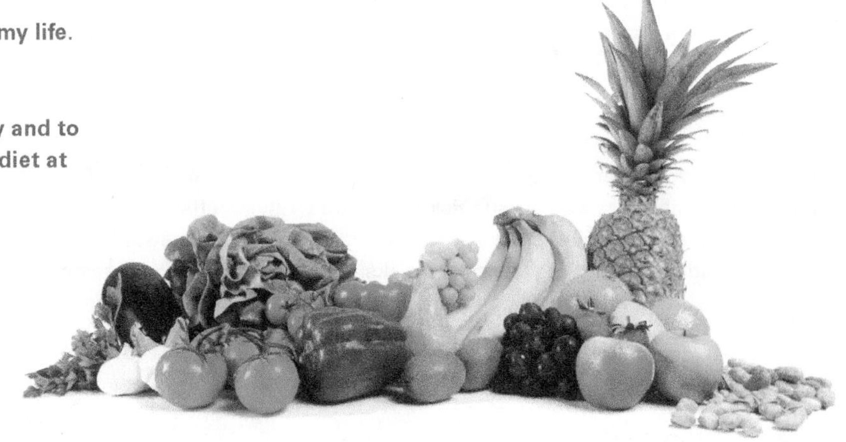

Scoring

If you score between 1 and 5 in any section, consider your risk. The higher the number you've scored, the greater your risk. If you answered "don't know" for any question, talk to your parents or other family members as soon as possible to find out if you have any unknown risks.

Your Plan for Change

The Assess Yourself activity evaluated your risk of heart disease. Based on your results and the advice of your physician, you may need to take steps to reduce your risk of CVD.

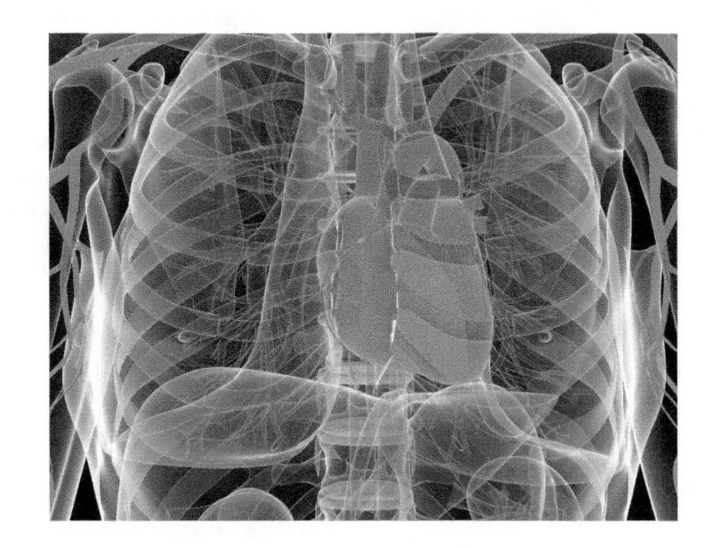

Today, you can:

◯ Get up and move! Take a walk in the evening, use the stairs instead of the escalator, or ride your bike to class. Start thinking of ways you can incorporate more physical activity into your daily routine.

◯ Begin improving your dietary habits by eating a healthier dinner. Replace the meat and processed foods you might normally eat with a serving of fresh fruit or soy-based protein and green leafy vegetables. Think about the amounts of saturated and *trans* fats you consume—which foods contain them, and how can you reduce consumption of these items?

Within the next 2 weeks, you can:

◯ Begin a regular exercise program, even if you start slowly. Set small goals and try to meet them.

◯ Practice a new stress management technique. For example, learn how to meditate.

◯ Get enough rest. Make sure you get at least 8 hours of sleep per night.

By the end of the semester, you can:

◯ Find out your hereditary risk for CVD. Call your parents and find out if your grandparents or aunts or uncles developed CVD. Ask if they know their latest cholesterol LDL/HDL levels. Do you have a family history of diabetes?

◯ Have your own cholesterol and blood pressure levels checked. Once you know your levels, you'll have a better sense of what risk factors to address. If your levels are high, talk to your doctor about how to reduce them.

Assessyourself

5.26

What's Your Personal Risk for Cancer?

An interactive version of this assessment is available online in MasteringHealth.

There are many cancer risk factors that you have the power to change. Once you carefully assess your risks, you can make lifestyle changes and pursue risk-reduction strategies that may lessen your susceptibility to various cancers.

Read each question and circle the number corresponding to each Yes or No. Be honest and accurate to get the most complete understanding of your cancer risks. Individual scores for specific questions should not be interpreted as a precise measure of relative risk, but the totals in each section give a general indication.

1 Breast Cancer

	Yes	No
1. Do you do a monthly breast self-exam?	1	2
2. Do you look at your breasts in the mirror regularly, checking for any irregular indentations/lumps, discharge from the nipples, or other noticeable changes?	1	2
3. Has your mother, sister, or daughter been diagnosed with breast cancer?	2	1
4. Have you ever been pregnant?	1	2
5. Have you had lumps or cysts in your breasts or underarm?	2	1

Total points: __________

2 Skin Cancer

	Yes	No
1. Do you spend a lot of time outdoors, either at work or at play?	2	1
2. Do you use sunscreens with an SPF rating of 15 or more?	1	2
3. Do you use tanning beds or sun booths regularly to maintain a tan?	2	1
4. Do you examine your skin once a month, checking any moles or other irregularities, and using a hand mirror to check hard-to-see areas such as your back, buttocks, genitals, and neck, and under your hair?	1	2
5. Do you purchase and wear sunglasses that filter out harmful sun rays?	1	2

Total points: __________

3 Cancers of the Reproductive System

Men

	Yes	No
1. Do you examine your penis regularly for unusual bumps or growths?	1	2
2. Do you perform regular testicular self-exams?	1	2
3. Do you have a family history of prostate or testicular cancer?	2	1
4. Do you practice safe sex and wear condoms with every sexual encounter?	1	2
5. Do you avoid exposure to harmful environmental hazards such as mercury, coal tars, benzene, chromate, and vinyl chloride?	1	2

Total points: __________

Women

	Yes	No
1. Do you have regularly scheduled Pap tests?	1	2
2. Have you been infected with the human papillomavirus, Epstein-Barr virus, or other viruses believed to increase cancer risk?	2	1
3. Has your mother, sister, or daughter been diagnosed with breast, cervical, endometrial, or ovarian cancer (particularly at a young age)?	2	1
4. Do you practice safe sex and use condoms with every sexual encounter?	1	2
5. Are you obese, taking estrogen, or consuming a diet that is very high in saturated fats?	2	1

Total points: __________

4 Cancers in General

		Yes	No
1.	Do you smoke cigarettes on most days of the week?	2	1
2.	Do you consume a diet that is rich in fruits and vegetables?	1	2
3.	Are you obese, or do you lead a primarily sedentary lifestyle?	2	1
4.	Do you live in an area with high air pollution levels or work in a job where you are exposed to several chemicals on a regular basis?	2	1
5.	Are you careful about the amount of animal fat in your diet, substituting olive oil or canola oil for animal fat whenever possible?	1	2
6.	Do you limit your overall consumption of alcohol?	1	2
7.	Do you eat foods rich in lycopenes (such as tomatoes) and antioxidants?	1	2
8.	Are you "body aware" and alert for changes in your body?	1	2
9.	Do you have a family history of ulcers or of colorectal, stomach, or other digestive-system cancers?	2	1
10.	Do you avoid unnecessary exposure to radiation, cell phone emissions, and microwave emissions?	1	2

Total points: __________

Analyzing Your Scores

Look carefully at each question for which you circled a 2. Are there any areas in which you received mostly 2s? Did you receive total points of 6 or higher in parts 1 through 3? Did you receive total points of 11 or higher in part 4? If so, you have at least one identifiable risk. The higher your score, the more risks you may have.

Your Plan for Change

The Assess Yourself activity identifies certain behaviors that can contribute to increased cancer risks. If you have identified particular risky behaviors, consider steps you can take to change these behaviors and improve your future health.

Today, you can:

◯ Perform a breast or testicular self-exam and commit to doing one every month.

◯ Take advantage of the salad bar in your dining hall for lunch or dinner and load up on greens, or request veggies such as steamed broccoli or sautéed spinach.

Within the next 2 weeks, you can:

◯ Buy a bottle of sunscreen (with SPF 15 or higher) and begin applying it as part of your daily routine. (Be sure to check the expiration date, particularly on sale items!) Also, stay in the shade from 10 A.M. to 2 P.M., as this is when the sun is strongest.

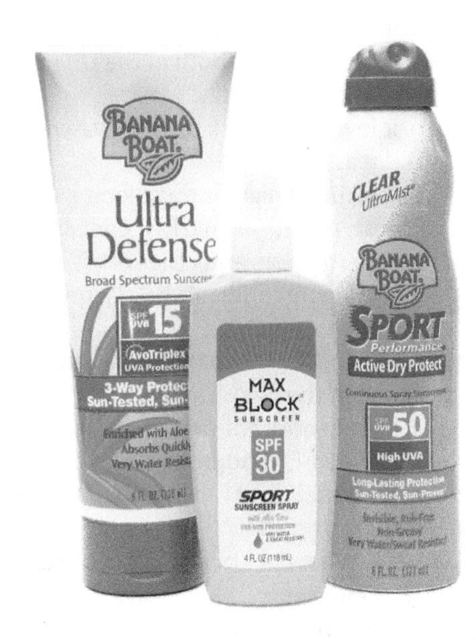

◯ Find out your family health history. Talk to your parents, grandparents, or an aunt or uncle to find out if family members have developed cancer. This will help you assess your own genetic risk.

By the end of the semester, you can:

◯ Work toward achieving a healthy weight. If you aren't already engaged in a regular exercise program, begin one now. Maintaining a healthy body weight and exercising regularly will lower your risk for cancer.

◯ Stop smoking, avoid secondhand smoke, and limit your alcohol intake.

Summary

To hear an MP3 Tutor session, scan here or visit the Study Area in **MasteringHealth**.

LO 5.1 The cardiovascular system consists of the heart and circulatory system, a network of vessels that supplies the body with nutrients and oxygen.

LO 5.2–5.7 Cardiovascular diseases include atherosclerosis, coronary artery disease, peripheral artery disease, coronary heart disease, stroke, hypertension, angina pectoris, arrhythmias, congestive heart failure, and congenital and rheumatic heart disease.

LO 5.8–5.10 Many risk factors for cardiovascular disease can be modified, such as cigarette smoking, high blood cholesterol and triglyceride levels, hypertension, lack of exercise, a diet high in saturated fat, obesity, diabetes, and emotional stress. Some risk factors, such as age, gender, and heredity, cannot be modified.

LO 5.11 Coronary bypass surgery is an established treatment for heart blockage; however, increasing numbers of angioplasty procedures and stents are being used with great success. Drug therapies can be used to prevent and treat CVD.

LO 5.12 Cancer is a group of diseases characterized by uncontrolled growth and spread of abnormal cells. These cells may create tumors.

LO 5.13 Cancers are grouped into four categories: carcinomas, sarcomas, lymphomas, and leukemias.

LO 5.14 Lifestyle factors for cancer include smoking, obesity, poor diet, lack of exercise, and stress. Biological factors include inherited genes, age, and gender. Infectious agents that may cause cancer are chronic hepatitis B and C, human papillomavirus, and genital herpes.

LO 5.15–5.20 There are many different types of cancer. Common cancers include those of the lung, breast, colon and rectum, skin, prostate, testis, ovary, and uterus; leukemia; and lymphomas.

LO 5.21 Early diagnosis improves survival rate. Self-exams for breast, testicular, and skin cancer aid early diagnosis.

LO 5.22 Diabetes mellitus is characterized by a persistently high level of glucose in the blood. In type 1 diabetes, the immune system attacks insulin-making cells in the pancreas, dangerously elevating insulin levels. In type 2 diabetes, the pancreas doesn't make sufficient insulin, or the cells don't use it efficiently.

LO 5.23 Risk factors for diabetes include age, ethnicity, genetics, and lifestyle. Prediabetes will eventually lead to diabetes if health risks are not addressed.

LO 5.24 Treatments for diabetes include improving lifestyle factors, taking medications, undergoing weight-loss surgery, and receiving insulin.

Pop Quiz

Visit MasteringHealth to personalize your study plan with Chapter Review Quizzes and Dynamic Study Modules.

LO 5.6 1. A stroke results
a. when a heart stops beating.
b. when cardiopulmonary resuscitation has failed to revive a stopped heart.
c. when blood flow in the brain has been compromised, either due to blockage or hemorrhage.
d. when blood pressure rises above 120/80 mm Hg.

LO 5.8 2. Which of the following is *correct* about metabolic syndrome?
a. It is decreasing among the general population both in the United States and globally.
b. It lowers your risk of cardiovascular disease.
c. It includes high fasting blood glucose, obesity, high triglyceride levels, hypertension, and other risks.
d. It is a nonmodifiable risk factor for CVD.

LO 5.9 3. The "bad" type of cholesterol found in the bloodstream is known as
a. high-density lipoprotein (HDL).
b. low-density lipoprotein (LDL).
c. total cholesterol.
d. triglycerides.

LO 5.9 4. What does a person's cholesterol level indicate?
a. The formation of fatty substances, called *plaque*, which can clog the arteries
b. The level of triglycerides in the blood, which can increase risk of coronary disease
c. Hypertension, which leads to thickening and hardening of the arteries
d. The level of *C-reactive proteins* in the blood, indicating inflammation

LO 5.12 5. When cancer cells have *metastasized*,
a. they have grown into a malignant tumor.
b. they have spread to other parts of the body.
c. the cancer is retreating and cancer cells are dying off.
d. the tumor is localized and considered in situ.

LO 5.12 6. A cancerous *neoplasm* is a
a. type of biopsy.
b. form of benign tumor.
c. type of treatment for a tumor.
d. malignant group of cells or tumor.

LO 5.14 7. "If you are male and smoke, your chances of getting lung cancer are 23 times greater than those of a nonsmoker." This statement refers to a type of risk assessed statistically, known as
a. relative risk.
b. comparable risk.
c. cancer risk.
d. genetic predisposition.

LO 5.18 8. The more serious and life-threatening type of skin cancer is
a. basal cell carcinoma.
b. squamous cell carcinoma.
c. melanoma.
d. lymphoma.

LO 5.22 9. Which of the following is true of type 2 diabetes?
a. It is an autoimmune disorder.
b. It is correlated with obesity and sedentary lifestyle.
c. It usually appears suddenly.
d. It is also referred to as insulin-dependent diabetes.

LO 5.22 10. By 2050, experts predict more than _____ Americans will have diabetes.
a. 1 in 3
b. 1 in 10
c. 1 in 100
d. 1 in 200

Answers to these questions can be found on page A-1. If you answered a question incorrectly, review the module identified by the Learning Outcome. For even more study tools, visit MasteringHealth.

Consumerism and Complementary and Alternative Medicine

6

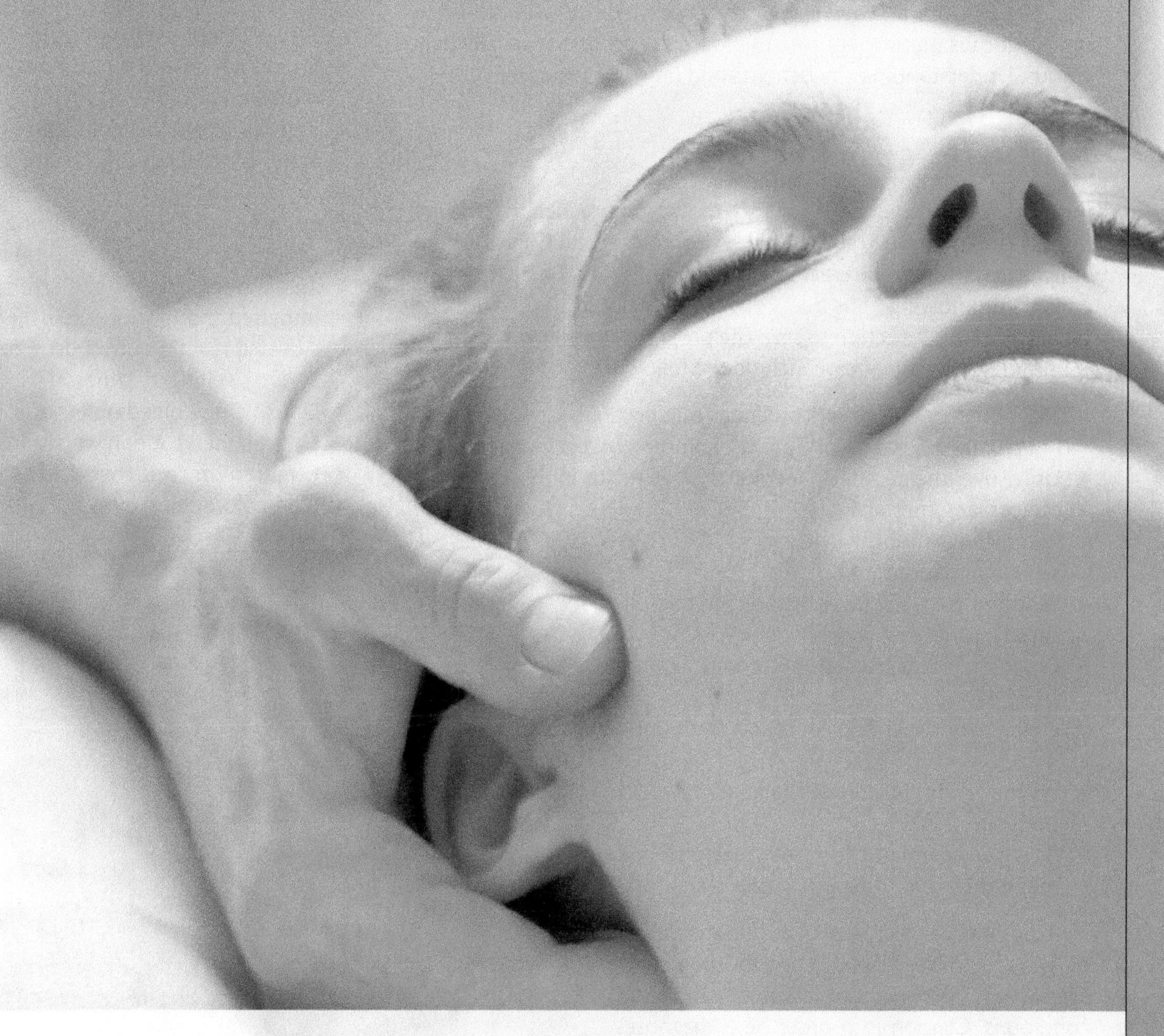

Have there been times when you wondered whether you were sick enough to go to your campus health clinic? Have you left medical visits feeling that you didn't get a thorough exam, or with more questions than when you arrived? Have you wondered about, or successfully used, alternative medical care? Have you ever had to help a loved one make health care decisions?

There are many reasons for you to learn to make better decisions about your health and health care. Most important, you only have one body. If you don't treat it with care, you will pay a major price in terms of monetary costs and consequences to your health. Doing everything you can to stay healthy and to recover rapidly when you do get sick will enhance every other part of your life. Throughout this book we have emphasized the importance of healthy preventive behaviors. Learning when and how to navigate the health care system are important parts of taking charge of your health.

6.1 Taking Responsibility for Your Health Care

learning outcome

6.1 Explain how to use the medical system and when to seek medical help.

As the health care industry has become more sophisticated in seeking your business, so must you become more sophisticated in purchasing its products and services. Acting responsibly in times of illness can be difficult, but the person best able to act on your behalf is you.

If you are not feeling well, you must first decide whether you need to seek medical advice. Not seeking treatment, whether because of high costs or limited coverage, or trying to medicate yourself when more rigorous methods of treatment are needed is potentially dangerous. Understanding the benefits and limits of self-care is critical for responsible consumerism.

Self-Care

Individuals can practice behaviors that promote health, prevent disease, and minimize reliance on the formal medical system. Minor afflictions can often be treated without professional help. Self-care consists of knowing your body, paying attention to its signals, and taking appropriate action to stop the progression of illness or injury. Common forms of self-care include the following:

- Diagnosing symptoms or conditions that occur frequently but may not require physician visits (e.g., the common cold, minor abrasions)
- Using over-the-counter remedies to treat minor infrequent pains, scrapes, or symptoms
- Performing monthly breast or testicular self-examinations
- Learning first aid for common, uncomplicated injuries and conditions
- Checking blood pressure, pulse, and temperature
- Doing periodic checks for blood cholesterol level
- Learning from reliable self-help books, websites, and DVDs
- Benefiting from nutrition, rest, exercise, and meditation and other relaxation techniques

In addition, a vast array of at-home diagnostic kits are now available to test for pregnancy, allergies, HIV, genetic disorders, and many other conditions. Caution is in order here: diagnoses from these devices and kits may not always be accurate—or you may not have the ability to understand the ramifications of what you learn without professional interpretation. Home health tests are not substitutes for regular, complete examinations by a trained practitioner.

Using self-care methods appropriately takes education and effort. Taking prescription drugs used for a previous illness to treat your current illness, using unproven self-treatment methods, or using other people's medications are examples of inappropriate self-care.

When to Seek Help

Effective self-care means paying attention to your body's warning signs and understanding when to seek medical attention. Deciding which conditions warrant professional advice is not always easy. Generally, you should consult a physician if you experience *any* of the following:

- A serious accident or injury
- Sudden or severe chest pains, especially if they cause breathing difficulties
- Trauma to the head or spine accompanied by persistent headache, blurred vision, loss of consciousness, vomiting, convulsions, or paralysis
- Sudden high fever or recurring high temperature (over 102°F for children and 103°F for adults) and/or sweats
- Tingling sensation in the arm accompanied by slurred speech or impaired thought processes
- Adverse reactions to a drug or insect bite (shortness of breath, severe swelling, dizziness)
- Unexplained bleeding or loss of fluid from any body opening
- Unexplained sudden weight loss
- Persistent or recurrent diarrhea or vomiting
- Blue-colored lips, eyelids, or nail beds

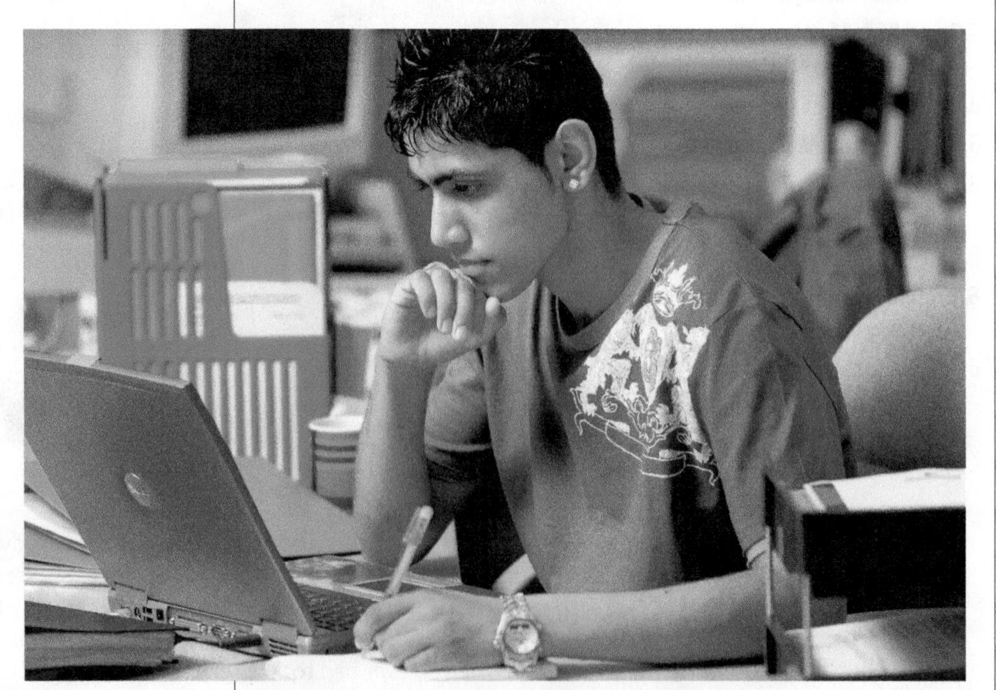

Deciding when to contact a physician can be difficult. Most people first research symptoms online and try to diagnose and treat a condition themselves.

- Any lump, swelling, thickness, or sore that does not subside or that grows for over a month
- Any marked change or pain in bowel or bladder habits
- Yellowing of the skin or the whites of the eyes
- Any symptom that is unusual and recurs over time
- Pregnancy

The Placebo Effect

The *placebo effect* is an apparent cure or improved state of health brought about by a substance, product, or procedure that has no generally recognized therapeutic value. Patients often report improvements in a condition based on what they expect, desire, or were told would happen after receiving a treatment, even though that treatment was, for example, simple sugar pills instead of powerful drugs.

There is also a *nocebo* effect, in which a practitioner's negative assessment of a patient's symptoms leads to a worsening of the condition, such as increased anxiety and pain. Similarly, a negative assessment of a treatment's potential efficacy induces a failure to respond to that treatment.

Researchers are investigating how and why expectation appears to change physiology. Evidence from pain studies suggests that use of a placebo for pain control causes the brain to release the same endogenous (natural) opioids it releases when the study participant uses a pain medication with an active ingredient.[1] But pain is not the only factor to respond to expectation: A study of resting tremor (such as involuntary finger-tapping) in patients with Parkinson's disease found that positive or negative expectations of a treatment's effectiveness reduced or increased patient tremor when they were given the same valid medication or the same placebo.[2] Similar chemical changes on brain imaging tests were seen with placebos in studies of depression and alcohol dependency treatment.[3]

See It! Videos

How do you avoid misdiagnosed medical advice online? Watch **Misdiagnosis on the Web** in the Study Area of MasteringHealth.

See It! Videos

Knowing your medical history can keep you informed of health risks. Watch **Your Medical History** in the Study Area of MasteringHealth.

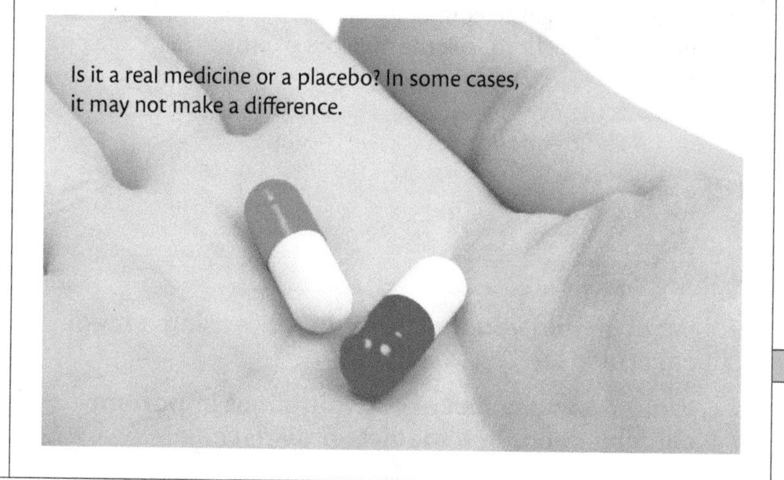
Is it a real medicine or a placebo? In some cases, it may not make a difference.

People who unknowingly use placebos when medical treatment is needed increase their risk for health problems. However, what we learn from the ways in which placebos work may someday help us harness the mind's power to treat certain diseases and conditions.

Skills for Behavior Change

BE PROACTIVE IN YOUR HEALTH CARE

Here are some tips for getting the most out of doctor visits and being proactive in your health care:

- Keep records of your own and your family's medical histories.
- Research your condition—causes, physiological effects, possible treatments, and prognosis. Don't rely on your health care provider for this information.
- If you use a complementary and alternative medicine (CAM) therapy such as acupuncture, choose a practitioner with care. Your insurer may also cover such services.
- Bring a friend or relative along to medical visits to help you review what the doctor says. If you go alone, take notes. Write down what happened and what was said.
- Ask the practitioner to explain the problem and possible treatments, tests, and drugs in a clear and understandable way. If you don't understand something, ask for clarification.
- If a health care provider prescribes any medications, ask whether you can take generic equivalents that cost less.
- Ask for a written summary of the results of your visit and any lab tests.
- Find out what studies have been done on the safety and effectiveness of any treatment in which you are interested. Consult only reliable sources—texts, journals, and government resources. Start with the websites listed at the end of this text.
- If you have any doubt about a recommended treatment, get a second opinion.
- Decisions regarding treatment should be made in consultation with your health care provider and based on your condition and needs.
- If you use any CAM therapy, inform your primary health care provider. It is particularly important to talk with your provider if you are thinking about replacing your prescribed treatment with one or more supplements, are currently taking a prescription drug, have a chronic medical condition, are planning to have surgery, are pregnant or nursing, or are thinking about giving supplements to children.
- When filling prescriptions, ask the pharmacist to show you the package inserts that list medical considerations. Request detailed information about potential drug and food interactions.
- Remember that *natural* and *safe* are not necessarily the same. You can become seriously ill from seemingly harmless "natural" products. Be cautious about combining herbal medications, just as you would about combining other drugs. Seek help if you notice any unusual side effects.

check yourself

- **What are four instances in which you should seek medical help?**

6.2 Assessing Health Professionals

learning outcome

6.2 List factors to consider when choosing a medical provider.

The most satisfied patients are those who feel their health care provider explains diagnosis and treatment options thoroughly and communicates competency and caring.[4] When evaluating health care providers, consider the following questions:

- Does the provider listen to you and give you time to ask questions? Does the provider return your calls? Is he or she available to answer questions between visits?
- What professional education and training has the provider had? What license or board certification(s) does he or she hold? Note that *board-certified* indicates that a physician has passed the national board examination for his or her specialty (e.g., pediatrics) and has been certified as competent in that specialty; *board-eligible* means that the physician is eligible to take a specialty board's exam, but not necessarily that he or she has passed it.
- Is the provider a specialist in family or internal medicine, or does the provider have another specialty? Is this right for you?
- Is the provider affiliated with an accredited medical facility or institution? The Joint Commission is an independent nonprofit organization that evaluates and accredits more than 15,000 health care organizations and programs in the United States. Accreditation requires that these institutions verify all education, licensing, and training claims of affiliated practitioners.
- Is the provider open to complementary or alternative strategies? Would he or she refer you for different treatments if appropriate?
- Does the provider indicate clearly how long a given treatment may last, what side effects you might expect, and what problems you should watch for?
- Who will be responsible for your care when your provider is on vacation or off call?
- Are professional reviews and information on any lawsuits involving the provider available online?
- If you have health insurance, is the provider in-network? You will most likely end up paying less out of pocket with an in-network doctor.

Ask yourself the following questions about the quality of care you are receiving:

- Did your health care provider take a thorough health history and ask for any recent updates to it? Was your examination thorough?
- Did your provider listen to you?
- Did you feel comfortable asking questions? Did your provider answer thoroughly, in a way that was easy to understand?

Asking the right questions at the right time may save you suffering and expense. Many patients find that writing their questions down before an appointment helps.

Active participation in your treatment is the only sensible course in a health care environment that encourages **defensive medicine**, or the use of medical practices designed to avert the possibility of malpractice suits. In a recent survey of physicians, 58 percent indicated that they have ordered a test or procedure for primarily defensive medicine reasons.[5] Unwarranted treatment such as the overuse of antibiotics and use of diagnostic tests to protect against malpractice exposure are driving up the cost of medicine.[6]

In addition to asking the suggested questions above, being proactive in your health care also means that you should be aware of your rights as a patient:[7]

1. The right of informed consent means that before receiving any care you should be fully informed of what is planned, the risks and potential benefits, and possible alternative forms of treatment, including the option to refuse treatment. Your consent must be voluntary and without any form of coercion. It is critical that you read any consent forms carefully and amend them as necessary before signing.
2. You have the right to know whether the treatment you are receiving is standard or experimental. In experimental conditions, you have the legal and ethical right to know if any drug is being used in the research project for a purpose not approved by the Food and Drug Administration (FDA) and whether the study is one in which some people receive treatment while others receive a placebo.
3. You have the right to make decisions regarding the health care that is recommended by the physician.
4. You have the right to confidentiality. This means that you do not have an obligation to reveal the source of payment for your treatment. It also means you have the right to make personal decisions concerning all reproductive matters.
5. You have the right to receive adequate health care, as well as to refuse treatment and to cease treatment at any time.
6. You are entitled to have access to all of your medical records and to have those records remain confidential.
7. You have the right to continuity of health care.
8. You have the right to seek the opinions of other health care professionals regarding your condition.
9. You have the right to courtesy, respect, dignity, responsiveness, and timely attention to your health needs.

check yourself

- **What should you look for when choosing a medical provider?**
- **What do you consider the four most important characteristics in a medical provider?**

Types of Allopathic Health Care Providers

learning outcome

6.3 Identify the main types of allopathic health care providers.

Conventional health care, also called **allopathic medicine,** mainstream medicine, or traditional Western medical practice, is based on the premise that illness is a result of exposure to harmful environmental agents, such as infectious microorganisms and pollutants or organic changes in the body. The prevention of disease and the restoration of health involve vaccines, drugs, surgery, and other treatments.

Allopathic health care providers use **evidence-based medicine,** in which decisions regarding patient care are based on a combination of clinical expertise, patient values, and current best scientific evidence.

Selecting a **primary care practitioner (PCP)**—a medical practitioner you can visit for routine ailments, preventive care, general medical advice, and referrals—is not easy. The PCP for most people is a family practitioner, internist, pediatrician, or obstetrician-gynecologist (ob-gyn). Some people see nurse practitioners or physician assistants who work for individual doctors or medical groups, whereas others use nontraditional providers as their primary source of care. As a college student, you may opt to visit a PCP at your campus health center.

Doctors undergo rigorous training before they can begin practicing. After 4 years of undergraduate work, students typically spend 4 years studying for the medical degree (MD). Some students then choose a specialty, such as pediatrics, cardiology, or surgery, spending a 1-year internship and several years in residency with that emphasis.

Specialists include **osteopaths,** general practitioners who receive training similar to that of MDs, but who place special emphasis on the skeletal and muscular systems. Their treatments may involve manipulation of muscles and joints. Osteopaths receive the degree of doctor of osteopathy (DO) rather than MD.

Eye care specialists can be either ophthalmologists or optometrists. An **ophthalmologist** holds a medical degree and can perform surgery and prescribe medications. An **optometrist** typically evaluates visual problems and fits glasses but is not a trained physician. If you have an eye infection, glaucoma, or other eye condition that requires diagnosis and treatment, you need to see an ophthalmologist.

Dentists are specialists who diagnose and treat diseases of the teeth, gums, and oral cavity. They attend dental school for 4 years and receive the title of doctor of dental surgery (DDS) or doctor of medical dentistry (DMD). *Orthodontists* specialize in the alignment of teeth. *Oral surgeons* perform surgical procedures to correct problems of the mouth, face, and jaw.

Nurses are highly trained and strictly regulated health professionals who provide a wide range of services, including patient education, counseling, community health and disease prevention information, and administration of medications. Registered nurses (RNs) in the United States complete either a 4-year program leading to a bachelor of science in nursing (BSN) degree or a 2-year associate degree program. Lower-level licensed practical or vocational nurses (LPNs or LVNs) complete a 1- to 2-year training program based in a community college or a hospital.

Nurse practitioners (NPs) are nurses with advanced training obtained through either a master's degree program or a specialized nurse practitioner program. Nurse practitioners have the training and authority to conduct diagnostic tests and prescribe medications (in some states).

Physician assistants (PAs) examine and diagnose patients, offer treatment, and write prescriptions under a physician's supervision. Unlike an NP, a PA must practice under a physician's supervision.

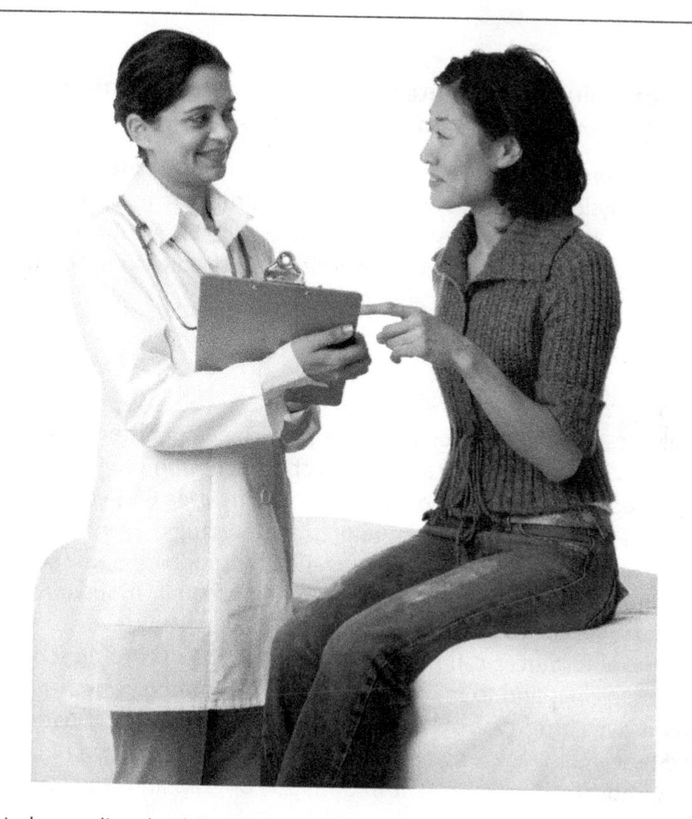

Understanding the differences among different types of health care providers is important. In some cases, you may need to see a doctor with a particular specialty; in other cases, a nurse practitioner or physician assistant may be satisfactory.

check yourself

- **What is allopathic medicine?**
- **What are some of the major types of allopathic health care providers?**

6.4 Choosing Health Products: Prescription and OTC Drugs

learning outcome

6.4 Explain how to determine the risks and benefits of prescription and over-the-counter medicines.

Prescription drugs can be obtained only with a written prescription from a physician, whereas over-the-counter drugs can be purchased without a prescription. Just as making wise decisions about providers is an important aspect of responsible health care, so is making wise decisions about medications.

Prescription Drugs

In about 3 out of 4 doctor visits, the physician administers or prescribes at least one medication.[8] In fact, prescription drug use has increased steadily over the past decade, and over 68 percent of Americans now use one or more prescription drugs.[9] Even though these drugs are administered under medical supervision, the wise consumer still takes precautions. Hazards and complications arising from the use of prescription drugs are common.

Several resources can help you determine the risks of prescription medicines and to make educated decisions about whether to take a given drug. One of the best is the Center for Drug Evaluation and Research (www.fda.gov). This consumer-specific section of the FDA website provides current information on risks and benefits of prescription drugs.

Generic drugs, medications sold under a chemical name rather than a brand name, contain the same active ingredients as brand-name drugs but are less expensive. If your doctor prescribes a drug, always ask if a generic equivalent exists and if it would be safe and effective for you to try. There is some controversy about effectiveness of generic drugs: Substitutions sometimes are made in minor ingredients that can affect the way the drug is absorbed, potentially causing discomfort or even allergic reactions in some patients.[10] Tell your doctor about any reactions you have to medications.

Medications Online: Buyer Beware Consumers may choose to have prescriptions filled online for convenience and to save money. Although many websites operate legally and observe the traditional safeguards for dispensing drugs, be wary of rogue websites that sell unapproved or counterfeit drugs or that sidestep practices meant to protect consumers.

The Verified Internet Pharmacy Practice Sites (VIPPS) seal is given to online pharmacy sites that meet state licensure requirements. Follow these tips to protect yourself from fraudulent sites:[11]

- Buy only from state-licensed pharmacy sites based in the United States (preferably from VIPPS-certified sites).
- Don't buy from sites that sell prescription drugs without a prescription or that offer to prescribe a medication for the first time without a physical exam by your doctor or by answering an online questionnaire.
- Use legitimate websites that have a licensed pharmacist to answer your questions.
- Don't provide personal information, such as a Social Security number, credit card information, or medical or health history, unless you are sure the website will keep your information safe and private.

48.5% of Americans report taking at least one prescription drug in the past month; 21.7% report taking three or more such drugs.

Over-the-Counter (OTC) Drugs

Over-the-counter (OTC) drugs are nonprescription substances used for self-medication. American consumers spend billions of dollars yearly on OTC preparations for relief of everything from runny noses to ingrown toenails. Despite a common belief that OTC products are safe and effective, indiscriminate use and abuse can occur with these drugs as with all others. For example, people who frequently drop medication into their eyes to "get the red out" or pop antacids after every meal are likely to become dependent on these remedies. Many experience adverse side effects because they ignore or don't read the warnings on OTC drug labels. The FDA has developed a standard label that appears on most OTC products (Figure 6.1).

Understanding the actions and side effects of OTC drugs is part of being a smart consumer. *Pain relievers* can be useful for counteracting localized or general pain and for reducing fever. They exist in several general formulations (common brand names follow each): *aspirin* (Bayer, Bufferin), *acetaminophen* (Tylenol), *ibuprofen* (Advil, Motrin), and *naproxen sodium* (Aleve, Naprosyn). Possible side effects include stomach problems ranging from simple stomach upset to worsening of ulcers; overdose or prolonged overuse can cause liver damage. Aspirin and ibuprofen also

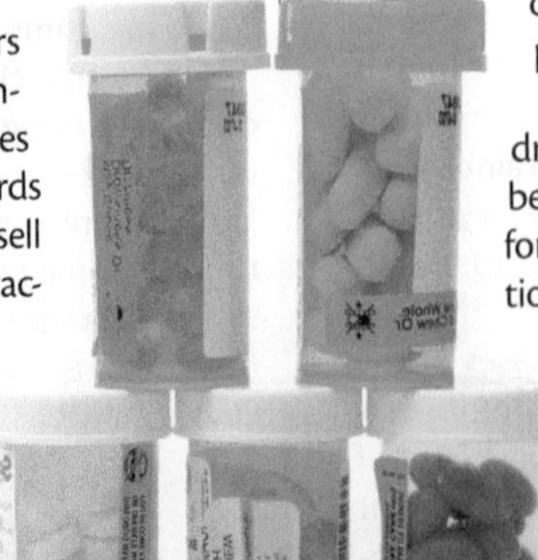

Be very cautious if you consider ordering medications from an online pharmacy.

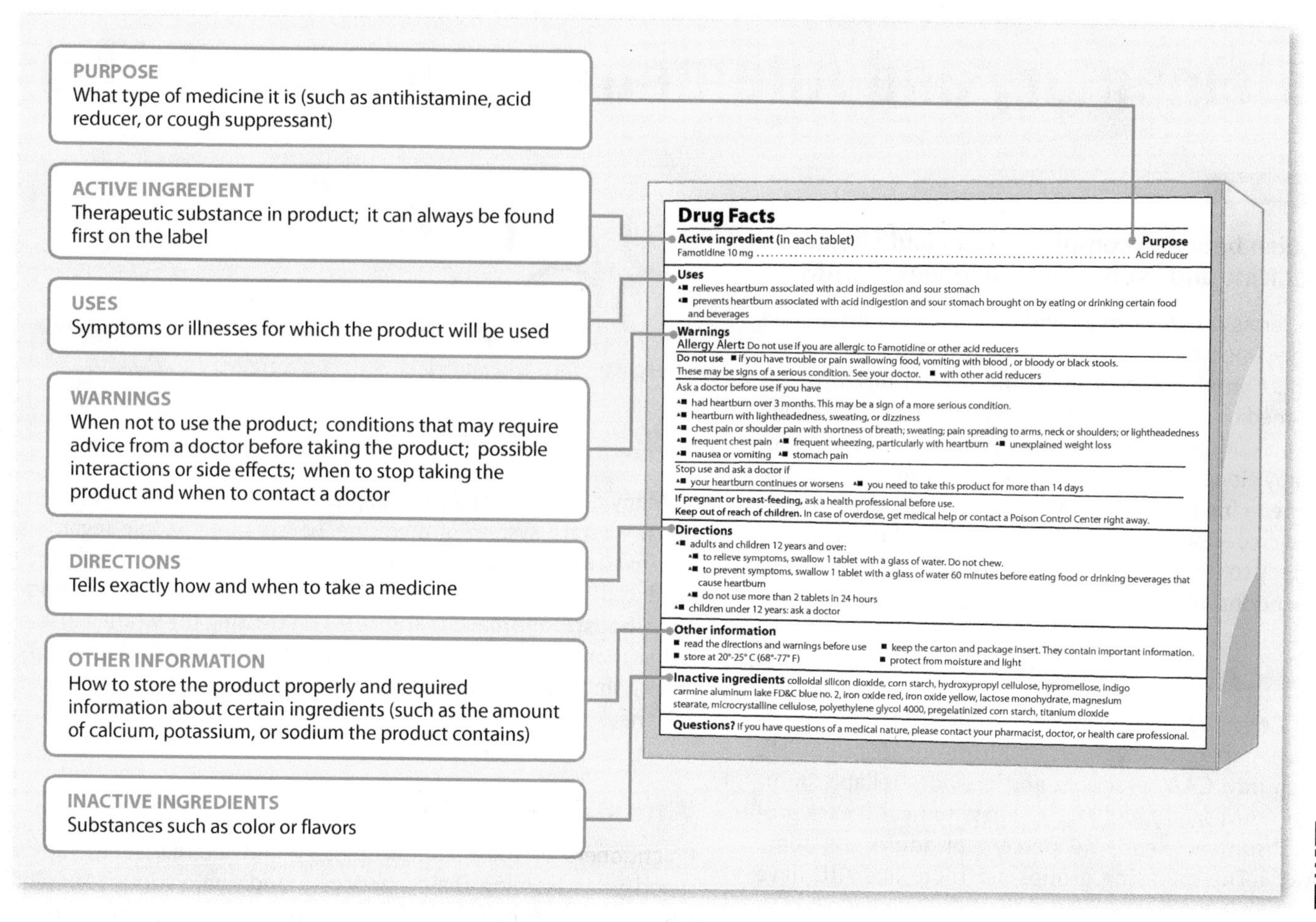

Figure 6.1 The Over-the-Counter Medicine Label

Source: Consumer Healthcare Products Association, OTC Label, www.otcsafety.org. Used with permission.

VIDEO TUTOR
Being a Good Health Care Consumer

reduce blood clotting ability (which can be a problem for those taking anticlotting medications) and, for a few users, can trigger severe allergic reactions. Finally, aspirin should not be taken by anyone under 18, because it has been associated with Reye's syndrome in children and teenagers.

Cold and allergy medicines mask (but don't eliminate) symptoms in a variety of ways. *Antihistamines* (Claritin, Benadryl, Xyzal) dry runny noses, clear postnasal drip and sinus congestion, and reduce tears. They are mild central nervous system depressants and, as such, can cause drowsiness, dizziness, and disturbed coordination in many people. *Decongestants* (Sudafed, DayQuil, Allermed) reduce nasal stuffiness due to colds. In terms of side effects, different people react differently to these medications: Some may exhibit nervousness, restlessness, and sleep problems, whereas others may feel drowsy or nauseated.

Antacids (Tums, Maalox) relieve "heartburn," usually by combating stomach acid with a chemical base such as calcium or aluminum. Occasional use is safe, but chronic use can lead to reduced mineral absorption from food; possible concealment of ulcer; reduced effectiveness of anticlotting medications; interference with the function of certain antibiotics (for antacids that contain aluminum); worsened high blood pressure (for antacids that contain sodium); and aggravated kidney problems.

Laxatives (Ex-lax, Citrucel) are designed to relieve constipation. Although safe with limited and occasional use, long-term regular use can lead to reduced absorption of minerals from food, dehydration, and even dependency (the user's body becoming dependent on the drug for regular bowel movement).

Sleep aids and relaxants (Nytol, Sleep-Eze, Sominex) are designed to help relieve occasional sleeplessness. Short-term side effects include drowsiness and reduced mental alertness, dry mouth and throat, constipation, dizziness, and lack of coordination. Long-term use can lead to dependency.

check yourself

- **What factors should you consider when ordering prescription drugs online?**
- **What are the benefits and potential side effects for three OTC drugs that you use or might use in the future?**

6.5 Complementary and Alternative Medicine (CAM)

learning **outcome**

6.5 Distinguish between complementary and alternative medicine and list the four categories of CAM.

Although the terms *complementary* and *alternative* are often used interchangeably when referring to therapies, there is a distinction between them. **Complementary medicine** is used *together with* conventional medicine as part of a modern integrative-medicine approach.[12] An example of complementary medicine is the use of massage therapy along with prescription medicine to treat anxiety. **Alternative medicine** has traditionally been used *in place of* conventional medicine—for example, following a special diet or using an herbal remedy to treat cancer *instead* of using radiation, surgery, or other conventional treatments.

Who Uses CAM and Why?

The National Center for Complementary and Alternative Medicine (NCCAM), part of the National Institutes of Health (NIH), funds research into CAM practices and provides reliable information about CAM safety and effectiveness to health care providers and consumers. Nearly 40 percent of adults use some form of CAM.[13] The following groups are more likely to have used CAM:

- More women than men
- People with higher educational levels
- People who have been hospitalized in the past year
- Former smokers (compared with current smokers or those who have never smoked)
- People with back, neck, head, or joint aches or other painful conditions
- People with gastrointestinal disorders or sleeping problems

36% of 18- to 29-year-olds report having used some form of CAM.

Many people seek CAM therapies as alternatives to the conventional Western system of medicine, which some people regard as too invasive, too high-tech, and too toxic in terms of laboratory-produced medications. In contrast, most CAM therapies incorporate a **holistic** approach that focuses on treating the whole person, rather than just an isolated part of the body. Some CAM patients believe that alternative practices will give them greater control over their health care.

Who Can Provide CAM Treatments?

Practitioners of most complementary and alternative therapies spend years learning their practice. In addition, various forms of CAM are increasingly being taught in U.S. medical schools. Similar to conventional medicine, there is no national training, certification, or licensure standard for CAM practitioners, and state regulations differ. Whereas practitioners of conventional medicine have graduated from U.S.-sanctioned schools of medicine or are licensed medical practitioners recognized by the American Medical Association (AMA)—the governing body for all physicians—each CAM domain has a different set of training standards, guidelines for practice, and licensure procedures.

Figure 6.2 The Ten Most Common Complementary and Alternative Medicine (CAM) Therapies among U.S. Adults

Source: Data from P. M. Barnes, B. Bloom, and R. Nahin, "Complementary and Alternative Medicine Use among Adults and Children: United States, 2007," *CDC National Health Statistics Report*, no. 12 (December 2008).

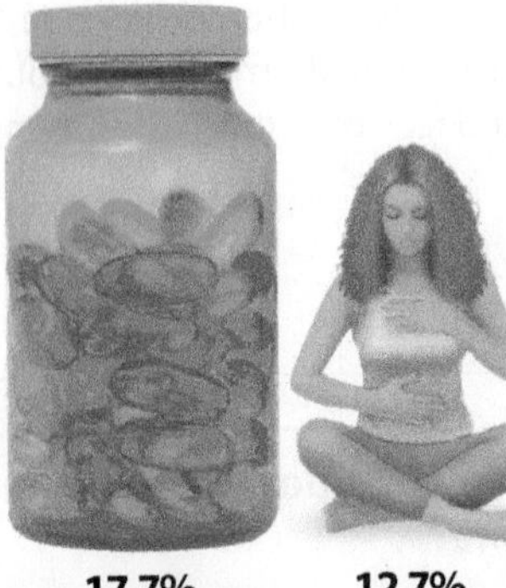

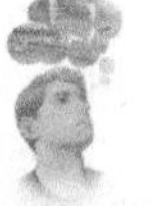

17.7% Natural products
12.7% Deep breathing
9.4% Meditation
8.6% Chiropractic & osteopathic
8.3% Massage
6.1% Yoga
3.6% Diet-based therapies
2.9% Progressive relaxation
2.2% Guided imagery
1.8% Homeopathic treatment

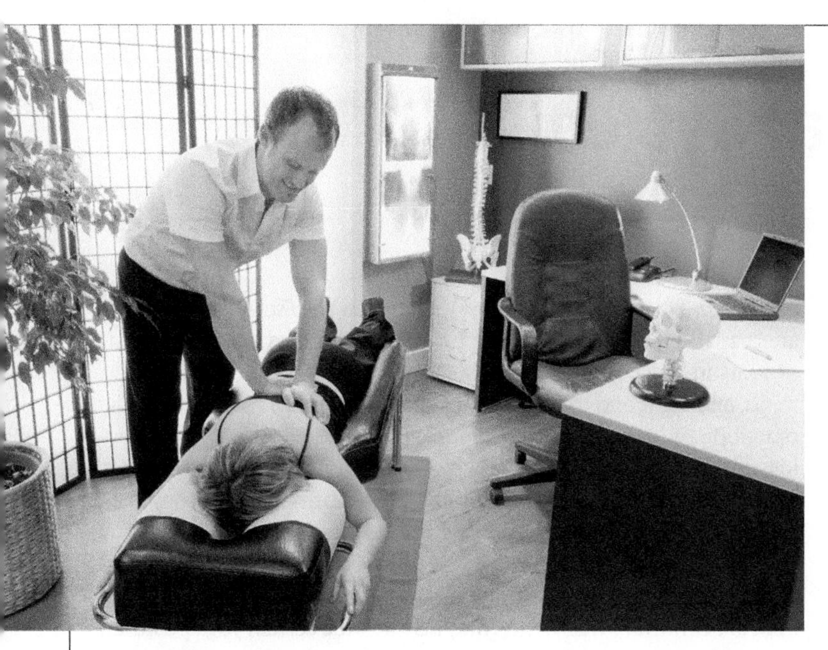

Why are so many people using alternative medicine?

People use alternative medicine for multiple reasons, and many treatments can benefit a variety of physical and mental ailments. For example, chiropractic medicine has shown positive results among people with back and neck pain and headaches.

Nearly all health insurance providers cover at least one form of CAM, with acupuncture, chiropractic, and massage therapy being the most common. However, people who choose CAM often must pay the full cost of services themselves.

What Are the Major Therapies and Categories of CAM?

The ten most common CAM therapies are identified in Figure 6.2. CAM therapies vary widely in terms of the nature and extent of the treatment and the types of problems for which they offer help. They also vary in effectiveness. Research has shown some to be effective for specific conditions, whereas others simply have not been adequately studied or research indicates they are not effective for any specific condition.[14]

Before considering any treatments, consult reliable resources to thoroughly evaluate risks, the scientific basis of claimed benefits, and any contraindications to using the product or service. Avoid practitioners who promote their treatments as a cure-all for every health problem or who seem to promise remedies for ailments that have thus far defied the best scientific efforts of mainstream medicine. In short, apply the same strategies to researching CAM as you would to choosing allopathic care.

The NCCAM has grouped the many varieties of CAM into five general domains of practice, recognizing that domains may overlap (Figure 6.3).

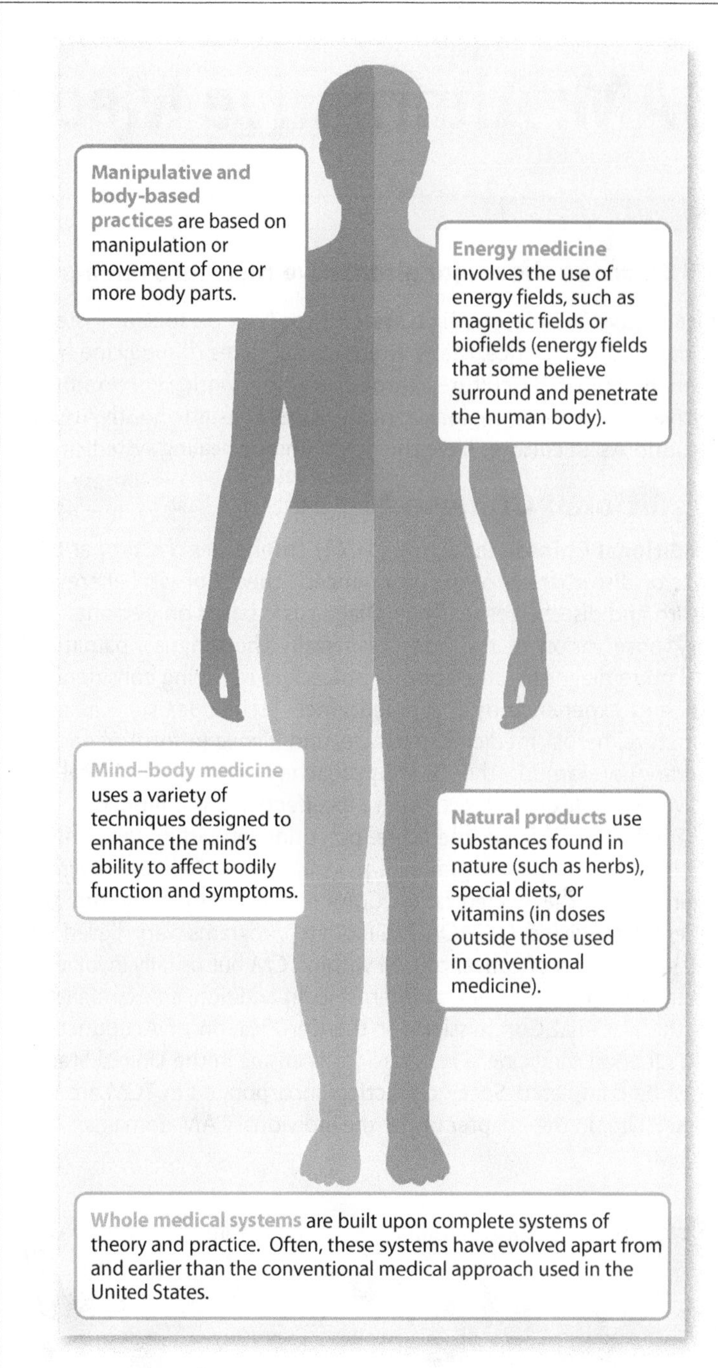

Figure 6.3 The Categories of Complementary and Alternative Medicine (CAM)

NCCAM groups CAM practices into four types, recognizing that there can be some overlap. In addition, NCCAM studies entire CAM medical systems, which cut across all categories.

Source: National Center for Complementary and Alternative Medicine, "The Use of Complementary and Alternative Medicine in the United States," NCCAM Publication no. D434, 2010.

VIDEO TUTOR
CAM: Risks vs. Benefits

check yourself

- **What is the difference between complementary and alternative medicine?**
- **What are the five categories of CAM?**

6.6 CAM: Alternative Medical Systems

learning outcome

6.6 Describe the major alternative medical systems.

Alternative (whole) medical systems are built on specific systems of theory and practice. Many alternative systems of medicine have been practiced by cultures throughout the world. For example, Native American, aboriginal, African, Middle Eastern, South American, and Asian cultures have their own unique healing systems.

Traditional Chinese Medicine

Traditional Chinese medicine (TCM) emphasizes the proper balance or disturbances of **qi** (pronounced "chee"), or vital energy, in health and disease, respectively. Diagnosis is based on personal history, observation of the body (especially the tongue), palpation, and pulse diagnosis, an elaborate procedure requiring considerable skill and experience by the practitioner. Techniques such as acupuncture, herbal medicine, massage, and *qigong* (a form of energy therapy) are among the TCM approaches to health and healing. TCM is complex, and research into its effectiveness is limited.[15]

Traditional Chinese medicine practitioners within the United States must complete a graduate program at a college or university approved by the Accreditation Commission for Acupuncture and Oriental Medicine (ACAOM). Graduate programs vary based on the specific area of concentration within TCM but usually involve an extensive 3- or 4-year clinical internship. In addition, an examination by the National Commission for the Certification of Acupuncture and Oriental Medicine, a standard for licensing in the United States, must be completed. Specific practices incorporated in TCM are discussed later in this chapter under the individual CAM domains.

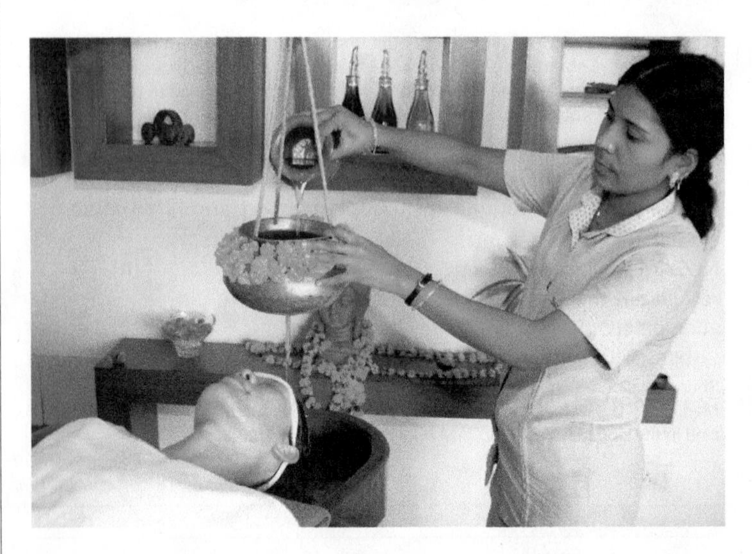

Shirodhara—a traditional Ayurvedic treatment in which warm herbalized oil is poured over the forehead in guided rhythmic patterns—is said to relieve stress and anxiety, treat insomnia and chronic headaches, and improve memory.

Ayurveda

Ayurveda (Ayurvedic medicine) relates to the "science of life," an alternative medical system that began and evolved over thousands of years in India. Ayurveda seeks to integrate and balance the body, mind, and spirit and to restore harmony in the individual.[16] Ayurvedic practitioners use various techniques, including questioning, observing, and touching patients and classifying patients into one of three body types, or *doshas*, before establishing a treatment plan. They then establish a treatment plan to bring the doshas into balance, thereby reducing the patient's symptoms. Dietary modification and herbal remedies drawn from the botanical wealth of the Indian subcontinent are common. Treatments may also include certain yoga postures, meditation, massage, steam baths, changes in sleep patterns and sun exposure, and controlled breathing. Research into Ayurveda is limited, but studies have shown some of the herbal remedies to be effective.[17]

Training of Ayurvedic practitioners varies. At present, no national standard exists for certifying or training Ayurvedic practitioners, although professional groups are working toward creating licensing guidelines.

Homeopathy

Homeopathic medicine, developed in Germany in the late 1700s, is an unconventional Western system based on the principle that "like cures like"—in other words, the same substance that in large doses produces the symptoms of an illness will in very small doses cure the illness. Many homeopathic remedies are derived from toxic substances such as arsenic and belladonna; however, the preparation of the remedy may be so diluted that no actual molecules of the original substance remain.[18] Little evidence supports homeopathy being effective in terms of treating any specific condition.[19]

Homeopathic training varies considerably and is offered through diploma programs, certificate programs, short courses, and correspondence courses. Laws that detail requirements to practice vary from state to state.

Naturopathy

Naturopathic medicine views disease as a manifestation of the body's effort to ward off impurities and harmful substances from the environment. Naturopathic physicians emphasize restoring health rather than curing disease. They employ an array of healing practices, including nutrition; homeopathy; acupuncture; herbal medicine; spinal and soft-tissue manipulation; physical therapies involving electric currents, ultrasound, water, magnets, and light therapy; therapeutic counseling; and pharmacology.

Several major naturopathic schools in the United States and Canada provide training, conferring the *naturopathic doctor* (*ND*) degree on students who have completed a 4-year graduate program that emphasizes humanistically oriented family medicine.

check yourself

- **Describe three alternative medical systems.**

6.7 CAM: Manipulative and Body-Based Practices

learning outcome

6.7 Describe major manipulative and body-based CAM practices.

The CAM category of **manipulative and body-based practices** includes methods based on manipulation or movement of the body.

Chiropractic Medicine

Chiropractic medicine has been practiced for more than 100 years and focuses on manipulation of the spine and other neuromuscular structures.[20] The goals of chiropractic medicine are to correct alignment problems, alleviate pain, and support the body's self-healing abilities. Today, many health care organizations work closely with chiropractors, and many insurance companies pay for chiropractic treatment, particularly if it is recommended by a medical doctor.

Chiropractic medicine is based on the idea that a life-giving energy flows through the spine by way of the nervous system. If the spine is partly misaligned, that force is disrupted. Chiropractors use a variety of techniques to manipulate the spine into proper alignment so energy can flow unimpeded. Therapies may combine spinal adjustments with treatments such as heat and ice, electrical stimulation, exercise, and relaxation techniques. Chiropractic treatment can be effective for back pain, neck pain, and headaches.[21]

The average chiropractic training program requires 4 years of intensive courses in biochemistry, anatomy, physiology, diagnostics, pathology, nutrition, and related topics, plus hands-on clinical training. Many chiropractors then obtain certification in neurology, geriatrics, or pediatrics. Although states vary, increasing numbers require a 4-year undergraduate degree prior to entrance into a 4-year chiropractic program. Applicants must then pass an examination given by the National Board of Chiropractic Examiners. Chiropractic practice is licensed and regulated in all 50 states.[22]

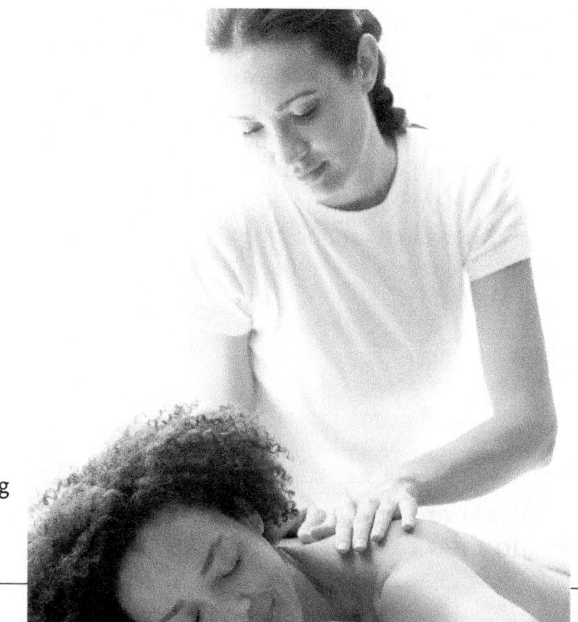

Oh, my aching back? Try massage!

Massage Therapy

Massage therapy is soft tissue manipulation by trained therapists for relaxation and healing. Therapists manipulate the patient's muscles and connective tissues to loosen the fibers and break up adhesions, improve the body's circulation, and remove waste products. Massage is used to treat painful conditions, promote relaxation, reduce stress and anxiety, and relieve depression. Some of the more popular types of massage therapy are the following:

- *Swedish massage* uses long strokes, kneading, and friction on the muscles and moves the joints to aid flexibility.
- *Deep tissue massage* uses strokes and pressure on areas where muscles are tight or knotted, focusing on layers of muscle deep under the skin.
- *Sports massage* is performed to prevent athletic injury and keep the body flexible. It is also used to help athletes recover from injuries.
- *Trigger point massage* (or *pressure point massage*) applies deep, focused pressure on myofascial trigger points—"knots" that can form in the muscles, are painful when pressed, and can cause symptoms throughout the body.
- *Shiatsu massage* uses varying, rhythmic pressure on parts of the body believed important for the flow of vital energy.

The course of study in massage schools typically covers sciences such as anatomy and physiology as well as massage techniques and business, ethical, and legal considerations.[23] The programs vary in length, quality, and whether they are accredited. For licensing, many states require a minimum of 500 hours of training and a passing grade on a national certification exam. Massage therapists work in private studios and health spas, as well as in medical and chiropractic offices, studios, hospitals, nursing homes, and fitness centers.[24]

Bodywork

CAM encompasses a broad range of movement-based approaches used to promote physical, emotional, mental, and spiritual well-being. The *Alexander Technique* is a movement education method designed to release harmful tension in the body to improve ease of movement, balance, and coordination. The *Feldenkrais method* is a system of gentle movements and exercises. It is designed to improve movement, flexibility, coordination, and overall functioning through techniques that enhance awareness and retrain the nervous system. *Pilates* is a popular exercise method focused on improving flexibility, strength, and body awareness. It involves a series of controlled movements, some of which are performed using special equipment.

check yourself

- **What are two manipulative and body-based CAM practices? What treatments do they involve?**

6.8 CAM: Energy Medicine

learning outcome

6.8 Describe major energy-based CAM practices.

Energy medicine therapies focus either on energy fields thought to originate within the body (biofields) or on fields from other sources (electromagnetic fields). The existence of these fields has not been experimentally proven. Some forms of energy therapy manipulate biofields by applying pressure and/or manipulating the body by placing the hands in, or through, these fields.[25] Popular examples of biofield therapy include acupuncture, acupressure, qigong, Reiki, and therapeutic touch.

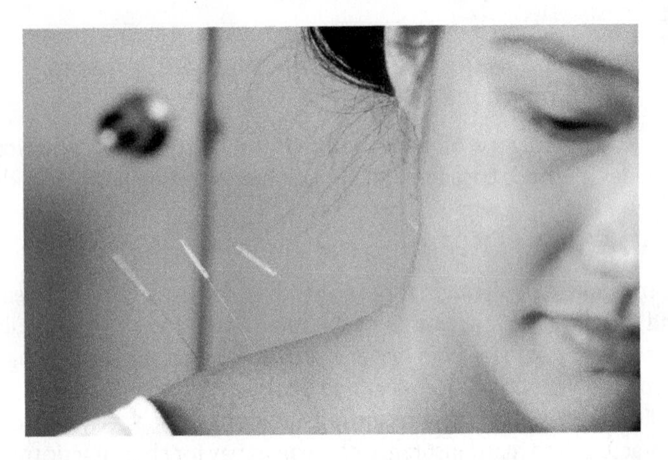

How does acupuncture work?

In acupuncture, long, thin needles are inserted into specific points along the body. This is thought to increase the flow of life-force energy, providing many physical and mental benefits.

Acupuncture and Acupressure

Acupuncture, one of the oldest forms of traditional Chinese medicine (and one of the most popular among Americans), is sought for a wide variety of health conditions, including musculoskeletal dysfunction, mood enhancement, and wellness promotion. It describes a family of procedures that involve stimulating anatomical points of the body with a series of precisely placed needles. The placement and manipulation of acupuncture needles is based on traditional Chinese theories of life-force energy (*qi*) flow through *meridians*, or energy pathways, in the body.

Following acupuncture, most participants in clinical studies report high levels of satisfaction with the treatment and improvement in their condition; however, extensive research has been inconclusive, and there is significant controversy over whether or not such results are simply a placebo response.[26] A 2012 study provided further evidence of a modest but significant reduction in chronic pain among people receiving acupuncture, particularly when they believe it will work and when needles are used in a specific way.[27]

Most U.S. acupuncturists are state licensed; however, licensing requirements vary by state. Many have completed a 2- to 3-year postgraduate program to obtain a master of traditional Oriental medicine (MTOM) degree. In addition, many conventional physicians and dentists practice acupuncture.[28]

Acupressure is based on the same principles of energy flow as acupuncture. Instead of inserting needles, however, the therapist applies pressure to points critical to balancing *yin* and *yang*, the two complementary principles that influence overall harmony (health) of the body. The goal of the therapy is for *qi* to be evenly distributed and flow freely throughout the body. Practitioners must have the same basic training and understanding of meridians and acupuncture points as do acupuncturists.

Other Forms of Energy Therapy

Qigong, a traditional Chinese medicine technique, brings together movement, meditation, and regulation of breathing to increase the flow of *qi*, enhance blood circulation, and improve immune function. Recent research shows that qigong, and the related practice *tai chi*, are effective for promoting bone health, cardiopulmonary fitness, and balance.[29]

Reiki is a hands-on energy therapy that originated in Japan. The name is derived from the Japanese words representing "universal" and "vital energy," or *ki*. Reiki is based on the belief that by channeling *ki* to the patient, the practitioner facilitates healing. In two related therapies, *therapeutic touch* and *healing touch*, the therapist attempts to perceive, through his or her hands held just above the patient's body, imbalances in the patient's energy. The therapist promotes healing by increasing the flow of the body's energies and bringing them into balance. Research supporting the effectiveness of these therapies is limited.[30]

See It! Videos

Is acupuncture right for you? Watch **Health Benefits of Acupuncture** in the Study Area of MasteringHealth.

check yourself

- **What are two energy-based CAM practices? What do their treatments involve?**

6.9 Other CAM Practices

learning outcome

6.9 Describe several mind–body and biologically based CAM practices.

Mind–Body Medicine

Mind–body medicine employs a variety of techniques designed to facilitate the mind's capacity to affect bodily functions and symptoms. At present, mind-body techniques include deep breathing, meditation, yoga, progressive relaxation, and guided imagery—all commonly used CAM therapies in the United States.

Research on **psychoneuroimmunology (PNI)** supports the effectiveness of mind–body therapies. PNI studies the interrelationships among behavioral, neural, endocrine, and immune processes.[31] Scientists are exploring how relaxation, biofeedback, meditation, yoga, laughter, exercise, and activities that involve mind "quieting" may counteract negative stressors and increase immune function.

A recent review study of PNI found that psychological support—including relaxation therapies—can improve wound healing,[32] whereas inflammatory molecules such as C-reactive protein, which is a risk factor for heart disease, were found to be reduced in older adults after 16 weeks of **tai chi**.[33]

Dietary Products

Dietary products, including specially formulated foods and dietary supplements, are perhaps the most controversial domain of CAM therapies because of the sheer number of options available and the many claims that are made about their effects. Many of these claims have not been thoroughly investigated, and many of the products are not currently regulated.

CAM therapies commonly involve increased intake of certain *functional foods*—foods said to improve some aspect of physical or mental functioning beyond the contribution of their specific nutrients. Both whole foods, such as broccoli and nuts, and modified foods, such as an energy bar said to enhance memory, are classified as functional foods.[34] Food producers sometimes refer to their functional foods as **nutraceuticals** to emphasize their combined nutritional and pharmaceutical benefits. For example, the label on a package of cocoa may state that the product provides antioxidants. The claim is backed up by research: Cocoa contains antioxidant phytochemicals called flavonoids, which have been shown to modestly reduce blood pressure.[35] The FDA regulates claims made on food labels; however, the FDA does not test functional foods prior to their coming to market and can only remove a product from the market if it is found to be unsafe.

Other common functional foods and their benefits include the following:

- **Plant stanols/sterols.** Reduces "bad" low-density lipoprotein (LDL) cholesterol.
- **Oat fiber.** Can lower LDL cholesterol; serves as a natural soother of nerves; stabilizes blood sugar levels.
- **Soy protein.** May lower heart disease risk by reducing LDL cholesterol and triglycerides.
- **Garlic.** Lowers cholesterol and reduces clotting tendency of blood; lowers blood pressure; may serve as a form of antibiotic.
- **Ginger.** May prevent motion sickness, stomach pain, and stomach upset; discourages blood clots; may relieve rheumatism.
- **Probiotics.** Yogurt and other fermented dairy foods that are labeled "Live and Active Cultures" contain active, friendly bacteria called *probiotics*. Normal residents of the large intestine, probiotics in foods are thought to reduce the risk for certain types of infections, including opportunistic yeast infections and those associated with acute diarrhea. The National Institutes of Health (NIH) is currently funding extensive research into the therapeutic effects of probiotics on human health.[36]

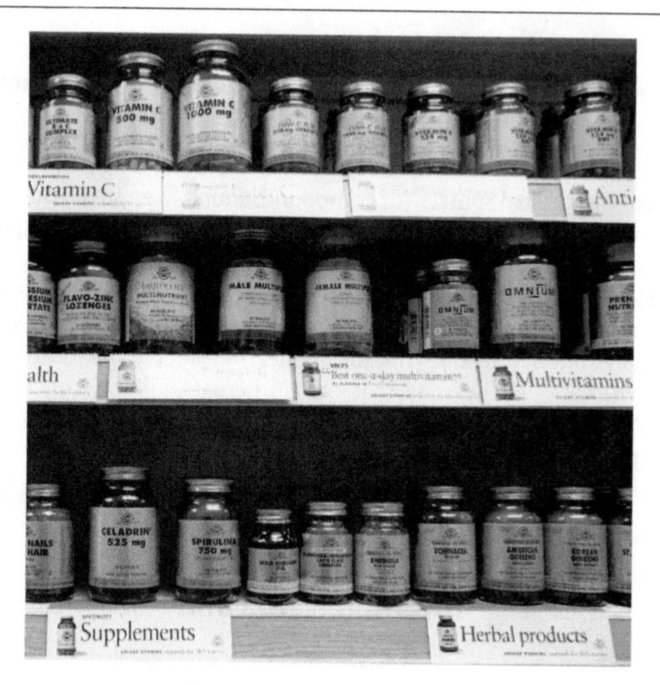

Do herbal remedies have any risks or side effects?

Herbs do have the potential to cause negative side effects. St. John's wort, for example, has potentially dangerous interactions with some prescription antidepressants and should never be taken with them. Other herbs, such as kava, can have negative effects even when taken alone.

check yourself

- **What are several mind–body practices used in complementary medicine?**
- **What are functional foods?**

6.10

Herbal Remedies and Supplements

learning outcome

6.10 Describe how to evaluate the safety and efficacy of herbal remedies and supplements.

People have been using herbal remedies for thousands of years. Herbs were the original sources for compounds found in approximately 25 percent of the pharmaceutical drugs we use today, including aspirin (white willow bark), the heart medication digitalis (foxglove), and the cancer treatment Taxol (Pacific yew).

It's tempting to assume herbal remedies are safe because they are natural, but natural does not mean safe. For example, in recent years the NCCAM has warned that certain herbal products containing kava may be associated with severe liver damage.[37] Even rigorously tested products can be risky. Many plants are poisonous, and some can be toxic if ingested in high doses. Others may be dangerous when combined with prescription or over-the-counter drugs, could disrupt the normal action of the drugs, or could cause unusual side effects.[38] Table 6.1 gives an overview of some of the most common herbal supplements on the market.

In general, herbal medicines tend to be milder than synthetic medications and produce their effects more slowly. But too much of any herb, particularly from nonstandardized extracts, can cause problems.

Not all the supplements on the market today are directly derived from plant sources. In recent years, there have been increasing media claims on the health benefits of various hormones, enzymes, and other biological and synthetic compounds. Although a few products have been widely studied, there is little quality research to support the claims of many others. Table 6.2 lists popular nonherbal supplements and their risks and benefits.

TABLE 6.1 Common Herbs and Herbal Supplements: Benefits, Research, and Risks

Herb	Claims of Benefits	Research Findings	Potential Risks
Echinacea (purple coneflower, *Echinacea purpurea, E. angustifolia, E. pallida*)	Stimulates the immune system and helps fight infection. Used to both prevent and treat colds and flu.	Some studies have provided preliminary evidence of its effectiveness in treating respiratory infections, but two recent studies found no benefit either for prevention or treatment.	Allergic reactions, including rashes, increased asthma, gastrointestinal problems, and anaphylaxis (a life-threatening allergic reaction).
Flaxseed (*Linum usitatissimum*) and flaxseed oil	Used as a laxative and for hot flashes and breast pain, as well as to reduce cholesterol levels and risk of heart disease and cancer.	Flaxseed contains soluble fiber and may have a laxative effect. Study results are mixed on whether flaxseed decreases hot flashes. Insufficient data is available on the effect of flaxseed on cholesterol levels, heart disease, or cancer risks.	Delays absorption of medicines, but otherwise has few side effects. Oil taken in excess could cause diarrhea. Should be taken with plenty of water.
Ginkgo (*Ginkgo biloba*)	Popularly used to prevent cognitive decline, dementia, and Alzheimer's disease, and general vascular disease.	Although some small studies have had promising results, the large Ginkgo Evaluation of Memory study found ginkgo did not reduce Alzheimer's disease or dementia, slow cognitive decline, or reduce blood pressure.	Gastric irritation, headache, nausea, dizziness, difficulty thinking, memory loss, and allergic reactions. Ginkgo seeds are highly toxic; only products made from leaf extracts should be used.
Ginseng (*Panax ginseng*)	Claimed to increase resistance to stress, boost the immune system, lower blood glucose and blood pressure, and improve stamina and sex drive.	Some studies suggest that ginseng may improve immune function and lower blood glucose; however, research overall is inconclusive.	Headaches, insomnia, and gastrointestinal problems are the most commonly reported adverse effects.
Green tea (*Camellia sinensis*)	Useful for lowering cholesterol and risk of some cancers, protecting the skin from sun damage, bolstering mental alertness, and boosting heart health.	Although some studies have shown promising links between green and white tea consumption and cancer prevention, recent research questions the ability of tea to significantly reduce the risk of breast, lung, or prostate cancer.	Insomnia, liver problems, anxiety, irritability, upset stomach, nausea, diarrhea, or frequent urination.

Sources: National Center for Complementary and Alternative Medicine, "Herbs at a Glance," January 2014, http://nccam.nih.gov; American Cancer Society, "Green Tea," May 2012, www.cancer.org.

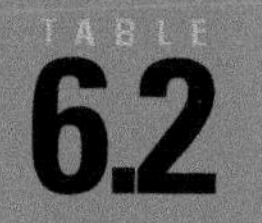

TABLE 6.2 Common Nonherbal Supplements: Benefits, Research, and Risks

Supplement	Claims	Research Findings	Potential Risks
Coenzyme Q10 (antioxidant enzyme found in the heart, liver, kidneys, and pancreas)	Used to improve heart function and reduce blood pressure; also used to increase male fertility and to prevent cancer.	Appears to improve heart function in patients with heart failure. Research on blood-pressure reduction is mixed. May improve sperm quality and count. No proven cancer-prevention benefits.	Does not appear to be associated with serious side effects. Some common side effects include nausea, headaches, insomnia, and heartburn. May reduce effectiveness of anticoagulant medications.
Vitamin E	Claimed to reduce risk of heart disease and age-related vision impairment and slow cognitive decline.	Research into the role of vitamin E in heart disease and vision loss is mixed. There is no evidence supporting its use for improving brain function.	High doses cause bleeding when taken with blood thinners.
Glucosamine (biological substance that helps the body grow cartilage)	Used to relieve pain and inflammation in arthritis and related degenerative joint diseases.	Research shows no significant difference in effectiveness between glucosamine and a placebo. For moderate-to-severe joint pain, glucosamine may be effective when taken with chondroitin sulfate.	Few side effects noted.
Carnitine (amino acid derivative)	Used to improve athletic performance and slow cognitive decline.	Extensive research finds no evidence it improves performance in healthy athletes. Limited evidence suggests that it may enhance mental function in older adults with mild cognitive impairment.	Interacts with some drugs. Common side effects include nausea, vomiting, abdominal cramps, diarrhea, "fishy" body odor. Some evidence of increased risk for cardiovascular disease.
Melatonin (hormone)	Used to regulate circadian rhythms (to prevent jet lag) and treat insomnia; claims of antiaging benefits.	Some evidence supports its usefulness in regulating sleep patterns. No scientific support for antiaging claims.	Nausea, headaches, dizziness, blood vessel constriction; possibly a danger for people with high blood pressure or other cardiovascular problems.
SAMe (pronounced "sammy") (biological compound that aids over 40 functions in the body)	Used in treatment of mild to moderate depression and in treatment of arthritis pain.	Studies have supported its usefulness in treating depression and arthritis pain.	Fewer side effects than prescription antidepressants, but questions remain over correct dosage, form, and long-term side effects.
Zinc (mineral)	Supports immune system; lozenges used to lessen duration and severity of cold symptoms.	Some research suggests that zinc lozenges can reduce the severity and duration of a cold if taken within 24 hours of onset of symptoms.	Use of zinc lozenges can cause nausea. Excessive use can reduce immune function.

Source: Office of Dietary Supplements, National Institutes of Health, "Dietary Supplement Fact Sheets," April 2014, http://ods.od.nih.gov.

Strategies to Protect Supplement Consumers' Health

The burgeoning popularity of functional foods and dietary supplements concerns many scientists and consumers. It is important to gather whatever information you can on both the safety and efficacy of any CAM treatment you are considering. In the case of functional foods and dietary supplements, start your own research with NCCAM (www.nccam.nih.gov) and the Cochrane Collaboration's review on complementary and alternative medicine (www.cochrane.org).

Dietary supplements can currently be sold without FDA approval. This raises issues of consumer safety. Even when products are dispensed by CAM practitioners, the situation can be risky. Products sold in "health food" stores and over the Internet may have varying levels of the active ingredient or may contain additives to which the consumer may have an adverse reaction.

As a result of such concerns, pressure has mounted to establish an approval process for dietary supplements similar to the process the FDA uses for drugs. In the meantime, if you're considering purchasing a dietary supplement, look for the USP Verified Mark on the label (Figure 6.4). The USP (United States Pharmacopeia) is a nonprofit, scientific organization. It does not regulate or determine the safety of medications, foods, or dietary supplements, but it does offer verification services to manufacturers of dietary supplement products. Dietary supplement products must meet stringent quality and manufacturing criteria to earn the USP Verified Mark.[39]

Figure 6.4 The U.S. Pharmacopeia Verified Mark

Source: Used with permission of The United States Pharmacopeial Convention, 12601 Twinbrook Parkway, Rockville, MD 20857.

check yourself

- **What factors should you consider when evaluating herbs or supplements?**

6.11 Health Insurance

learning outcome

6.11 Outline the structure of the U.S. health insurance system.

Whether you're visiting your regular doctor, consulting a specialist, or preparing for a hospital stay, chances are you'll be using some form of health insurance to pay for your care. The fundamental principle of insurance underwriting is that the cost of health care can be predicted for large populations, with the total resulting cost determining health care premiums (payments). Policyholders pay **premiums** into a pool, which is held in reserve until needed. When you are sick or injured, the insurance company pays out of the pool, regardless of your total contribution. Depending on circumstances, you may never pay for what your medical care costs, or you may pay much more. The idea is that you pay affordable premiums so that you never have to face catastrophic bills.

In today's profit-oriented system, insurers prefer to have healthy people in their plans who pour money into risk pools without taking money out. Unfortunately, not everyone has health insurance. In total, about 31 million Americans—15.8 percent—are *uninsured*; that is, they have no private health insurance and are not eligible for Medicare, Medicaid, or other subsidized government health programs.[40] The vast majority of the uninsured work or are dependents of employed people.

Not having health insurance has been associated with individuals delaying health care, as well as increased mortality. *Underinsurance*—the inability to pay for expenses despite being covered—can also cause poor health outcomes. In a 2013 national survey of college students, 6 percent of respondents said they did not have health insurance.[41] However, those who are covered only under their school's health care plan—18.9 percent according to the same survey—may not realize that such plans are usually short term and have a low upper limit of benefits, which would be problematic if the student were to have a severe illness or injury. Few students buy higher-level catastrophic plans.

Racial and ethnic minorities are overly represented in the number of uninsured Americans. Almost a third of all Hispanic Americans are uninsured compared to 18.7 percent of African Americans and 11.5 percent of whites.[42] Issues such as citizenship and language barriers contribute to some of the disparities in access to health insurance for many in our country.

Why should all Americans be concerned about those who are uninsured and underinsured? People without adequate health care coverage are less likely than other Americans to have their children immunized, seek early prenatal care, obtain annual blood pressure checks and other screenings, and seek attention for symptoms of health problems. Experts believe that this ultimately leads to higher system costs because their conditions go undetected at their earliest, most treatable stage, deteriorating to a more debilitating and costly stage before they are forced to seek help, often in an emergency room. Because emergency care is far more expensive than clinic care, uninsured and underinsured patients are often unable to pay, and the cost is absorbed by "the system" in the form of higher hospital costs, insurance premiums, and taxes.

Private Health Insurance

Originally, health insurance consisted solely of coverage for hospital costs (it was called *major medical*), but gradually it was extended to cover routine treatment and other areas, such as dental services and pharmaceuticals. These payment mechanisms, which provided no incentive to contain costs, laid the groundwork for today's steadily rising health care costs. At the same time, because most insurance did not cover routine or preventive services, consumers were encouraged to wait until illness developed to seek care instead of seeking preventive care. Consumers were also free to choose any provider or service, including inappropriate—and often very expensive—care.

To limit potential losses, private insurance companies began increasingly employing several mechanisms: cost sharing (in the form of deductibles, co-payments, and coinsurance), waiting periods, exclusions, "preexisting condition" clauses, and upper limits on payments:

- *Deductibles* are payments (commonly about $1,000 annually) you make for health care before insurance coverage kicks in to pay for eligible services.

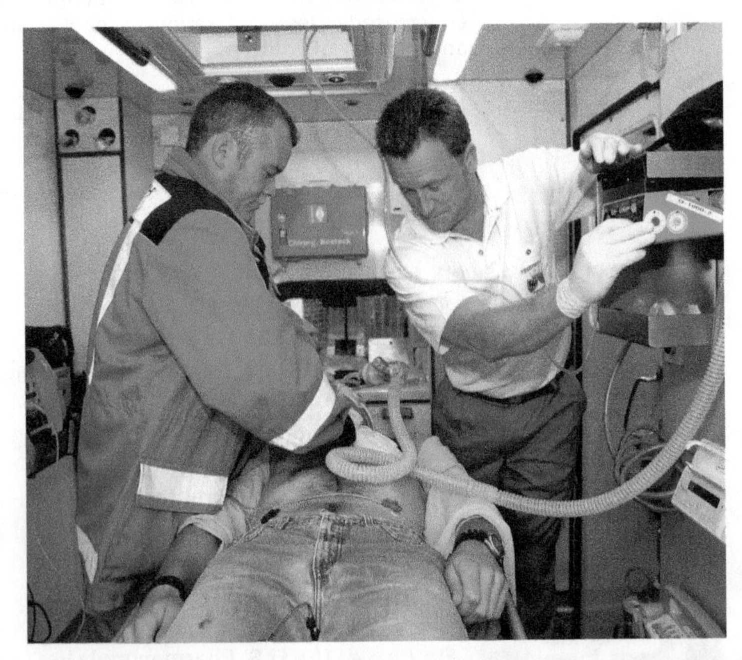

People without insurance can't gain access to preventive care, so they seek care only in an emergency or crisis. Because emergency care is extraordinarily expensive, they often are unable to pay, and the cost is absorbed by those who can pay—the insured or taxpayers.

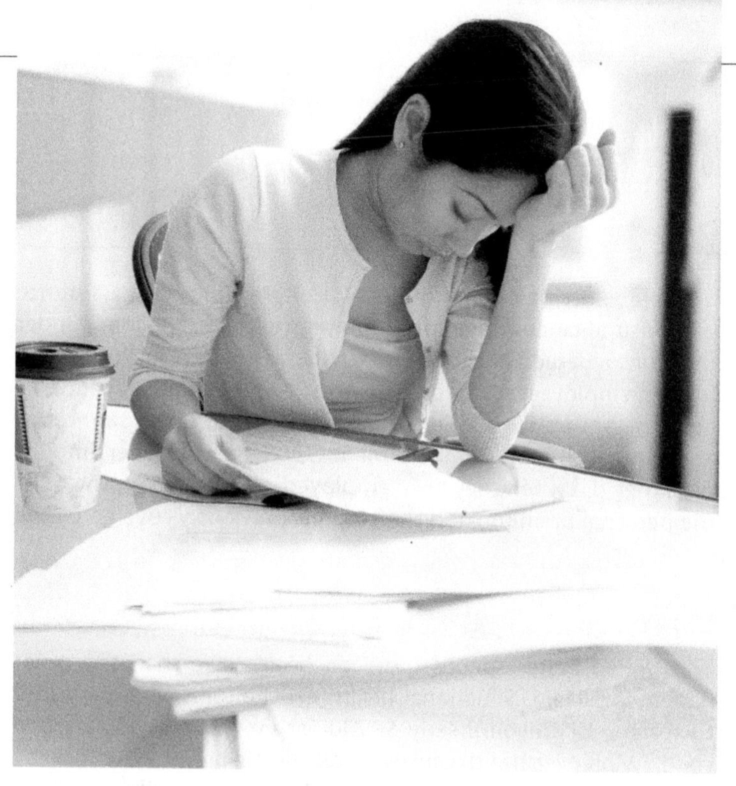

What should I consider when choosing health insurance?

Choosing a health insurance plan can be confusing. Some things to think about include how comprehensive your coverage needs to be, how convenient your care must be, how much you are willing to spend on premiums and co-payments, what the overall cost will be, and whether the services of the plan meet your needs.

- *Co-payments* are set amounts that you pay per service or product received, regardless of the total cost (e.g., $20 per doctor visit or per prescription filled).
- *Coinsurance* is the percentage of costs that you must pay based on the terms of the policy (e.g., 20% of the total bill).
- Some group plans specify a *waiting period* that cannot exceed 90 days before they will provide coverage. Waiting periods do not apply to plans purchased by individuals.
- All insurers set some limits on the types of *covered services* (e.g., most exclude cosmetic surgery, private rooms, and experimental procedures).
- *Preexisting condition clauses* once limited the insurance company's liability for medical conditions that a consumer had before obtaining coverage. For example, if a person applying for insurance had cancer, the insurer could deny the application entirely, or agree to cover the applicant, but only for conditions unrelated to the cancer. Under the 2010 Patient Protection and Affordable Care Act (ACA) no one can be discriminated against because of a preexisting condition.
- Some insurance plans also imposed an *annual upper limit* or *lifetime limit*, after which coverage would end. The ACA makes this practice illegal.

Managed Care

Managed care describes a health care delivery system consisting of a network of providers and facilities linked contractually to deliver health benefits within a set annual budget, sharing economic risk, with membership rules for participating patients. More than 73 million Americans are enrolled in health maintenance organizations (HMOs), the most common type.[43] Managed care plans have grown steadily over the past decade—indemnity insurance, which pays providers on a fee-for-service basis, has become unaffordable or unavailable for most Americans.

Health maintenance organizations provide a range of covered benefits (e.g., checkups, surgery, lab tests) for a fixed prepaid amount. This is both the least expensive form of managed care and the most restrictive—patients are typically required to use the plan's doctors and hospitals and to see a PCP for treatment and referrals.

Preferred provider organizations (PPOs) are networks of independent doctors and hospitals. Members may see doctors not on the preferred list, for an additional cost.

In point of service (POS) plans—offered by many HMOs—a patient selects a PCP from a list of participating providers; this physician becomes the patient's "point of service." If referrals are made outside the network, the patient is still partially covered.

Medicare and Medicaid

The government, through programs such as Medicare and Medicaid, currently funds 45 percent of total U.S. health care spending.[44]

Medicare covers 99 percent of Americans over age 65, all totally and permanently disabled people (after a waiting period), and all people with end-stage kidney failure—together, these groups comprise over 60 million people, or 1 in 6 Americans.[45] As the costs of care have soared, Medicare has placed limits on provider reimbursements. As a result, some physicians and managed care programs have stopped accepting Medicare patients.

To control hospital costs, in 1983 the federal government set up a Medicare payment system based on *diagnosis-related groups (DRGs)*. Nearly 500 groupings of diagnoses were created to establish how much a hospital would be reimbursed for a particular patient. This system motivates hospitals to discharge patients quickly, to provide more ambulatory care, and to admit patients classified into the most favorable (profitable) DRGs. Many private health insurance companies have also adopted reimbursement rates based on DRGs.

Medicaid is a federal–state welfare program covering approximately 62 million people defined as low income, including many who are blind, disabled, elderly, pregnant, or eligible for Temporary Assistance for Needy Families (TANF). Because each state determines eligibility and payments to providers, the way Medicaid operates from state to state varies widely.

check yourself

- **What are four common barriers to adequate health insurance?**
- **What structures and limits do private insurers use to control costs?**

6.12 Issues Facing the Health Care System

learning outcome

6.12 Identify the major challenges facing the U.S. health care system.

In recent decades, the number of Americans without health insurance increased dramatically as costs and restrictions on eligibility for coverage rose. In 2010, Congress passed the Patient Protection and Affordable Care Act (ACA) to provide a means for these and all Americans to obtain affordable heath care. In addition to increasing access to care, the ACA is expected to address America's high cost of care and to improve the overall quality of care.

Access

Access to care is one of the challenges facing the U.S. health care system. In 2012, there were almost 700,000 physicians in the United States.[46] However, there is an oversupply of higher-paid specialists and a shortage of lower-paid primary care physicians (family practitioners, internists, pediatricians, etc.). Likewise, of the nearly 5,000 non-federal hospitals in the United States, over 60 percent serve urban areas, leaving many rural communities without readily accessible care.[47]

Managed care health plans determine access on the basis of participating providers, health plan benefits, and administrative rules. Often this means that consumers do not have the freedom to choose specialists, facilities, or treatment options beyond those contracted with the health plan and recommended by their primary care provider, even if care providers and facilities are only a few miles away. Quality of the patient's health insurance plan matters, too: patients with excellent insurance coverage may be encouraged to undergo expensive tests and treatments, whereas patients with poor insurance may not be informed of the full variety of diagnostic and treatment options.[48]

Key provisions in the ACA aim to increase access to quality health insurance among Americans:

- Insurers are now required to cover several preventive services, such as health screenings for cancer and counseling on topics such as losing weight, quitting smoking, and reducing alcohol use.
- Insurers are required to cover young adults on a parent's plan through age 26.
- Coverage is required for prescription medications, including psychotropic medications.
- Americans with preexisting conditions cannot be denied coverage.
- No annual and lifetime limits on benefits are allowed.
- Affordable Insurance Exchanges (AIEs) facilitate consumer shopping and enrollment in plans with the same kinds of choices that members of Congress have.
- Small businesses, which typically paid as much as 18 percent more than large businesses for health insurance coverage for their employees, now qualify for special tax credits to help fund insurance plans.

Even before passage of the ACA, Congress provided assistance with insurance coverage for employees who change jobs. Under the Consolidated Omnibus Budget Reconciliation Act (COBRA), former employees, retirees, and their spouses and dependents have the option to continue their insurance for up to 18 months at group rates. People who enroll in COBRA pay a higher amount than they did when they were employed, as they're covering both the personal premium and the amount previously covered by the employer.

Cost

The United States spends more on health care than any other nation. In 2014, U.S. national health expenditures were projected to reach \$3.1 trillion, nearly \$9,700 for every man, woman, and child.[49] Moreover, health care expenditures are projected to grow by 5.8 percent each year, reaching over \$5 trillion annually by 2022—nearly 20 percent of our projected gross domestic product (GDP; see Figure 6.5).[50]

Why are America's health care costs so high? Many factors are involved: a for-profit health industry; excess administrative costs; duplication of services; an aging population; growing rates of obesity, inactivity, and related health problems; demand for new medical technologies; an emphasis on crisis-oriented care instead of prevention; and inappropriate use of services.

Our system's more than 2,000 health insurance companies prevents *economies of scale* (bulk purchasing at a reduced cost) and administrative efficiency realized in countries with single-payer systems. Commercial insurance companies commonly experience administrative costs greater than 12 percent of the total health care insurance premium.[51] These administrative expenses contribute to the high cost of

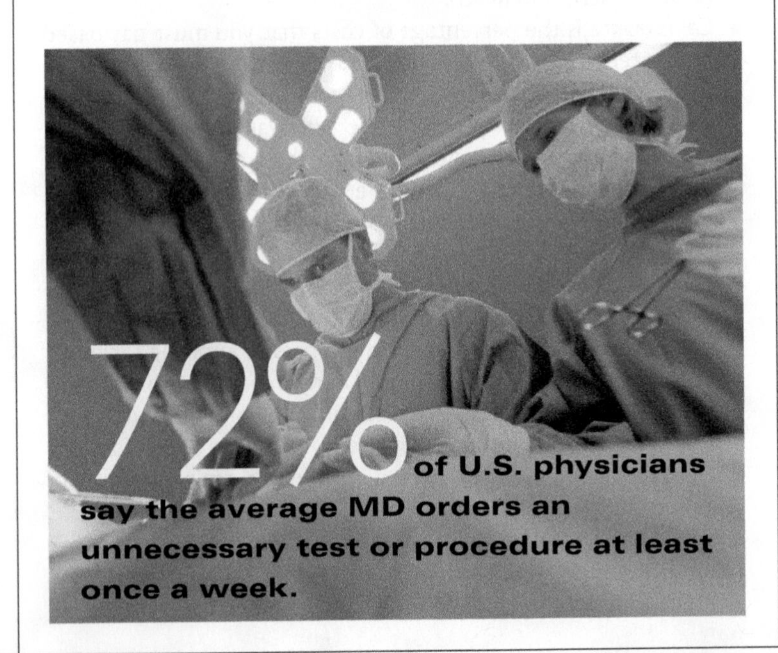

health care and are largely passed on to consumers in the form of higher prices for goods and services.

The ACA mandates the following cost-control measures:

- Insurance companies that spend less than 80 percent of premium dollars on medical care in a given year have to send enrollees a rebate.
- All insurance companies have to publicly justify their actions if they plan to raise rates by 10 percent or more.
- Tougher screening procedures and penalties are helping to reduce health care fraud.

2014 estimated total expenditures = $3.1 trillion

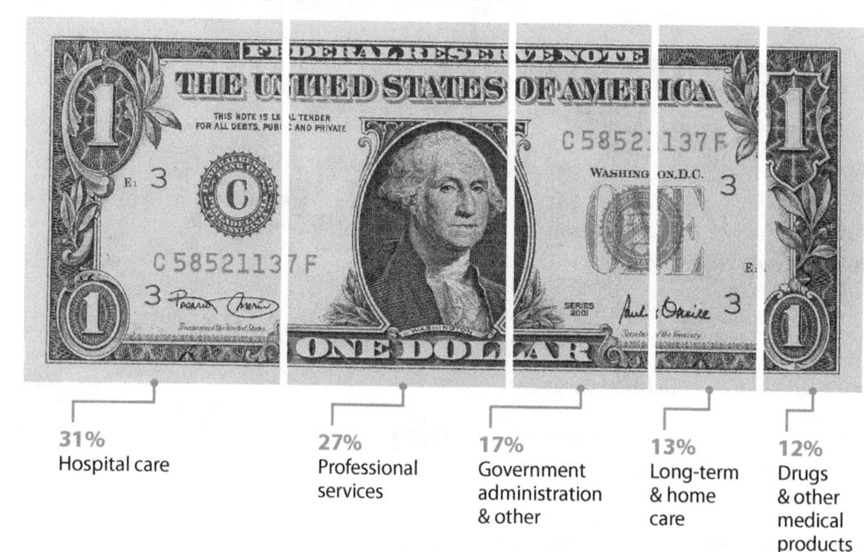

Figure 6.5 Where Do We Spend Our Health Care Dollars?

Source: Data are from Centers for Medicare & Medicaid Services, "National Health Expenditure Projections 2012–2022: Forecast Summary," November 2013, www.cms.gov.

The Debate over Universal Coverage

Whether universal health care coverage will—or should—be achieved in the United States and through what mechanism remain hotly debated topics. Proponents of reform argue that health care is a basic human right and should be available and affordable for everyone. Opponents of health care reform feel that health care is not a right, but a commodity. They contend that the high cost of changing the system is more than the United States can afford and that the government should not interfere in what has been largely a free-market industry. In addition, lobbying efforts by the insurance industry, pharmaceutical manufacturers, and special interest groups have all played a role in thwarting comprehensive reform.

The ACA does not provide for a system of national health care but is merely a set of initial steps toward increasing the number of insured Americans. Although it has reduced the number of uninsured Americans by an estimated 9 million, it has been subjected to intense and often rancorous debate. The reforms mandated by the ACA are currently being implemented, and their actual effects are uncertain.

Debate continues over the goal of universal coverage. Arguments for national health insurance include the following:[52]

- Health care is a human right. The United Nations Universal Declaration of Human Rights states that "everyone has the right to a standard of living adequate for the health and well-being of oneself and one's family, including ... medical care."[53]
- Americans would be more likely to engage in preventive health behaviors and clinicians would be encouraged to practice preventive medicine; people who are underinsured and uninsured often avoid preventive care checkups because of the cost.
- A national system of health care would further increase economic prosperity by enabling Americans to live longer and healthier lives, thus increasing their contributions to society.

Arguments against national health insurance include the following:[54]

- Health care is not a right, because it is not in the Bill of Rights in the U.S. Constitution, which lists rights the government cannot infringe upon, not services the government must ensure.
- It is the individual's responsibility to ensure personal health. Diseases and health problems can often be prevented by choosing to live healthier lifestyles.
- Expenses for health care would have to be paid for with higher taxes or spending cuts in other areas.
- Profit motives, competition, and ingenuity lead to cost control and effectiveness. These concepts should be brought to health care reform.

Quality

The U.S. health care system has several mechanisms for ensuring quality: education, licensure, certification/registration, accreditation, peer review, and malpractice litigation. Some of these are mandatory before a professional or organization may provide care; others are voluntary. Insurance companies and government payers may link payment to whether a practitioner is board certified or a facility is accredited by an appropriate agency. In addition, most insurance plans require prior authorization and/or second opinions, not only to reduce costs, but also to improve quality of care.

Although our health care spending far exceeds that of any other nation, we rank far below many other nations in key indicators of quality. In 2011, the Department of Health and Human Services released to Congress a National Strategy for Quality Improvement in Health Care. Its priorities include a new emphasis on promoting the safest, most preventive, and most effective care, increasing communication and coordination among providers, and ensuring that patients and families are engaged as partners in their care.[55]

check yourself

- **What are two arguments for and two against universal health care coverage?**
- **What are three challenges faced by the U.S. health care system?**

Assess yourself

6.13

Are You a Smart Health Care Consumer?

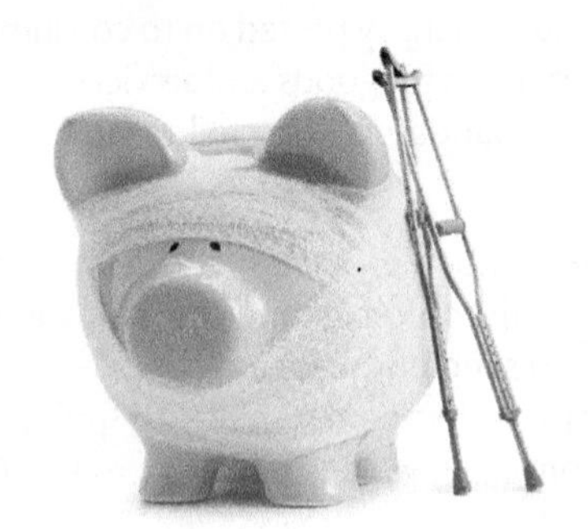

An interactive version of this assessment is available online in MasteringHealth.

Answer the following questions to determine what you might do to become a better health care consumer.

	Yes	No
1. Do you have health insurance?	◯	◯
2. If you answered yes to question 1, do you understand the coverage available to you under your plan?	◯	◯
3. Do you know which health care services are available for free or at a reduced cost at your student health center or local clinic?	◯	◯
4. When you receive a prescription, do you ask the doctor or pharmacist if a generic brand could be substituted?	◯	◯
5. When you receive a prescription, do you ask the doctor or pharmacist about potential side effects and interactions?	◯	◯
6. Do you report any unusual drug side effects to your health care provider?	◯	◯
7. Do you read labels carefully before buying over-the-counter (OTC) medications?	◯	◯
8. Do you take medication as directed?	◯	◯
9. When you receive a diagnosis, do you seek more information about the diagnosis and treatment?	◯	◯
10. When considering a CAM technique, do you research and identify scientific findings about the specific CAM therapy?	◯	◯
11. Do you research the credentials of your practitioner before receiving treatment?	◯	◯
12. Do you inform new practitioners of all the treatments you are currently receiving, including all CAM and traditional therapies?	◯	◯
13. Do you choose only supplements with the USP (United States Pharmacopeia) seal on their labels?	◯	◯
14. Do you consult a physician before taking a supplement?	◯	◯

Your Plan for Change

Once you have considered your responses to the Assess Yourself questions, you may want to change or improve certain behaviors in order to get the best treatment from your health care provider and the health care system.

Today, you can:

◯ Research your insurance plan. Find out which health care providers and hospitals you can visit, the amounts of co-payments and premiums you are responsible for, and the drug coverage offered.

◯ Update your medicine cabinet. Dispose properly of any expired prescriptions or OTC medications. Keep on hand a supply of basic items, such as pain relievers, antiseptic cream, bandages, cough suppressants, and throat lozenges.

Within the next 2 weeks, you can:

◯ Find a regular health care provider if you do not already have one and make an appointment for a general checkup.

◯ Check with your insurance provider and see what CAM practitioners and therapies are covered.

◯ Find out what alternative therapies your college's health clinic offers.

By the end of the semester, you can:

◯ Become an advocate for others' health. Write to your congressperson or state legislature to express your interest in health care reform.

◯ Make relaxation and mind–body stress-reducing techniques a part of your everyday life. This can simply mean practicing meditation or deep breathing, or even taking long walks in nature. You don't need to visit a CAM practitioner or follow a specific therapeutic practice to benefit from methods of relaxation, meditation, and spiritual awakening.

Summary

To hear an MP3 Tutor session, scan here or visit the Study Area in **MasteringHealth.**

LO 6.1 Self-care and individual responsibility are key factors in reducing rising health care costs and improving health status. Planning can help you navigate health care treatment in unfamiliar situations or emergencies.

LO 6.2 Evaluate health professionals by considering their qualifications, their record of treating similar problems, and their ability to work with you.

LO 6.3 Conventional Western (allopathic) medicine is based on scientifically validated methods and procedures. Medical doctors, specialists of various kinds, nurses, and physician assistants practice allopathic medicine.

LO 6.4 Consumers need to understand the risks and benefits of prescription drugs and over-the-counter (OTC) medications. Regulations governing drug labels help ensure that information about these products is available.

LO 6.5 People are using complementary and alternative medicine (CAM) in increasing numbers.

LO 6.6 Alternative medical systems include traditional Chinese medicine (TCM), Ayurveda, homeopathy, and naturopathy.

LO 6.7–LO 6.9 CAM also includes manipulative and body-based practices, energy medicine, mind–body medicine, and biologically based practices.

LO 6.10 The FDA does not study and approve dietary supplements before they are brought to market; thus there is no guarantee of their safety or effectiveness. However, the USP Verified Mark indicates that a supplement has met certain criteria for product purity and manufacturing standards.

LO 6.11 Health insurance is based on the concept of spreading risk. Insurance is provided by private insurance companies (which charge premiums) and government Medicare and Medicaid programs (which are funded by taxes). Managed care attempts to control costs by streamlining administration and stressing preventive care.

LO 6.12 Concerns about the U.S. health care system include access, cost, and quality. The Patient Protection and Affordable Care Act was passed by Congress in 2010 to address these issues.

Pop Quiz

Visit MasteringHealth to personalize your study plan with Chapter Review Quizzes and Dynamic Study Modules.

LO 6.1 1. Of the following conditions, which would be appropriately managed by self-care?
a. A persistent temperature of 104°F or higher
b. Sudden weight loss of more than a few pounds without changes in diet or exercise patterns
c. A sore throat, runny nose, and cough that persist for a few days
d. Yellowing of the skin or the whites of the eyes

LO 6.3 2. What medical practice is based on procedures whose objective is to heal by countering the patient's symptoms?
a. Allopathic medicine
b. Nonallopathic medicine
c. Osteopathic medicine
d. Chiropractic medicine

LO 6.5 3. CAM therapies focus on treating both the mind and the whole body, which makes them part of a
a. natural approach.
b. psychological approach.
c. holistic approach.
d. gentle approach.

LO 6.6 4. What type of medicine addresses imbalances of *qi*?
a. Chiropractic medicine
b. Naturopathic medicine
c. Traditional Chinese medicine
d. Homeopathic medicine

LO 6.6 5. The alternative system of medicine based on the principle that "like cures like" is
a. naturopathic medicine.
b. homeopathic medicine.
c. Ayurvedic medicine.
d. chiropractic medicine.

LO 6.9 6. The use of techniques to improve the psychoneuroimmunology of the human body is called
a. acupressure.
b. mind–body medicine.
c. Reiki.
d. bodywork.

LO 6.6 7. What system places equal emphasis on body, mind, and spirit and strives to restore the innate harmony of the individual?
a. Ayurvedic medicine
b. Homeopathic medicine
c. Naturopathic medicine
d. Traditional Chinese medicine

LO 6.10 8. The "USP Dietary Supplement Verified" seal indicates that a supplement is
a. safe and pure.
b. effective.
c. low cost.
d. child safe.

LO 6.11 9. What mechanism used by private insurance companies requires that the subscriber pay a certain amount directly to the provider before the insurance company will begin paying for services?
a. Coinsurance
b. Cost sharing
c. Co-payments
d. Deductibles

LO 6.11 10. Andrea, 28, is a single parent on welfare. Her medical bills are paid by a federal health insurance program for the poor. This program is
a. an HMO.
b. Social Security.
c. Medicaid.
d. Medicare.

Answers to these questions can be found on page A-1. If you answered a question incorrectly, review the module identified by the Learning Outcome. For even more study tools, visit MasteringHealth.

Web Links for Health and Wellness

Chapter 1 Fitness

- **ACSM Online.** The American College of Sports Medicine and all its resources. www.acsm.org
- **American Council on Exercise.** Information on exercise and disease prevention. www.acefitness.org

Chapter 2 Weight Management and Body Image

- **ChooseMyPlate.gov.** USDA's ChooseMyPlate.gov offers extensive information about meal planning and physical activity for healthy living. www.choosemyplate.gov
- **The Rudd Center for Food Policy and Obesity.** The latest in obesity research, public policy, and ways to stop obesity at the community level. www.yaleruddcenter.org
- **National Eating Disorders Association.** Information for eating disorder sufferers and those wishing to help others with eating and body image issues. www.nationaleatingdisorders.org

Chapter 3 Nutrition

- **Academy of Nutrition and Dietetics.** Provides information on a range of dietary topics, including sports nutrition, healthful cooking, and nutritional eating. www.eatright.org
- **U.S. Food and Drug Administration (FDA).** The FDA provides information for consumers and professionals in the areas of food safety, supplements, and medical devices. www.fda.gov
- **Food and Nutrition Information Center.** This site offers a wide variety of information related to food and nutrition. http://fnic.nal.usda.gov
- **U.S. Department of Agriculture (USDA).** The USDA offers a full discussion of the USDA's Dietary Guidelines for Americans. www.usda.gov

Chapter 4 Stress

- **American College Health Association.** This site provides information and data from the National College Health Assessment survey. www.acha.org
- **Higher Education Research Institute.** This organization provides annual surveys of first-year and senior college students that cover academic, financial, and health-related issues. www.heri.ucla.edu
- **American College Counseling Association.** The website of the professional organization for college counselors offers useful links and articles. www.collegecounseling.org

Chapter 5 CVD, Cancer, and Diabetes

- **American Heart Association.** Information, statistics, and resources regarding cardiovascular care, including an opportunity to test your risk for CVD. www.heart.org
- **American Cancer Society.** Information, statistics, and resources regarding cancer. www.cancer.org
- **American Diabetes Association.** Information and resources for those with diabetes. www.diabetes.org

Chapter 14 Environmental Health

- **Environmental Protection Agency (EPA).** The government agency responsible for overseeing environmental regulation and protection issues in the United States. www.epa.gov
- **National Center for Environmental Health (NCEH).** Information on a wide variety of environmental health issues; includes a series of helpful fact sheets. www.cdc.gov/nceh
- **National Environmental Health Association (NEHA).** Educational resources and opportunities for environmental health professionals. www.neha.org

Chapter 6 Consumerism and Complementary and Alternative Medicine

- **Agency for Healthcare Research and Quality (AHRQ).** Links to sites that address health care concerns and provide information on making critical decisions about personal care. www.ahrq.gov
- **National Committee for Quality Assurance (NCQA).** Assessments and reports on managed care plans, including HMOs. www.ncqa.org
- **HealthCare.Gov.** Information regarding the Patient Protection and Affordable Care Act. www.healthcare.gov
- **National Center for Complementary and Alternative Medicine (NCCAM).** Information and research on complementary and alternative practices. http://nccam.nih.gov

Answers to Pop Quiz Questions

Chapter 1

1. c; 2. b; 3. d; 4. c; 5. a; 6. a; 7. b; 8. a; 9. d; 10. a

Chapter 2

1. a; 2. c; 3. b; 4. b; 5. c; 6. b; 7. a; 8. a; 9. b; 10. b

Chapter 3

1. a; 2. b; 3. b; 4. a; 5. d; 6. c; 7. b; 8. d; 9. a; 10. d

Chapter 4

1. c; 2. c; 3. d; 4. b; 5. c; 6. d; 7. c; 8. c; 9. d; 10. c

Chapter 5

1. c; 2. c; 3. b; 4. a; 5. b; 6. d; 7. a; 8. c; 9. b; 10. a

Chapter 6

1. c; 2. a; 3. c; 4. c; 5. b; 6. b; 7. a; 8. a; 9. d; 10. c

Glossary

abortion The termination of a pregnancy by expulsion or removal of an embryo or fetus from the uterus.
abstinence Refraining from a behavior.
accountability Accepting responsibility for personal decisions, choices, and actions.
acid deposition The acidification process that occurs when pollutants are deposited by precipitation, clouds, or directly on the land.
acquaintance rape A rape in which the rapist is known to the victim (replaces the formerly used term *date rape*).
acquired immunodeficiency syndrome (AIDS) A disease caused by a retrovirus, the human immunodeficiency virus (HIV), that attacks the immune system, reducing the number of helper T cells and leaving the victim vulnerable to infections, malignancies, and neurological disorders.
acupressure Technique of traditional Chinese medicine related to acupuncture that uses the application of pressure to selected points along the meridians to balance energy.
acupuncture Branch of traditional Chinese medicine that uses the insertion of long, thin needles to affect flow of energy (*qi*) along energy pathways (meridians) within the body.
acute stress The short-term physiological response to an immediate perceived threat.
adaptive response Form of adjustment in which the body attempts to restore homeostasis.
adaptive thermogenesis Theoretical mechanism by which the brain regulates metabolic activity according to caloric intake.
addiction Persistent, compulsive dependence on a behavior or substance, including mood-altering behaviors or activities, despite ongoing negative consequences.
aerobic capacity (or power) The functional status of the cardiorespiratory system; refers specifically to the volume of oxygen the muscles consume during exercise.
aerobic exercise Any type of exercise that requires oxygen to make energy for activity.
aggravated rape Rape that involves one or multiple attackers, strangers, weapons, or physical beating.
alcohol abuse Use of alcohol that interferes with work, school, or personal relationships or that entails violations of the law.
alcohol poisoning A potentially lethal blood alcohol concentration that inhibits the brain's ability to control consciousness, respiration, and heart rate; usually occurs as a result of drinking a large amount of alcohol in a short period of time. Also known as *acute alcohol intoxication*.
alcoholic hepatitis A condition resulting from prolonged use of alcohol in which the liver is inflamed; can be fatal.
Alcoholics Anonymous (AA) An organization whose goal is to help alcoholics stop drinking; includes auxiliary branches such as Al-Anon and Alateen.
alcoholism (alcohol dependency) Condition in which personal and health problems related to alcohol use are severe and stopping alcohol use results in withdrawal symptoms.
allopathic medicine Conventional, Western medical practice; in theory, based on scientifically validated methods and procedures.
allostatic load Wear and tear on the body caused by prolonged or excessive stress responses.
alternative (whole) medical systems Specific theories of health and balance that have developed outside the influence of conventional medicine.
alternative insemination A fertilization procedure accomplished by depositing semen from a partner or donor into a woman's vagina via a thin tube.
alternative medicine Treatment used in place of conventional medicine.
altruism The giving of oneself out of genuine concern for others.
Alzheimer's disease (AD) A chronic condition involving changes in nerve fibers of the brain that results in mental deterioration.
amino acids The nitrogen-containing building blocks of protein.
amniocentesis A medical test in which a small amount of fluid is drawn from the amniotic sac to test for Down syndrome and other genetic diseases.
amniotic sac The protective pouch surrounding the fetus.
amphetamines A large and varied group of synthetic agents that stimulate the central nervous system.
anabolic steroids Artificial forms of the hormone testosterone that promote muscle growth and strength.
anal intercourse The insertion of the penis into the anus.
androgyny High levels of traditional masculine and feminine traits in a single person.
aneurysm A weakened blood vessel that may bulge under pressure and, in severe cases, burst.
angina pectoris Chest pain occurring as a result of reduced oxygen flow to the heart.
angiography A technique for examining blockages in heart arteries.
angioplasty A technique in which a catheter with a balloon at the tip is inserted into a clogged artery; the balloon is inflated to flatten fatty deposits against artery walls and a stent is typically inserted to keep the artery open.
anorexia nervosa An eating disorder characterized by deliberate food restriction, self-starvation or extreme exercising to achieve weight loss, and an extremely distorted body image.
antagonism A drug interaction in which two drugs compete for the same available receptors, potentially blocking each other's actions.
antibiotic resistance The ability of bacteria or other microbes to withstand the effects of an antibiotic.
antibiotics Medicines used to kill microorganisms, such as bacteria.
antibodies Substances produced by the body that are individually matched to specific antigens.
antigen Substance capable of triggering an immune response.
antioxidants Substances believed to protect against oxidative stress and resultant tissue damage at the cellular level.
anxiety disorders Mental illnesses characterized by persistent feelings of threat and worry in coping with everyday problems.
appetite The desire to eat; normally accompanies hunger but is more psychological than physiological.
appraisal The interpretation and evaluation of information provided to the brain by the senses.
arrhythmia An irregularity in heartbeat.
arteries Vessels that carry blood away from the heart to other regions of the body.
arterioles Branches of the arteries.
asbestos A mineral compound that separates into stringy fibers and lodges in the lungs, where it can cause various diseases.
asthma A long-term, chronic inflammatory disorder that causes tiny airways in the lung to spasm in response to triggers. Many cases of asthma are triggered by environmental pollutants.

atherosclerosis Condition characterized by deposits of fatty substances (plaque) on the inner lining of an artery.

atria (singular: *atrium*) The heart's two upper chambers, which receive blood.

attention-deficit/hyperactivity disorder (ADHD) A learning disability characterized by hyperactivity and distraction.

autism spectrum disorder (ASD) A neurodevelopmental disorder characterized by difficulty mastering communication and social behavior skills.

autoerotic behaviors Sexual self-stimulation.

autoimmune disease Disease caused by an overactive immune response against the body's own cells.

autoinoculate Transmission of a pathogen from one part of your body to another part.

autonomic nervous system (ANS) The portion of the central nervous system regulating body functions that a person does not normally consciously control.

Ayurveda (Ayurvedic medicine) A comprehensive system of medicine, derived largely from ancient India, that places equal emphasis on the body, mind, and spirit, and strives to restore the body's innate harmony through diet, exercise, meditation, herbs, massage, exposure to sunlight, and controlled breathing.

background distressors Environmental stressors of which people are often unaware.

bacteria (singular: *bacterium*) Simple, single-celled microscopic organisms; about 100 known species of bacteria cause disease in humans.

barbiturates Drugs that depress the central nervous system and have sedating, hypnotic, and anesthetic effects.

barrier methods Contraceptive methods that block the meeting of egg and sperm by means of a physical barrier (such as condom, diaphragm, or cervical cap), a chemical barrier (such as spermicide), or both.

basal metabolic rate (BMR) The rate of energy expenditure by a body at complete rest in a neutral environment.

belief Appraisal of the relationship between some object, action, or idea and some attribute of that object, action, or idea.

benign Harmless; refers to a noncancerous tumor.

benzodiazepines A class of central nervous system depressant drugs with sedative, hypnotic, and muscle relaxant effects.

bereavement The loss or deprivation experienced by a survivor when a loved one dies.

bidis Hand-rolled flavored cigarettes.

binge drinking A *binge* is a pattern of drinking alcohol that brings blood alcohol concentration (BAC) to 0.08 gram-percent or above; for a typical adult, this pattern corresponds to consuming five or more drinks (male) or four or more drinks (female) in about 2 hours.

binge-eating disorder A type of eating disorder characterized by gorging on food once a week or more, but not typically followed by a purge.

biofeedback A technique using a machine to self-monitor physical responses to stress.

biopsy Removal and examination of a tissue sample to determine if a cancer is present.

biopsychosocial model of addiction Theory of the relationship between an addict's biological (genetic) nature and psychological and environmental influences.

bipolar disorder A form of mood disorder characterized by alternating mania and depression; also called *manic depression*.

bisexual Experiencing attraction to and preference for sexual activity with people of both sexes.

blood alcohol concentration (BAC) The ratio of alcohol to total blood volume; the factor used to measure the physiological and behavioral effects of alcohol.

body composition Describes the relative proportions of fat and fat-free (muscle, bone, water, organs) tissues in the body.

body dysmorphic disorder (BDD) A psychological disorder characterized by an obsession with one's appearance and a distorted view of one's body or with a minor or imagined flaw in appearance.

body image How you see yourself in your mind, what you believe about your appearance, and how you feel about your body.

body mass index (BMI) A number calculated from a person's weight and height that is used to assess risk for possible present or future health problems.

bulimia nervosa An eating disorder characterized by binge eating followed by inappropriate purging measures or compensatory behavior, such as vomiting or excessive exercise, to prevent weight gain.

caffeine A stimulant drug that is legal in the United States and found in many coffees, teas, chocolates, energy drinks, and certain medication.

calorie A unit of measure that indicates the amount of energy obtained from a particular food.

cancer A large group of diseases characterized by the uncontrolled growth and spread of abnormal cells.

candidiasis Yeast-like fungal infection often transmitted sexually; also called moniliasis or yeast infection.

capillaries Minute blood vessels that branch out from the arterioles and venules; their thin walls permit exchange of oxygen, carbon dioxide, nutrients, and waste products among body cells.

carbohydrates Basic nutrients that supply the body with glucose, the energy form most commonly used to sustain normal activity.

carbon dioxide (CO_2) Gas created by the combustion of fossil fuels, exhaled by animals, and used by plants for photosynthesis; the primary greenhouse gas in Earth's atmosphere.

carbon footprint The amount of greenhouse gases produced by an individual, nation, or other entity, usually expressed in equivalent tons of carbon dioxide emissions.

carbon monoxide A gas found in cigarette smoke that binds at oxygen receptor sites in the blood.

carcinogens Cancer-causing agents.

cardiometabolic risks Physical and biochemical changes that are risk factors for the development of cardiovascular disease and type 2 diabetes.

cardiorespiratory fitness The ability of the heart, lungs, and blood vessels to supply oxygen to skeletal muscles during sustained physical activity.

cardiovascular disease (CVD) Diseases of the heart and blood vessels.

cardiovascular system Organ system, consisting of the heart and blood vessels, that transports nutrients, oxygen, hormones, metabolic wastes, and enzymes throughout the body.

carotenoids Fat-soluble plant pigments with antioxidant properties.

carpal tunnel syndrome (CTS) A common occupational injury in which the median nerve in the wrist becomes irritated, causing numbness, tingling, and pain in the fingers and hands.

carrying capacity of the earth The largest population that can be supported indefinitely given the resources available in the environment.

celiac disease An inherited autoimmune disorder affecting the digestive process of the small intestine and triggered by the consumption of gluten.

celibacy State of abstaining from sexual activity.

cell-mediated immunity Aspect of immunity that is mediated by specialized white blood cells that attack pathogens and antigens directly.

cervical cap A small cup made of latex or silicone that is designed to fit snugly over the entire cervix.

cervix Lower end of the uterus that opens into the vagina.

cesarean section (C-section) Surgical birthing procedure in which a baby is removed through an incision made in the mother's abdominal wall and uterus.

chancre Sore often found at the site of syphilis infection.

chemotherapy The use of drugs to kill cancerous cells.

chewing tobacco A stringy type of tobacco that is placed in the mouth and then sucked or chewed.
chickenpox A highly infectious disease caused by the herpes varicella zoster virus.
child abuse Deliberate, intentional words or actions that cause harm, potential for harm, or threat of harm to a child.
child maltreatment Any act or series of acts of commission or omission by a parent or caregiver that results in harm, potential for harm, or threat of harm to a child.
chiropractic medicine Manipulation of the spine and neuromuscular structure to promote proper energy flow.
chlamydia Bacterially caused STI of the urogenital tract; most commonly reported STI in the United States.
chlorofluorocarbons (CFCs) Chemicals that contribute to the depletion of the atmospheric ozone layer.
cholesterol A form of fat circulating in the blood that can accumulate on the inner walls of arteries, causing a narrowing of the channel through which blood flows.
chorionic villus sampling (CVS) A prenatal test that involves snipping tissue from the fetal sac to be analyzed for genetic defects.
chronic disease A disease that typically begins slowly, progresses, and persists, with a variety of signs and symptoms that can be treated but not cured by medication.
chronic mood disorder Experience of persistent emotional states, such as sadness, despair, and hopelessness.
chronic stress An ongoing state of physiological arousal in response to ongoing or numerous perceived threats.
cirrhosis The last stage of liver disease associated with chronic heavy alcohol use, during which liver cells die and damage becomes permanent.
climate change A shift in typical weather patterns that includes fluctuations in seasonal temperatures, rain or snowfall amounts, and the occurrence of catastrophic storms.
clitoris A pea-sized nodule of tissue located at the top of the labia minora; central to sexual arousal in women.
club drugs Synthetic analogs (drugs that produce similar effects) of existing illicit drugs.
codependence A self-defeating relationship pattern in which a person is controlled by an addict's addictive behavior.
cognitive restructuring The modification of thoughts, ideas, and beliefs that contribute to stress.
cohabitation Living together without being married.
collateral circulation Adaptation of the heart to partial damage accomplished by rerouting needed blood through unused or underused blood vessels while the damaged heart muscle heals.
collective violence Violence perpetrated by groups against other groups.
common-law marriage Cohabitation lasting a designated period of time (usually 7 years) that is considered legally binding in some states.
comorbidities The presence of one or more diseases at the same time.
complementary medicine Treatment used in conjunction with conventional medicine.
complete (high-quality) proteins Proteins that contain all nine of the essential amino acids.
complex carbohydrates A major type of carbohydrate that provides sustained energy.
compulsion Preoccupation with a behavior and an overwhelming need to perform it.
compulsive buying disorder People who are preoccupied with shopping and spending.
compulsive exercise Disorder characterized by a compulsion to engage in excessive amounts of exercise and feelings of guilt and anxiety if the level of exercise is perceived as inadequate.
compulsive shoppers People who are preoccupied with shopping and spending.
computerized axial tomography (CAT) scan A scan by a machine that uses radiation to view internal organs not normally visible in X-rays.
conception The fertilization of an ovum by a sperm.
conflict An emotional state that arises when the behavior of one person interferes with the behavior of another.
conflict resolution A concerted effort by all parties to constructively resolve points of contention.
congeners Forms of alcohol that are metabolized more slowly than ethanol and produce toxic by-products.
congenital cardiovascular defect Cardiovascular problem that is present at birth.
congestive heart failure (CHF) or heart failure (HF) An abnormal cardiovascular condition that reflects impaired cardiac pumping and blood flow; pooling blood leads to congestion in body tissues.
consummate love A relationship that combines intimacy, compassion, and commitment.
contemplation A practice of concentrating the mind on a spiritual or ethical question or subject, a view of the natural world, or an icon or other image representative of divinity.
contraception (birth control) Methods of preventing conception.
contraceptive sponge Contraceptive device, made of polyurethane foam and containing nonoxynol-9, that fits over the cervix to create a barrier against sperm.
coping Managing events or conditions to lessen the physical or psychological effects of excess stress.
core strength Strength in the body's core muscles, including deep back and abdominal muscles that attach to the spine and pelvis.
coronary artery disease (CAD) A narrowing or blockage of coronary arteries, usually caused by atherosclerotic plaque buildup.
coronary bypass surgery A surgical technique whereby a blood vessel taken from another part of the body is implanted to bypass a clogged coronary artery.
coronary heart disease (CHD) A narrowing of the small blood vessels that supply blood to the heart.
coronary thrombosis A blood clot occurring in a coronary artery.
corpus luteum A body of cells that forms from the remains of the graafian follicle following ovulation; it secretes estrogen and progesterone during the second half of the menstrual cycle.
cortisol Hormone released by the adrenal glands that makes stored nutrients more readily available to meet energy demands.
countering Substituting a desired behavior for an undesirable one.
Cowper's glands Glands that secrete a fluid that lubricates the urethra and neutralizes any acid remaining in the urethra after urination.
cross-tolerance Development of a physiological tolerance to one drug that reduces the effects of another, similar drug.
cunnilingus Oral stimulation of a woman's genitals.
Daily Values (DVs) Percentages listed as "% DV" on food and supplement labels; made up of the RDIs and DRVs together.
defensive medicine The use of medical practices designed to avert the possibility of malpractice suits in the future.
dehydration Abnormal depletion of body fluids; a result of lack of water.
delirium tremens (DTs) A state of confusion brought on by withdrawal from alcohol; symptoms include hallucinations, anxiety, and trembling.
dementias Progressive brain impairments that interfere with memory and normal intellectual functioning.
denial Inability to perceive or accurately interpret the self-destructive effects of the addictive behavior.
dentist Specialist who diagnoses and treats diseases of the teeth, gums, and oral cavity.

Depo-Provera, Depo-subQ Provera Injectable method of birth control that lasts for 3 months.
depressants Drugs that slow down the activity of the central nervous and muscular systems and cause sleepiness or calmness.
determinants of health The range of personal, social, economic, and environmental factors that influence health status.
detoxification The early abstinence period during which an addict adjusts physically and cognitively to being free from the influences of the addiction.
diabetes mellitus A group of diseases characterized by elevated blood glucose levels.
diaphragm A latex, cup-shaped device designed to cover the cervix and block access to the uterus; should always be used with spermicide.
diastolic blood pressure The lower number in the fraction that measures blood pressure, indicating pressure on arterial walls during the relaxation phase of heart activity.
dietary supplements Vitamins and minerals taken by mouth that are intended to supplement existing diets.
digestive process The process by which the body breaks down foods and either absorbs or excretes them.
dilation and evacuation (D&E) An abortion technique that uses a combination of instruments and vacuum aspiration.
dioxins Highly toxic chlorinated hydrocarbons found in herbicides and produced during certain industrial processes.
dipping Placing a small amount of chewing tobacco between the front lip and teeth for rapid nicotine absorption.
disaccharides Combinations of two monosaccharides.
discrimination Actions that deny equal treatment or opportunities to a group, often based on prejudice.
disease prevention Actions or behaviors designed to keep people from getting sick.
disordered eating A pattern of atypical eating behaviors that is used to achieve or maintain a lower body weight.
gambling disorder Compulsive gambling that cannot be controlled.
distillation The process whereby mash is subjected to high temperatures to release alcohol vapors, which are then condensed and mixed with water to make the final product.
distress Stress that can have a detrimental effect on health; negative stress.
domestic violence The use of force to control and maintain power over another person in the home environment, including both actual harm and the threat of harm.
downshifting Taking a step back and simplifying a lifestyle that has become focused on trying to keep up, is hectic, and is packed with pressure and stress; also known as voluntary simplicity.
drug abuse Excessive use of a drug.
drug misuse Use of a drug for a purpose for which it was not intended.
drug resistance That which occurs when microbes, such as bacteria, viruses, or other pathogens, grow and proliferate in the presence of chemicals that would normally kill them or slow their growth.
dysfunctional families Families in which there is violence; physical, emotional, or sexual abuse; parental discord; or other negative family interactions.
dysmenorrhea Condition of pain or discomfort in the lower abdomen just before or after menstruation.
dyslexia A language-based learning disorder characterized by reading, writing, and spelling problems.
dyspareunia Pain experienced by women during intercourse.
dysthymic disorder (dysthymia) A type of depression that is milder and harder to recognize than major depression; chronic and often characterized by fatigue, pessimism, or a short temper.
eating disorder A psychiatric disorder characterized by severe disturbances in body image and eating behaviors.
ecological or public health model A view of health in which diseases and other negative health events are seen as the result of an individual's interaction with his or her social and physical environment.
ecosystem The collection of physical (nonliving) and biological (living) components of an environment and the relationships between them.
ectopic pregnancy Dangerous condition that results from the implantation of a fertilized egg outside the uterus, usually in a fallopian tube.
ejaculation The propulsion of semen from the penis.
ejaculatory duct Tube formed by the junction of the seminal vesicle and the vas deferens that carries semen to the urethra.
electrocardiogram (ECG) A record of the electrical activity of the heart; may be measured during a stress test.
embolus A blood clot that becomes dislodged from a blood vessel wall and moves through the circulatory system.
embryo The fertilized egg from conception through the eighth week of development.
emergency contraceptive pills (ECPs) Drugs taken within 3 to 5 days after unprotected intercourse to prevent fertilization or implantation.
emotional health The feeling part of psychosocial health; includes your emotional reactions to life.
emotional intelligence A person's ability to identify, understand, use, and manage emotional states effectively and interact positively with others in relationships.
emotions Intensified feelings or complex patterns of feelings.
emphysema A chronic lung disease in which the tiny air sacs in the lungs are destroyed, making breathing difficult.
enablers People who knowingly or unknowingly protect addicts from the natural consequences of their behavior.
endemic Describing a disease that is always present to some degree.
endometriosis Disorder in which endometrial tissue establishes itself outside the uterus.
endometrium Soft, spongy matter that makes up the uterine lining.
endorphins Opioid-like hormones that are manufactured in the human body and contribute to natural feelings of well-being.
energy medicine Therapies using energy fields, such as magnetic fields or biofields.
enhanced greenhouse effect The warming of Earth's surface as a direct result of human activities that release greenhouse gases into the atmosphere, trapping more of the sun's radiation than is normal.
environmental stewardship A responsibility for environmental quality shared by all those whose actions affect the environment.
environmental tobacco smoke (ETS) Smoke from tobacco products, including sidestream and mainstream smoke; commonly called *secondhand smoke*.
epidemic Disease outbreak that affects many people in a community or region at the same time.
epididymis The duct system atop the testis where sperm mature.
epinephrine Also called *adrenaline*, a hormone that stimulates body systems in response to stress.
episodic acute stress The state of regularly reacting with wild, acute stress about one thing or another.
erectile dysfunction (ED) Difficulty in achieving or maintaining a penile erection sufficient for intercourse.
ergogenic drug Substance believed to enhance athletic performance.
erogenous zones Areas of the body that, when touched, lead to sexual arousal.
essential amino acids Nine of the basic nitrogen-containing building blocks of protein, which must be obtained from foods to ensure health.
estrogens Hormones secreted by the ovaries that control the menstrual cycle.

ethnoviolence Violence directed at persons affiliated with a particular ethnic group.

ethyl alcohol (ethanol) An addictive drug produced by fermentation and found in many beverages.

eustress Stress that presents opportunities for personal growth; positive stress.

evidence-based medicine Decisions regarding patient care based on clinical expertise, patient values, and current best scientific evidence.

exercise Planned, structured, and repetitive bodily movement done to improve or maintain one or more components of physical fitness.

exercise addicts People who exercise compulsively to try to meet needs of nurturance, intimacy, self-esteem, and self-competency.

exercise metabolic rate (EMR) The energy expenditure that occurs during exercise.

extensively drug-resistant TB (XDR-TB) Form of TB that is resistant to nearly all existing antibiotics.

fallopian tubes (oviducts) Tubes that extend from near the ovaries to the uterus; site of fertilization and passageway for fertilized eggs.

family of origin People present in the household during a child's first years of life—usually parents and siblings.

fats Basic nutrients composed of carbon and hydrogen atoms; needed for the proper functioning of cells, insulation of body organs against shock, maintenance of body temperature, and healthy skin and hair.

fellatio Oral stimulation of a man's genitals.

female athlete triad A syndrome of three interrelated health problems seen in some female athletes: disordered eating, amenorrhea, and poor bone density.

female condom A single-use polyurethane sheath for internal use during vaginal or anal intercourse to catch semen on ejaculation.

female orgasmic disorder A woman's inability to achieve orgasm.

fermentation The process whereby yeast organisms break down plant sugars to yield ethanol.

fertility A person's ability to reproduce.

fertility awareness methods (FAMs) Several types of birth control that require alteration of sexual behavior rather than chemical or physical intervention in the reproductive process.

fertility rate Average number of births a female in a certain population has during her reproductive years.

fetal alcohol syndrome (FAS) A pattern of birth defects, learning, and behavioral problems in a child caused by the mother's alcohol consumption during pregnancy.

fetus A developing human from the ninth week until birth.

fiber The indigestible portion of plant foods that helps move food through the digestive system and softens stools by absorbing water.

fibrillation A sporadic, quivering pattern of heartbeat that results in extreme inefficiency in moving blood through the cardiovascular system.

fight-or-flight response Physiological arousal response in which the body prepares to combat or escape a real or perceived threat.

FITT Acronym for **F**requency, **I**ntensity, **T**ime, and **T**ype; the terms that describe the essential components of a program or plan to improve a health-related component of physical fitness.

flexibility The range of motion, or the amount of movement possible, at a particular joint or series of joints.

foams Spermicide packaged in aerosol cans and inserted into the vagina with an applicator.

food allergy Overreaction by the body to normally harmless proteins, which are perceived as allergens. In response, the body produces antibodies, triggering allergic symptoms.

food intolerance Adverse effects resulting when people who lack the digestive chemicals needed to break down certain substances eat those substances.

food irradiation Treating foods with gamma radiation from radioactive cobalt, cesium, or other sources of X-rays to kill microorganisms.

formaldehyde A colorless, strong-smelling gas released through off-gassing; causes respiratory and other health problems.

fossil fuels Carbon-based material used for energy; includes oil, coal, and natural gas.

frequency As part of the FITT prescription, refers to how many days per week a person should exercise to improve a component of physical fitness.

functional foods Foods believed to have specific health benefits and/or to prevent disease.

fungi A group of multicellular and unicellular organisms that obtain their food by infiltrating the bodies of other organisms, both living and dead; several microscopic varieties are pathogenic.

gay Sexual orientation involving primary attraction to people of the same sex.

gender The psychological condition of being feminine or masculine as defined by the society in which one lives.

gender identity Personal sense or awareness of being masculine or feminine, a male or a female.

gender roles Expressions of maleness or femaleness in everyday life.

gender-role stereotypes Generalizations concerning how men and women should express themselves and the characteristics each possesses.

gene Discrete segment of DNA in a chromosome that stores the code for assembling a particular body protein.

general adaptation syndrome (GAS) The pattern followed in the physiological response to stress, consisting of the alarm, resistance, and exhaustion phases.

generalized anxiety disorder (GAD) A constant sense of worry that may cause restlessness, difficulty in concentrating, tension, and other symptoms.

generic drugs Medications sold under chemical names rather than brand names.

genetically modified (GM) foods Foods derived from organisms whose DNA has been altered using genetic engineering techniques.

genital herpes STI caused by the herpes simplex virus.

genital warts Warts that appear in the genital area or the anus; caused by the human papillomavirus (HPV).

gestational diabetes Form of diabetes mellitus in which women who have never had diabetes before have high blood sugar (glucose) levels during pregnancy.

global warming A type of climate change in which average temperatures increase.

globesity High number of countries and large percentages of populations within countries who are classified as obese.

glycemic index (GI) Compares foods with the same amount of carbohydrates and determines how much each raises blood glucose levels.

glycemic load (GL) A food's glycemic index (potential to raise blood glucose) multiplied by the grams of carbohydrates it provides, divided by 100.

glycogen The polysaccharide form in which glucose is stored in the liver and, to a lesser extent, in muscles.

gonads The reproductive organs in a male (testes) or female (ovaries) that produce sperm (male), eggs (female), and sex hormones.

gonorrhea Second most common bacterial STI in the United States; if untreated, may cause sterility.

graafian follicle Mature ovarian follicle that contains a fully developed ovum, or egg.

greenhouse gases Gases that accumulate in the atmosphere, where they contribute to global warming by trapping heat near Earth's surface.

grief An individual's reaction to significant loss, including one's own impending death, the death of a loved one, or a quasi-death experience; grief can involve mental, physical, social, or emotional responses.

habit A repeated behavior in which the repetition may be unconscious.
hallucinogens Substances capable of creating auditory or visual distortions and unusual changes in mood, thoughts, and feelings.
hangover The physiological reaction to excessive drinking, including headache, upset stomach, anxiety, depression, diarrhea, and thirst.
hate crime A crime targeted against a particular societal group and motivated by bias against that group.
hazardous waste Waste that, due to its toxic properties, poses a hazard to humans or to the environment.
health The ever-changing process of achieving individual potential in the physical, social, emotional, mental, spiritual, and environmental dimensions.
health belief model (HBM) Model for explaining how beliefs may influence behaviors.
health disparities Differences in the incidence, prevalence, mortality, and burden of diseases and other health conditions among specific population groups.
health promotion The combined educational, organizational, procedural, environmental, social, and financial supports that help individuals and groups reduce negative health behaviors and promote positive change.
healthy life expectancy Expected number of years of full health remaining at a given age, such as at birth.
healthy weight Having a BMI of 18.5 to 24.9, the range of lowest statistical health risk.
heat cramps Involuntary and forcible muscle contractions that occur during or following exercise in hot and/or humid weather.
heat exhaustion A heat stress illness caused by significant dehydration resulting from exercise in hot and/or humid conditions.
heatstroke A deadly heat stress illness resulting from dehydration and overexertion in hot and/or humid conditions.
hepatitis A viral disease in which the liver becomes inflamed, producing symptoms such as fever, headache, and possibly jaundice.
herpes A general term for infections characterized by sores or eruptions on the skin caused by the herpes simplex virus.
herpes gladiatorum A skin infection caused by the herpes simplex type 1 virus and seen among athletes participating in contact sports.
heterosexual Experiencing primary attraction to and preference for sexual activity with people of the opposite sex.
high-density lipoproteins (HDLs) Compounds that facilitate the transport of cholesterol in the blood to the liver for metabolism and elimination from the body.
holistic Relating to or concerned with the whole body and the interactions of systems, rather than treatment of individual parts.
homeopathic medicine Unconventional Western system of medicine based on the principle that "like cures like."
homeostasis A balanced physiological state in which all the body's systems function smoothly.
homicide Death that results from intent to injure or kill.
homosexual Experiencing primary attraction to and preference for sexual activity with people of the same sex.
hormonal contraception Contraceptive methods that introduce synthetic hormones into the woman's system to prevent ovulation, thicken cervical mucus, or prevent a fertilized egg from implanting.
hormone replacement therapy or menopausal hormone therapy Use of synthetic or animal estrogens and progesterone to compensate for decreases in estrogens in a woman's body during menopause.
hostility Cognitive, affective, and behavioral tendencies toward anger and cynicism.
human chorionic gonadotropin (HCG) Hormone detectable in blood or urine samples of a mother within the first few weeks of pregnancy.
human immunodeficiency virus (HIV) The virus that causes AIDS by infecting helper T cells.
human papillomavirus (HPV) A group of viruses, many of which are transmitted sexually; some types of HPV can cause genital warts or cervical cancer.
humoral immunity Aspect of immunity that is mediated by antibodies secreted by white blood cells.
hunger The physiological impulse to seek food, prompted by the lack or shortage of basic foods needed to provide the energy and nutrients that support health.
hymen Thin tissue covering the vaginal opening in some women.
hyperglycemia Elevated blood glucose level.
hyperplasia A condition characterized by an excessive number of fat cells.
hypertension Sustained elevated blood pressure.
hypertrophy The act of swelling or increasing in size, as with cells.
hypnosis A trancelike state that allows people to become unusually responsive to suggestion.
hyponatremia or water intoxication The overconsumption of water, which leads to a dilution of sodium concentration in the blood with potentially fatal results.
hypothalamus An area of the brain located near the pituitary gland; works in conjunction with the pituitary gland to control reproductive functions. It also controls the sympathetic nervous system and directs the stress response.
hypothermia Potentially fatal condition caused by abnormally low body core temperature.
hysterectomy Surgical removal of the uterus.
hysterotomy The surgical removal of the fetus from the uterus.
imagined rehearsal Practicing, through mental imagery, to become better able to perform an event in actuality.
immunocompetence The ability of the immune system to respond to attack.
immunocompromised Having an immune system that is impaired.
Nexplanon (Implanon) A plastic capsule inserted in a woman's upper arm that releases a low dose of progestin to prevent pregnancy.
in vitro fertilization Fertilization of an egg in a nutrient medium and subsequent transfer back to the mother's body.
incomplete proteins Proteins that lack one or more of the essential amino acids.
incubation period The time between exposure to a disease and the appearance of symptoms.
induction abortion An abortion technique in which chemicals are injected into the uterus through the uterine wall; labor begins, and the woman delivers a dead fetus.
infection The state of pathogens being established in or on a host and causing disease.
infertility Inability to conceive after a year or more of trying.
influenza A common viral disease of the respiratory tract.
inhalants Products that are sniffed or inhaled in order to produce highs.
inhalation The introduction of drugs through the respiratory tract via sniffing, smoking, or inhaling.
inhibited sexual desire Lack of sexual appetite or lack of interest and pleasure in sexual activity.
inhibition A drug interaction in which the effects of one drug are eliminated or reduced by the presence of another drug at the same receptor site.
injection The introduction of drugs into the body via a hypodermic needle.
insulin Hormone secreted by the pancreas and required by body cells for the uptake and storage of glucose.
insulin resistance State in which body cells fail to respond to the effects of insulin; obesity increases the risk that cells will become insulin resistant.
intact dilation and extraction (D&X) A late-term abortion procedure in which the body of the fetus is extracted up to the head and then the contents of the cranium are aspirated.

intensity As part of the FITT prescription, refers to how hard or how much effort is needed when a person exercises to improve a component of physical fitness.

intentional injuries Injury, death, or psychological harm inflicted with the intent to harm.

Internet addiction The compulsive use of the computer, personal digital device, cell phone, or other forms of technology to access the Internet for activities such as e-mail, games, shopping, social networking, or blogging.

interpersonal violence Violence inflicted against one individual by another, or by a small group of others.

intersex General term for a variety of conditions in which a person is born with reproductive or sexual anatomy that doesn't seem to fit the typical definitions of female or male. Also termed disorders of sexual development (DSDs).

intervention A planned process of confronting an addict carried out by close family, friends, and a professional counselor.

intimate partner violence (IPV) Violent behavior, including physical violence, sexual violence, threats, and emotional abuse, occurring between current or former spouses or dating partners.

intimate relationships Relationships with family members, friends, and romantic partners, characterized by behavioral interdependence, need fulfillment, emotional attachment, and emotional availability.

intolerance A drug interaction in which the combination of two or more drugs in the body produces extremely uncomfortable reactions.

intrauterine device (IUD) A device, often T-shaped, that is implanted in the uterus to prevent pregnancy.

ionizing radiation Electromagnetic waves and particles having short wavelengths and energy high enough to ionize atoms.

ischemia Reduced oxygen supply to a body part or organ.

jealousy An aversive reaction evoked by a real or imagined relationship involving a person's partner and a third person.

jellies and creams Spermicide packaged in tubes and inserted into the vagina with an applicator.

labia majora "Outer lips," or folds of tissue covering the female sexual organs.

labia minora "Inner lips," or folds of tissue just inside the labia majora.

leach To dissolve and filter through soil.

lead A highly toxic metal found in emissions from lead smelters and processing plants; also sometimes found in pipes or paint in older houses.

learned helplessness Pattern of responding to situations by giving up because of repeated failure in the past.

learned optimism Teaching oneself to think positively.

lesbian Sexual orientation involving attraction of women to other women.

leukoplakia A condition characterized by leathery white patches inside the mouth; produced by contact with irritants in tobacco juice.

libido Sexual drive or desire.

life expectancy Expected number of years of life remaining at a given age, such as at birth.

locavore A person who primarily eats food grown or produced locally.

locus of control The location, *external* (outside oneself) or *internal* (within oneself), that an individual perceives as the source and underlying cause of events in his or her life.

loss of control Inability to reliably predict whether a particular instance of involvement with the addictive substance or behavior will be healthy or damaging.

low-density lipoproteins (LDLs) Compounds that facilitate the transport of cholesterol in the blood to the body's cells and cause the cholesterol to build up on artery walls.

low sperm count A sperm count below 20 million sperm per milliliter of semen.

lymphocyte A type of white blood cell involved in the immune response.

macrominerals Minerals that the body needs in fairly large amounts.

macrophage A type of white blood cell that ingests foreign material.

magnetic resonance imaging (MRI) A device that uses magnetic fields, radio waves, and computers to generate an image of internal tissues of the body for diagnostic purposes without the use of radiation.

mainstream smoke Smoke that is drawn through tobacco while inhaling.

major depression Severe depressive disorder that entails chronic mood disorder, physical effects such as sleep disturbance and exhaustion, and mental effects such as the inability to concentrate; also called *clinical depression*.

male condom A single-use sheath of thin latex or other material designed to fit over an erect penis and to catch semen upon ejaculation.

malignant Very dangerous or harmful; refers to a cancerous tumor.

malignant melanoma A virulent cancer of the melanocytes (pigment-producing cells) of the skin.

managed care Cost-control procedures used by health insurers to coordinate treatment.

manipulative and body-based practices Treatments involving manipulation or movement of one or more body parts.

marijuana Chopped leaves and flowers of *Cannabis indica* or *Cannabis sativa* (hemp); a psychoactive stimulant.

marital rape Any unwanted intercourse or penetration obtained by force, threat of force, or when the spouse is unable to consent.

massage therapy Soft tissue manipulation by trained therapists for relaxation and healing.

masturbation Self-stimulation of genitals.

measles A viral disease that produces symptoms such as an itchy rash and a high fever.

Medicaid A federal-state matching funds program that provides health insurance to low-income people.

Medicare A federal health insurance program that covers people age 65 and older, the permanently disabled, and people with end-stage kidney disease.

medical abortion The termination of a pregnancy during its first 9 weeks using hormonal medications that cause the embryo to be expelled from the uterus.

medical model A view of health in which health status focuses primarily on the individual and a biological or diseased organ perspective.

meditation A relaxation technique that involves concentrated focus to quiet the mind and increase awareness of the present moment.

menarche The first menstrual period.

meningitis An infection of the meninges, the membranes that surround the brain and spinal cord.

menopause The permanent cessation of menstruation, generally between the ages of 40 and 60.

mental health The thinking part of psychosocial health; includes your values, attitudes, and beliefs.

mental illnesses Disorders that disrupt thinking, feeling, moods, and behaviors, and that impair daily functioning.

metabolic syndrome (MetS) A group of metabolic conditions occurring together that increase a person's risk of heart disease, stroke, and diabetes.

metastasis Process by which cancer spreads from one area to different areas of the body.

methicillin-resistant *Staphylococcus aureus* (MRSA) Highly resistant form of staph infection that is growing in international prevalence.

migraine A condition characterized by localized headaches that possibly result from alternating dilation and constriction of blood vessels.

mind-body medicine Techniques designed to enhance the mind's ability to affect bodily functions and symptoms.

mindfulness A practice of purposeful, nonjudgmental observation in which we are fully present in the moment.

minerals Inorganic, indestructible elements that aid physiological processes.

miscarriage Loss of the fetus before it is viable; also called *spontaneous abortion*.

modeling Learning specific behaviors by watching others perform them.
monogamy Exclusive sexual involvement with one partner.
mononucleosis A viral disease that causes pervasive fatigue and other long-lasting symptoms.
monosaccharides Simple sugars that contain only one molecule of sugar.
mons pubis Fatty tissue covering the pubic bone in females; in physically mature women, the mons is covered with coarse hair.
morbidly obese Having a body weight 100 percent or more above healthy recommended levels; in an adult, having a BMI of 40 or more.
mortality The proportion of deaths to the total population, within a given period of time.
motivation A social, cognitive, and emotional force that directs human behavior.
multidrug-resistant TB (MDR-TB) Form of TB that is resistant to at least two of the best antibiotics available.
multifactorial disease Disease caused by interactions of several factors.
mumps A once common viral disease that is controllable by vaccination.
municipal solid waste (MSW) Solid wastes such as durable goods; nondurable goods; containers and packaging; food waste; yard waste; and miscellaneous wastes from residential, commercial, institutional, and industrial sources.
muscle dysmorphia Body image disorder in which men believe that their body is insufficiently lean or muscular.
muscular endurance A muscle's ability to exert force repeatedly without fatiguing or the ability to sustain a muscular contraction for a length of time.
muscular strength The amount of force that a muscle is capable of exerting in one contraction.
mutant cells Cells that differ in form, quality, or function from normal cells.
myocardial infarction (MI) or heart attack A blockage of normal blood supply to an area in the heart.
natural products Treatments using substances found in nature, such as herbs, special diets, or vitamin megadoses.
naturopathy (naturopathic medicine) System of medicine in which practitioners work with nature to restore people's health.
negative consequences Severe problems associated with addiction, such as physical damage, legal trouble, financial problems, academic failure, or family dissolution.
neglect Failure to provide for a child's basic needs such as food, shelter, medical care, and clothing.
neoplasm A new growth of tissue that results from uncontrolled, abnormal cellular development and serves no physiological function.
neurotransmitters Chemicals that relay messages between nerve cells or from nerve cells to other body cells.
nicotine The primary stimulant chemical in tobacco products; nicotine is highly addictive.
nicotine poisoning Symptoms often experienced by beginning smokers, including dizziness, diarrhea, lightheadedness, rapid and erratic pulse, clammy skin, nausea, and vomiting.
nicotine withdrawal Symptoms, including nausea, headaches, irritability, and intense tobacco cravings, suffered by addicted smokers who stop using tobacco.
nonionizing radiation Electromagnetic waves having relatively long wavelengths and enough energy to move atoms around or cause them to vibrate.
nonpoint source pollutants Pollutants that run off or seep into waterways from broad areas of land.
nonverbal communication All unwritten and unspoken messages, both intentional and unintentional.
nuclear meltdown An accident that results when the temperature in the core of a nuclear reactor increases enough to melt the nuclear fuel and the containment vessel housing it.
nurse Health professional who provides many services for patients and who may work in a variety of settings.
nurse practitioner (NP) Professional nurse with advanced training obtained through either a master's degree program or a specialized nurse practitioner program.
nutraceuticals Food or food-based supplements that have combined nutritional and pharmaceutical benefits; used interchangeably with the term *functional foods.*
nutrients The constituents of food that sustain humans physiologically: proteins, carbohydrates, fats, vitamins, minerals, and water.
nutrition The science that investigates the relationship between physiological function and the essential elements of foods eaten.
NuvaRing A soft, flexible ring inserted into the vagina that releases hormones, preventing pregnancy.
obesity A body weight more than 20 percent above healthy recommended levels; in an adult, a BMI of 30 or more.
obesogenic Characterized by environments that promote increased food intake, nonhealthful foods, and physical inactivity; refers to conditions that lead people to become excessively fat.
obsession Excessive preoccupation with an addictive object or behavior.
obsessive-compulsive disorder (OCD) A form of anxiety disorder characterized by recurrent, unwanted thoughts and repetitive behaviors.
oncogenes Suspected cancer-causing genes present on chromosomes.
one repetition maximum (1 RM) The amount of weight or resistance that can be lifted or moved only once.
open relationship A relationship in which partners agree that sexual involvement can occur outside the relationship.
ophthalmologist Physician who specializes in the medical and surgical care of the eyes, including prescriptions for glasses.
opioids Drugs that induce sleep and relieve pain; includes derivatives of opium and synthetics with similar chemical properties; also called *narcotics.*
opium The parent drug of the opioids; made from the seedpod resin of the opium poppy.
opportunistic infections Infections that occur when the immune system is weakened or compromised.
optometrist Eye specialist whose practice is limited to prescribing and fitting lenses.
oral contraceptives Pills containing synthetic hormones that prevent ovulation by regulating hormones.
oral ingestion Intake of drugs through the mouth.
organic Grown without use of pesticides, chemicals, or hormones.
Ortho Evra A patch that releases hormones similar to those in oral contraceptives; each patch is worn for 1 week.
osteopath General practitioner who receives training similar to a medical doctor's but with an emphasis on the skeletal and muscular systems; often uses spinal manipulation as part of treatment.
other specified feeding or eating disorder (OSFED) Eating disorders that are a true psychiatric illness but that do not fit the strict diagnostic criteria for anorexia nervosa, bulimia nervosa, or binge-eating disorder.
ovarian follicles Areas within the ovary in which individual eggs develop.
ovaries Almond-sized organs that house developing eggs and produce hormones.
overload A condition in which a person feels overly pressured by demands.
overuse injuries Injuries that result from the cumulative effects of day-after-day stresses placed on tendons, muscles, and joints.
overweight Having a body weight more than 10 percent above healthy recommended levels; in an adult, having a BMI of 25 to 29.
ovulation The point of the menstrual cycle at which a mature egg ruptures through the ovarian wall.
ovum A single mature egg cell.

pancreas Organ that secretes digestive enzymes into the small intestine, and hormones, including insulin, into the bloodstream.

pandemic Global epidemic of a disease that occurs in several countries at the same time.

panic attack Severe anxiety reaction in which a particular situation, often for unknown reasons, causes terror.

Pap test A procedure in which cells taken from the cervical region are examined for abnormal cellular activity.

parasitic worms The largest of the pathogens, most of which are more a nuisance than they are a threat.

parasympathetic nervous system Branch of the autonomic nervous system responsible for slowing systems stimulated by the stress response.

pathogen A disease-causing agent.

pelvic inflammatory disease (PID) Term used to describe various infections of the female reproductive tract; can be caused by chlamydia or gonorrhea.

penis Male sexual organ that releases sperm.

peptic ulcer Damage to the stomach or intestinal lining, usually caused by digestive juices; most ulcers result from infection by the bacterium *Helicobacter pylori*.

perfect-use failure rate The number of pregnancies (per 100 users) that are likely to occur in the first year of use of a particular birth control method if the method is used consistently and correctly.

perineum Tissue that forms the "floor" of the pelvic region in both men and women.

peripheral artery disease (PAD) Atherosclerosis occurring in the lower extremities, such as in the feet, calves, or legs, or in the arms.

personal flotation device A device worn to provide buoyancy and keep the wearer, conscious or unconscious, afloat with the nose and mouth out of the water; also known as a life jacket.

personality disorders A class of mental disorders that are characterized by inflexible patterns of thought and beliefs that lead to socially distressing behavior.

pesticides Chemicals that kill pests such as insects, weeds, and rodents.

phobia A deep and persistent fear of a specific object, activity, or situation that results in a compelling desire to avoid the source of the fear.

smog Brownish haze that is a form of pollution produced by the photochemical reaction of sunlight with hydrocarbons, nitrogen compounds, and other gases in vehicle exhaust.

physical activity Refers to all body movements produced by skeletal muscles resulting in substantial increases in energy expenditure, but generally refers to movement of the large muscle groups.

physical fitness Refers to a set of attributes that allow you to perform moderate- to vigorous-intensity physical activities on a regular basis without getting too tired and with energy left over to handle physical or mental emergencies.

physician assistant (PA) A midlevel practitioner trained to handle most standard cases of care under the supervision of a physician.

physiological dependence The adaptive state that occurs with regular addictive behavior and results in withdrawal syndrome.

pituitary gland The endocrine gland that controls the release of hormones from the gonads.

placenta The network of blood vessels connected to the umbilical cord that transports oxygen and nutrients to a developing fetus and carries away fetal wastes.

plant sterols Essential components of plant membranes that, when consumed in the diet, appear to help lower cholesterol levels.

plaque Buildup of deposits in the arteries.

platelet adhesiveness Stickiness of red blood cells associated with blood clots.

pneumonia Inflammatory disease of the lungs characterized by chronic cough, chest pain, chills, high fever, and fluid accumulation; may be caused by bacteria, viruses, fungi, chemicals, or other substances.

point source pollutants Pollutants that enter waterways at a specific location.

poison Any substance harmful to the body when ingested, inhaled, injected, or absorbed through the skin.

pollutant A substance that contaminates some aspect of the environment and causes potential harm to living organisms.

polychlorinated biphenyls (PCBs) Toxic chemicals that were once used as insulating materials in high-voltage electrical equipment.

polydrug use Taking several medications, vitamins, recreational drugs, or illegal drugs simultaneously.

polysaccharides Complex carbohydrates formed by the combination of long chains of monosaccharides.

positive reinforcement Presenting something positive following a behavior that is being reinforced.

positron emission tomography (PET) scan Method for measuring heart activity by injecting a patient with a radioactive tracer that is scanned electronically to produce a three-dimensional image of the heart and arteries.

postpartum depression A mood disorder experienced by women who have given birth; involves depression, fatigue, and other symptoms and may last for weeks or months.

post-traumatic stress disorder (PTSD) A collection of symptoms that may occur as a delayed response to a serious trauma.

power The ability to make and implement decisions.

prayer Communication with a transcendent Presence.

preconception care Medical care received prior to becoming pregnant that helps a woman assess and address potential maternal health issues.

prediabetes Condition in which blood glucose levels are higher than normal, but not high enough to be classified as diabetes.

preeclampsia A pregnancy complication characterized by high blood pressure, protein in the urine, and edema.

pre-gaming A strategy of drinking heavily at home before going out to an event or other location.

prehypertensive Blood pressure is above normal, but not yet in the hypertensive range.

prejudice A negative evaluation of an entire group of people that is typically based on unfavorable and often wrong ideas about the group.

premature ejaculation Ejaculation that occurs prior to or almost immediately following penile penetration of the vagina.

premenstrual dysphoric disorder (PMDD) Collective name for a group of negative symptoms similar to but more severe than PMS, including severe mood disturbances.

premenstrual syndrome (PMS) Comprises the mood changes and physical symptoms that occur in some women during the 1 or 2 weeks prior to menstruation.

premium Payment made to an insurance carrier, usually in monthly installments, that covers the cost of an insurance policy.

primary aggression Goal-directed, hostile self-assertion that is destructive in character.

primary care practitioner (PCP) A medical practitioner who treats routine ailments, advises on preventive care, gives general medical advice, and makes appropriate referrals when necessary.

prion A recently identified self-replicating, protein-based pathogen.

process addictions Behaviors such as disordered gambling, compulsive buying, compulsive Internet or technology use, work addiction, compulsive exercise, and sexual addiction that are known to be addictive because they are mood altering.

procrastinate To intentionally put off doing something.

progesterone Hormone secreted by the ovaries; helps the endometrium develop and helps maintain pregnancy.

proof A measure of the percentage of alcohol in a beverage.
prostate gland Gland that secretes nutrients and neutralizing fluids into the semen.
prostate-specific antigen (PSA) An antigen found in prostate cancer patients.
proteins The essential constituents of nearly all body cells; necessary for the development and repair of bone, muscle, skin, and blood; the key elements of antibodies, enzymes, and hormones.
protozoans Microscopic single-celled organisms that can be pathogenic.
psychoactive drugs Drugs that have the potential to alter mood or behavior.
psychological hardiness A personality trait characterized by control, commitment, and the embrace of challenge.
psychological resilience The process of adapting well in the face of adversity, trauma, tragedy, threats, or significant sources of stress, such as family and relationship problems, serious health problems, or workplace and financial stressors.
psychological health The mental, emotional, social, and spiritual dimensions of health.
psychoneuroimmunology (PNI) The study of the interrelationship between the mind and body on immune system functioning.
puberty The period of sexual maturation.
pubic lice Parasitic insects that can inhabit various body areas, especially the genitals.
qi Element of traditional Chinese medicine that refers to the vital energy force that courses through the body; when *qi* is in balance, health is restored.
radiation absorbed doses (rads) Units that measure exposure to radiation.
radiotherapy The use of radiation to kill cancerous cells.
radon A naturally occurring radioactive gas resulting from the decay of certain radioactive elements.
rape Sexual penetration without the victim's consent.
reactive aggression Hostile emotional reaction brought about by frustrating life experiences.
receptor sites Specialized areas of cells and organs where chemicals, enzymes, and other substances interact.
relapse The tendency to return to the addictive behavior after a period of abstinence.
religion A system of beliefs, practices, rituals, and symbols designed to facilitate closeness to the sacred or transcendent.
repetitive motion disorder (RMD) An injury to soft tissue, tendons, muscles, nerves, or joints due to the physical stress of repeated motions; sometimes called *overuse syndrome*, *cumulative trauma disorders*, or *repetitive stress injuries*.
resiliency The ability to adapt to change and stressful events in healthy and flexible ways.
resting metabolic rate (RMR) The energy expenditure of the body under BMR conditions plus other daily sedentary activities.
rheumatic heart disease A heart disease caused by untreated streptococcal infection of the throat.
RICE Acronym for the standard first aid treatment for virtually all traumatic and overuse injuries: **r**est, **i**ce, **c**ompression, and **e**levation.
rickettsia A small form of bacteria that live inside other living cells.
risk behaviors Actions that increase susceptibility to negative health outcomes.
rubella (German measles) A milder form of measles that causes a rash and mild fever in children and may damage a fetus or a newborn baby.
satiety The feeling of fullness or satisfaction at the end of a meal.
saturated fats Fats that are unable to hold any more hydrogen in their chemical structure; derived mostly from animal sources; solid at room temperature.
schizophrenia A mental illness with biological origins that is characterized by irrational behavior, severe alterations of the senses, and often an inability to function in society.
scrotum External sac of tissue that encloses the testes.
seasonal affective disorder (SAD) A type of depression that occurs in the winter months, when sunlight levels are low.
secondary sex characteristics Characteristics associated with sex but not directly related to reproduction, such as vocal pitch, degree of body hair, and location of fat deposits.
self-disclosure Sharing personal feelings or information with others.
self-efficacy Describes a person's belief about whether he or she can successfully engage in and execute a specific behavior.
self-esteem Refers to one's realistic sense of self-respect or self-worth.
self-injury Intentionally causing injury to one's own body in an attempt to cope with overwhelming negative emotions; also called *self-mutilation*, *self-harm*, or *nonsuicidal self-injury* (NSSI).
self-nurturance Developing individual potential through a balanced and realistic appreciation of self-worth and ability.
self-talk The customary manner of thinking and talking to yourself, which can affect your self-image.
semen Fluid containing sperm and nutrients that increase sperm viability and neutralize vaginal acid.
seminal vesicles Glandular ducts that secrete nutrients for the semen.
serial monogamy A series of monogamous sexual relationships.
set point theory Theory that a form of internal thermostat controls our weight and fights to maintain this weight around a narrowly set range.
sexual abuse of children Sexual interaction between a child and an adult or older child.
sexual addiction Compulsive involvement in sexual activity.
sexual assault Any act in which one person is sexually intimate with another without that person's consent.
sexual aversion disorder Desire dysfunction characterized by sexual phobias and anxiety about sexual contact.
sexual dysfunction Problems associated with achieving sexual satisfaction.
sexual fantasies Sexually arousing thoughts and dreams.
sexual harassment Any form of unwanted sexual attention related to any condition of employment, education, or performance evaluation.
sexual identity Recognition of oneself as a sexual being; a composite of biological sex characteristics, gender identity, gender roles, and sexual orientation.
sexual orientation A person's enduring emotional, romantic, sexual, or affectionate attraction to other persons.
sexual performance anxiety A condition of sexual difficulties caused by anticipating some sort of problem with the sex act.
sexual prejudice Negative attitudes and hostile actions directed at sexually identified social groups; also referred to as sexual bias.
sexuality All the thoughts, feelings, and behaviors associated with being male or female, experiencing attraction, being in love, and being in relationships that include sexual intimacy and activity.
sexually transmitted infections (STIs) Infectious diseases caused by pathogens transmitted through some form of intimate, usually sexual, contact.
shaping Using a series of small steps to gradually achieve a particular goal.
shift and persist A strategy of reframing appraisals of current stressors and focusing on a meaningful future that protects a person from the negative effects of too much stress.
shingles A disease characterized by a painful rash that occurs when the chickenpox virus is reactivated.
sick building syndrome (SBS) Occurs when occupants of a building experience acute health effects linked to time spent in a building, but no specific illness or cause can be identified; symptoms diminish when occupants are away from the building.
sidestream smoke The cigarette, pipe, or cigar smoke breathed by nonsmokers.
simple carbohydrates A major type of carbohydrate that provides short-term energy; also called *simple sugars*.

simple rape Rape by one person, usually known to the victim, that does not involve physical beating or use of a weapon.

sinoatrial node (SA node) Cluster of electric pulse-generating cells that serves as a natural pacemaker for the heart.

situational inducement Attempt to influence a behavior through situations and occasions that are structured to exert control over that behavior.

sleep debt The difference between the number of hours of sleep an individual needed in a given time period and the number of hours he or she actually slept.

snuff A powdered form of tobacco that is sniffed or absorbed through the mucous membranes in the nose or placed inside the cheek and sucked.

social bonds The level of closeness and attachment with other individuals.

social cognitive model (SCM) Model of behavior change emphasizing the role of social factors and thought processes (cognition) in behavior change.

social health Aspect of psychosocial health that includes interactions with others, ability to use social supports, and ability to adapt to various situations.

social learning theory Theory that people learn behaviors by watching role models—parents, caregivers, and significant others.

social phobia A phobia characterized by fear and avoidance of social situations; also called *social anxiety disorder*.

social physique anxiety (SPA) A desire to look good that has a destructive effect on a person's ability to function well in social interactions and relationships.

social support Network of people and services with whom you share ties and from whom you get support.

socialization Process by which a society communicates behavioral expectations to its individual members.

spermatogenesis The development of sperm.

spermicides Substances designed to kill sperm.

spiritual health The aspect of psychosocial health that relates to having a sense of meaning and purpose to one's life, as well as a feeling of connection with others and with nature.

spiritual intelligence (SI) The ability to access higher meanings, values, abiding purposes, and unconscious aspects of the self, a characteristic that helps us find a moral and ethical path to guide us through life.

spirituality An individual's sense of purpose and meaning in life, beyond material values.

stalking The willful, repeated, and malicious following, harassing, or threatening of another person.

standard drink The amount of any beverage that contains about 14 grams of pure alcohol (about 0.6 fluid ounce or 1.2 tablespoons).

staphylococci A group of round bacteria, usually found in clusters, that cause a variety of diseases in humans and other animals.

starch Polysaccharide that is the storage form of glucose in plants.

static stretching Stretching techniques that slowly and gradually lengthen a muscle or group of muscles and their tendons.

stent A stainless steel, mesh-like tube that is inserted to prop open the artery.

sterilization Permanent fertility control achieved through surgical procedures.

stereotactic radiosurgery A type of radiation therapy that can be used to zap tumors; also known as gamma knife surgery.

stillbirth A fetus that is dead at birth.

stimulants Drugs that increase activity of the central nervous system.

Streptococcus A round bacterium, usually found in chain formation.

stress A series of mental and physiological responses and adaptations to a real or perceived threat to one's well-being.

stress inoculation A stress-management technique in which a person consciously anticipates and prepares for potential stressors.

stressor A physical, social, or psychological event or condition that upsets homeostasis and produces a stress response.

stroke A condition occurring when the brain is damaged by disrupted blood supply; also called *cerebrovascular accident*.

subjective well-being An uplifting feeling of inner peace.

suction curettage An abortion technique that uses gentle suction to remove fetal tissue from the uterus.

sudden cardiac death Death that occurs as a result of abrupt, profound loss of heart function.

sudden infant death syndrome (SIDS) The sudden death of an infant under 1 year of age for no apparent reason.

suicidal ideation A desire to die and thoughts about suicide.

Superfund Fund established under the Comprehensive Environmental Response, Compensation, and Liability Act to be used for cleaning up toxic waste dumps.

suppositories Waxy capsules that are inserted deep into the vagina, where they melt and release a spermicide.

sustainable development Development that meets the needs of the present without compromising the ability of future generations to meet their own needs.

sympathetic nervous system Branch of the autonomic nervous system responsible for stress arousal.

sympathomimetics Food substances that can produce stresslike physiological responses.

synergism The interaction of two or more drugs that produce more profound effects than would be expected if the drugs were taken separately; also called *potentiation*.

syphilis One of the most widespread bacterial STIs; characterized by distinct phases and potentially serious results.

systolic blood pressure The upper number in the fraction that measures blood pressure, indicating pressure on the walls of the arteries when the heart contracts.

tar A thick, brownish substance condensed from particulate matter in smoked tobacco.

target heart rate The heart rate range of aerobic exercise that leads to improved cardiorespiratory fitness (i.e., 64% to 96% of maximal heart rate).

temperature inversion A weather condition occurring when a layer of cool air is trapped under a layer of warmer air, preventing the air from circulating.

teratogenic Causing birth defects; may refer to drugs, environmental chemicals, radiation, or diseases.

terrorism The unlawful use of force or violence against persons or property to intimidate or coerce a government, the civilian population, or any segment thereof in furtherance of political or social objectives.

testes Male sex organs that manufacture sperm and produce hormones.

testosterone The male sex hormone manufactured in the testes.

tetrahydrocannabinol (THC) The chemical name for the active ingredient in marijuana.

thrombolysis Injection of an agent to dissolve clots and restore some blood flow, thereby reducing the amount of tissue that dies from ischemia.

thrombus Blood clot attached to a blood vessel's wall.

time As part of the FITT prescription, refers to how long a person needs to exercise each time to improve a component of physical fitness.

tolerance Phenomenon in which progressively larger doses of a drug or more intense involvement in a behavior is needed to produce the desired effects.

toxic shock syndrome (TSS) A potentially life-threatening disease that occurs when specific bacterial toxins multiply and spread to the bloodstream, most commonly through improper use of tampons or diaphragms.

toxins Poisonous substances produced by certain microorganisms that cause various diseases.

toxoplasmosis A disease caused by an organism found in cat feces that, when contracted by a pregnant woman, may result in stillbirth or an infant with mental retardation or birth defects.

trace minerals Minerals that the body needs in only very small amounts.

traditional Chinese medicine (TCM) Ancient comprehensive system of healing that uses herbs, acupuncture, and massage to bring vital energy, *qi*, into balance and to remove blockages of qi that lead to disease.

trans fats (trans fatty acids) Fatty acids that are produced when polyunsaturated oils are hydrogenated to make them more solid.

transdermal The introduction of drugs through the skin.

transgendered Having a gender identity that does not match one's biological sex.

transient ischemic attack (TIA) Brief interruption of the blood supply to the brain that causes only temporary impairment; often an indicator of impending major stroke.

transsexual A person who is psychologically of one sex but physically of the other.

transtheoretical model Model of behavior change that identifies six distinct stages people go through in altering behavior patterns; also called the *stages of change model*.

traumatic injuries Injuries that are accidental and occur suddenly and violently.

traumatic stress A physiological and mental response that occurs for a prolonged period of time after a major accident, war, assault, natural disaster, or an event in which one may be seriously hurt, or killed, or witness horrible things.

trichomoniasis Protozoan STI characterized by foamy, yellowish discharge and unpleasant odor.

triglycerides The most common form of fat in the body; excess calories consumed are converted into triglycerides and stored as body fat.

trimester A 3-month segment of pregnancy; used to describe specific developmental changes that occur in the embryo or fetus.

triple marker screen (TMS) A common maternal blood test that can be used to identify fetuses with certain birth defects and genetic abnormalities.

tubal ligation Sterilization of the woman that involves the cutting and tying off or cauterizing of the fallopian tubes.

tuberculosis (TB) A disease caused by bacterial infiltration of the respiratory system.

tumor A neoplasmic mass that grows more rapidly than surrounding tissue.

type As part of the FITT prescription, refers to what kind of exercises a person needs to do to improve a component of physical fitness.

type 1 diabetes Form of diabetes mellitus in which the pancreas is not able to make insulin and therefore blood glucose cannot enter the cells to be used for energy.

type 2 diabetes Form of diabetes mellitus in which the pancreas does not make enough insulin or the body is unable to use insulin correctly.

typical-use failure rate The number of pregnancies (per 100 users) that are likely to occur in the first year of use of a particular birth control method if the method's use is not consistent or always correct.

ultrasonography (ultrasound) A common prenatal test that uses high-frequency sound waves to create a visual image of the fetus.

underweight Having a body weight more than 10 percent below healthy recommended levels; in an adult, having a BMI below 18.5.

unintentional injuries Injury, death, or psychological harm caused unintentionally or without premeditation.

unsaturated fats Fats that have room for more hydrogen in their chemical structure; derived mostly from plants; liquid at room temperature.

urethral opening The opening through which urine is expelled.

urinary tract infection (UTI) Infection, more common among women than men, of the urinary tract; causes include untreated STIs.

uterus (womb) Hollow, pear-shaped muscular organ whose function is to contain the developing fetus.

vaccination Inoculation with killed or weakened pathogens or similar, less dangerous antigens in order to prevent or lessen the effects of a disease.

vagina The passage in females leading from the vulva into the uterus.

vaginal intercourse The insertion of the penis into the vagina.

vaginismus A state in which the vaginal muscles contract so forcefully that penetration cannot occur.

values Principles that influence our thoughts and emotions and guide the choices we make in our lives.

variant sexual behavior A sexual behavior that is not practiced by most people.

vas deferens Tube that transports sperm from the epididymis to the ejaculatory duct.

vasectomy Sterilization of the man that involves the cutting and tying off of both vasa deferentia.

vasocongestion The engorgement of the genital organs with blood.

vegetarian A person who follows a diet that excludes some or all animal products.

veins Vessels that transport waste and carry blood back to the heart from other regions of the body.

ventricles The heart's two lower chambers, which pump blood through the blood vessels.

venules Branches of the veins.

very-low-calorie diets (VLCDs) Diets with a daily caloric value of 400 to 700 calories.

violence Aggressive behaviors that produce injuries and can result in death.

virulent Strong enough to overcome host resistance and cause disease.

viruses Pathogens that invade and inject their own DNA or RNA into a host cell, take it over, and force it to make copies of the pathogen.

visualization The creation of mental images to promote relaxation.

vitamins Essential organic compounds that promote growth and reproduction and help maintain life and health.

vulva Collective term for the external female genitalia.

waist-to-hip ratio Waist circumference divided by hip circumference; a high ratio indicates increased health risks due to unhealthy fat distribution.

wellness The achievement of the highest level of health possible in each of several dimensions.

whole grains Grains that are milled in their complete form, and thus include the bran, germ, and endosperm, with only the husk removed.

withdrawal 1 A method of contraception that involves withdrawing the penis from the vagina before ejaculation; also called coitus interruptus.

withdrawal 2 A series of temporary physical and biopsychosocial symptoms that occurs when an addict abruptly abstains from an addictive chemical or behavior.

work addiction The compulsive use of work and the work persona to fulfill needs for intimacy, power, and success.

yoga A system of physical and mental training involving controlled breathing, physical postures (*asanas*), meditation, chanting, and other practices that are believed to cultivate unity with the *Atman*, or spiritual life principle of the universe.

yo-yo diets Cycles in which people diet and regain weight.

zoonotic diseases Diseases of animals that may be transmitted to humans.

References

Chapter 1

1. Centers for Disease Control and Prevention, " Behavioral Risk Factor Surveillance System Prevalence and Trends Data," Accessed March 2014, http://apps.nccd.cdc.gov/BRFSS/display.asp?yr=2012&state=US&qkey=8041&grp=0&SUBMIT3=Go.
2. C. E. Garber et al., "American College of Sports Medicine Position Stand: Quantity and Quality of Exercise for Developing and Maintaining Cardiorespiratory, Musculoskeletal and Neuromotor Fitness in Apparently Healthy Adults: Guidance for Prescribing Exercise," *Medicine and Science in Sports and Exercise* 33, no. 7 (2011): 1334–59, DOI: 10.1249/MSS.0b013e318213fefb.
3. American College Health Association, *American College Health Association-National College Health Assessment II (ACHA-NCHA II) Reference Group Executive Summary, Fall 2013* (Hanover, MD: American College Health Association, 2014), Available at www.acha-ncha.org/reports_ACHA-NCHAII.html.
4. National Heart, Lung, and Blood Institute, U.S. Department of Health and Human Services, National Institutes of Health, "What Is Physical Activity," Updated September 2011, www.nhlbi.nih.gov/health/health-topics/topics/phys/; Office of Disease Prevention and Health Promotion, *2008 Physical Activity Guidelines for Americans, 2008,* Available at www.health.gov/paguidelines.
5. P. Kokkinos, H. Sheriff, and R. Kheirbek, "Physical Inactivity and Mortality Risk," *Cardiology Research and Practice,* 11 (2011): 924–49. www.hindawi.com/journals/crp/2011/924945. (Epub ahead of print.)
6. I. Lee et al., "Impact of Physical Inactivity on the World's Major Non-communicable Diseases," *Lancet* 380, no. 9838 (2012): 219–29.
7. S. Plowman and D. Smith, *Exercise Physiology for Health, Fitness, and Performance*, 3rd ed. (Philadelphia, PA: Lippincott Williams & Wilkins, 2011).
8. S. Grover et al., "Estimating the Benefits of Patient and Physician Adherence to Cardiovascular Prevention Guidelines: The MyHealthCheckup Survey," *Canadian Journal of Cardiology* 27, no. 2 (2011): 159–66.
9. American Heart Association, "About Cholesterol," Updated May 2013, www.heart.org/HEARTORG/Conditions/Cholesterol/AboutCholesterol/AboutCholesterol_UCM_001220_Article.jsp.
10. L. Montesi et al., "Physical Activity for the Prevention and Treatment of Metabolic Disorders," *Internal and Emergency Medicine* 8, no. 8 (2013): 655–66.
11. Ibid.
12. D. C. Lee et al. "Changes in Fitness and Fatness on the Development of Cardiovascular Disease Risk Factors Hypertension, Metabolic Syndrome, and Hypercholesterolemia," *Journal of the American College of Cardiology* 59, no. 7 (2012): 665–72.
13. M. Uusitupa, J. Tuomilehto, and P. Puska, "Are We Really Active in the Prevention of Obesity and Type 2 Diabetes at the Community Level?," *Nutrition and Metabolism in Cardiovascular Diseases* 21, no. 5 (2011): 380–89, DOI: 10.1016/j.numecd.2010.12.007.
14. National Diabetes Information Clearinghouse, U.S. Department of Health and Human Services, *Diabetes Prevention Program (DPP),* NIH Publication no. 09–5099 (Bethesda, MD: National Diabetes Information Clearinghouse, 2008), Available at http://diabetes.niddk.nih.gov/dm/pubs/preventionprogram.
15. N. Magné et al., "Recommendations for a Lifestyle Which Could Prevent Breast Cancer and Its Relapse: Physical Activity and Dietetic Aspects," *Critical Reviews in Oncology and Hematology* 80, no. 3 (2011): 450–59, DOI: 10.1016/j.critrevonc.2011.01.013.
16. L. H. Kushi et al., "American Cancer Society Guidelines on Nutrition and Physical Activity for Cancer Prevention," *CA: A Cancer Journal for Clinicians* 62, no. 1 (2012): 30–67.
17. World Cancer Research Fund/American Institute for Cancer Research, Policy and Action for Cancer Prevention, "Food, Nutrition, and Physical Activity: A Global Perspective" (Washington DC: AICR, 2009); A. Shibata, K. Ishii, and K. Oka, "Psychological, Social, and Environmental Factors of Meeting Recommended Physical Activity Levels for Colon Cancer Prevention among Japanese Adults," *Journal of Science and Medicine in Sport* 12, no. 2 (2010): e155–56; K. Y. Wolin et al., "Physical Activity and Colon Cancer Prevention: A Meta-Analysis," *British Journal of Cancer* 100, no. 4 (2009): 611–16.
18. C. M. Friedenreich and A. E. Cust, "Physical Activity and Breast Cancer Risk: Impact of Timing, Type, and Dose of Activity and Population Subgroup Effects," *British Journal of Sports Medicine* 42, no. 8 (2008): 636–47.
19. M. Nilsson et al., "Increased Physical Activity Is Associated with Enhanced Development of Peak Bone Mass in Men: A Five Year Longitudinal Study," *Journal of Bone and Mineral Research* 27, no. 5 (2012): 1206–14, DOI: 10.1002/jbmr.1549; M. Callréus et al., "Self-Reported Recreational Exercise Combining Regularity and Impact Is Necessary to Maximize Bone Mineral Density in Young Adult Women: A Population-Based Study of 1,061 Women 25 Years of Age," *Osteoporosis International* 23, no. 10 (2012): 2517–26, DOI: 10.1007/s00198-011-1886-5.
20. R. Rizzoli, C. A. Abraham, and M. L. Brandi, "Nutrition and Bone Health: Turning Knowledge and Beliefs in Healthy Behavior," *Current Medical Research & Opinion* 30, no. 1 (2014): 131–41.
21. V. A. Catenacci et al., "Physical Activity Patterns Using Accelerometry in the National Weight Control Registry," *Obesity* 19, no. 6 (2011): 1163N70, DOI: 10.1038/oby.2010.264.
22. T. L. Gillum et al., "A Review of Sex Differences in Immune Function after Aerobic Exercise," *Exercise Immunology Review* 17 (2011): 104–20.
23. MedLine Plus, National Institutes of Health, "Exercise and Immunity," May 2012, www.nlm.nih.gov/medlineplus/ency/article/007165.htm.
24. N. P. Walsh et al., "Position Statement. Part Two: Maintaining Immune Health," *Exercise and Immunology Review* 17 (2011): 64–103.
25. T. L. Gillum et al., "A Review of Sex Differences in Immune Function after Aerobic Exercise," *Exercise Immunology Review* 17 (2011): 104–20.
26. C. Huang et al., "Cardiovascular Reactivity, Stress, and Physical Activity," *Frontiers in Physiology* 4(2013): 1–13, DOI:10.3389/fphys.201300314.
27. T. M. Burkhalter and C. H. Hillman, "A Narrative Review of Physical Activity, Nutrition, and Obesity to Cognitive and Scholastic Performance across the Human Lifespan," *Advances in Nutrition: An International Review Journal* 2, no. 2 (2011): 201S–206S.
28. J. E. Ashlskog, Y. E. Geda, N. R. Graff-Radford, and R. C. Petersen, "Physical Exercise as a Preventive or Disease-Modifying Treatment of Dementia and Brain Aging," *Mayo Clinic Proceedings* 86, no. 9 (2011): 876–84.
29. J. Berry et al., "Lifetime Risks for Cardiovascular Disease Mortality by Cardiorespiratory Fitness Levels Measured at Ages 45, 55, and 65 Years in Men: The Cooper Center Longitudinal Study," *Journal of the American College of Cardiology* 57, no. 15 (2011): 1604–10; J. Woodcock et al., "Non-Vigorous Physical Activity and All-Cause Mortality: Systematic Review and Meta-Analysis of Cohort Studies," *International Journal of Epidemiology* 40, no. 1 (2011): 121–38.
30. C. E. Garber et al., "American College of Sports Medicine Position Stand," 2011.
31. Ibid.
32. T. Gotschi and K. Mills, *Active Transportation for America: The Case for Increased Federal Investment in Bicycling and Walking* (Washington, DC: Rails to Trails Conservancy, 2008), Available at www.railstotrails.org/ourwork/advocacy/activetransportation/makingthecase; D. Shinkle and A. Teigens, *Encouraging Bicycling and Walking: The State Legislative Role* (Washington, DC: National Conference of State Legislatures, 2008), Updated April 2009, Available at www.americantrails.org/resources/trans/Encourage-Bicycling-Walking-State-Legislative-Role.html.
33. Ibid; U.S. Environmental Protection Agency, "Climate Change: What You Can Do—On the Road," Updated September 2013, www.epa.gov/climatechange/wycd/road.html.
34. C. E. Garber et al., "American College of Sports Medicine Position Stand," 2011.
35. American College of Sports Medicine, *ACSM's Resource Manual for Guidelines for Exercise Testing and Prescription* (Philadelphia, PA: Lippincott Williams & Wilkins, 2014).
36. W. Micheo, L. Baerga, and G. Miranda, "Basic Principles Regarding Strength, Flexibility, Flexibility, and Stability Exercises," *Physical Medicine & Rehabilitation* 4, no. 11 (2012): 805–11, DOI: 10.1016/j.pmrj.2012.09.583; C. E. Garber et al., "American College of Sports Medicine Position Stand," 2011.
37. C. E. Garber et al., "American College of Sports Medicine Position Stand," 2011.
38. Ibid.
39. D. G. Behm and A. Chaouachi, "A Review of the Acute Effects of Static and Dynamic Stretching on Performance," *European Journal of Applied Physiology*, March 4, 2011, 21373870. (Epub ahead of print.)

40. K. C. Huxel Bliven and B. E. Anderson, "Core Stability Training for Injury Prevention," *Sports Health: A Multidisciplinary Approach* 5, no. 6 (2013): 514–22.
41. V. Baltzpoulos, "Isokinetic Dynamometry," in *Biomechanical Evaluation of Movement in Sport and Exercise: The British Association of Sport and Exercise Sciences Guidelines,* eds. C. Payton and R. Bartlett (New York, NY: Routledge, 2008), 105.
42. D. G. Behm and J. C. Colao Sanchez, "Instability Resistance Training across the Exercise Continuum," *Sports Health: A Multidisciplinary Approach* 5, no. 6 (2013): 500–503.
43. Ibid.
44. P. Williamson, *Exercise for Special Populations* (Philadelphia, PA: Lippincott Williams & Wilkins, 2011).
45. Ibid.
46. Ibid.
47. Ibid.
48. W. J. Chodzko-Zajko et al., "American College of Sports Medicine Position Stand: Exercise and Physical Activity for Older Adults," *Medicine and Science in Sports and Exercise* 41, no. 7 (2009): 1510–30.
49. M. N. Sawka et al., "American College of Sports Medicine Position Stand: Exercise and Fluid Replacement," *Medicine and Science in Sports and Exercise* 39, no. 2 (2007): 377–90.
50. Ibid.
51. S. Cutts, N. Obi, C. Pasapula, and W. Chan, "Plantar Fasciitis," *Annals of the Royal College of Surgeons of England* 94, no.8 (2012): 539–42.
52. P. Newman et al., "Risk Factors Associated with Medial Tibial Stress Syndrome in Runners: A Systematic Review and Meta-analysis," *Open Access Journal of Sports Medicine* 4 (2013): 229–41.
53. J. A. Rixe et al., "A Review of the Management of Patellofemoral Pain Syndrome," *The Physician and Sports Medicine* 41, no. 3 (2013): 19–28.
54. K. B. Fields et al., "Prevention of Running Injuries," *Current Sports Medicine Reports* 9, no. 3 (2010): 176–82.
55. American Academy of Ophthalmology, "Eye Health in Sports and Recreation," March 2014, www.aao.org/eyesmart/injuries/eyewear.cfm.
56. Ibid.
57. Bicycle Helmet Safety Institute, "Helmet-Related Statistics from Many Sources," January 2014, www.helmets.org/stats.htm.
58. American College Health Association, *American College Health Association-National College Health Assessment II: Reference Group Executive Summary, Fall 2013,* 2014.
59. Bicycle Helmet Safety Institute, "Helmet-Related Statistics from Many Sources," January 2014, www.helmets.org/stats.htm.
60. N. G. Nelson et al., "Exertional Heat-Related Injuries Treated in Emergency Departments in the U.S., 1997–2006," *American Journal of Preventive Medicine* 40, no. 1 (2011): 54–60.
61. L. E. Armstrong et al., "The American Football Uniform: Uncompensable Heat Stress and Hyperthermic Exhaustion," *Journal of Athletic Training* 45, no. 2 (2010): 117–27.
62. E. E. Turk, "Hypothermia," *Forensic Science Medical Pathology* 6, no. 2 (2010): 106–15.
63. Ibid.

Pulled Statistic

page 230, C. E. Garber et al., "American College of Sports Medicine Position Stand: Quantity and Quality of Exercise for Developing and Maintaining Cardiorespiratory, Musculoskeletal and Neuromotor Fitness in Apparently Healthy Adults: Guidance for Prescribing Exercise," *Medicine and Science in Sports and Exercise* 43, no. 7 (2011): 1334–59.

Chapter 2

1. D. Spruijt-Metz, "Etiology, Treatment, and Prevention of Obesity in Childhood and Adolescence: A Decade in Review," *Journal of Research on Adolescence* 21 (2011): 129–52, DOI: 10.1111/j.1532-7795.2010.00719.x; S. A. Affenito et al., "Behavioral Determinants of Obesity: Research Findings and Policy Implications," *Journal of Obesity* 2012 (2012), http://dx.doi.org/10.1155/2012/150732.
2. S. A. Affenito et al., "Behavioral Determinants of Obesity: Research Findings and Policy Implications," 2012.
3. C. L. Ogden et al., "Prevalence of Childhood and Adult Obesity in the United States, 2011–2012," *Journal of the American Medical Association* 311, no. 8 (2014): 806–14, DOI:10.1001/jama.2014.732; C. L. Ogden et al, "Prevalence of Obesity Among Adults: United States, 2011–2012," *NCHS Data Brief* 131 (2013), www.cdc.gov/nchs/data/databriefs/db131.htm.
4. U.S. Department of Health and Human Services, *The Surgeon General's Vision for a Healthy and Fit Nation* (Rockville, MD: U.S. Department of Health and Human Services, Office of the Surgeon General, 2010), Available at www.surgeongeneral.gov/library/obesityvision.
5. C. L. Ogden et al., "Prevalence of Childhood and Adult Obesity in the United States, 2011–2012," 2014.
6. A. Go et al., "AHA Statistical Update Heart Disease and Stroke Statistics—2014 Update: A Report from the American Heart Association," *Circulation* 129 (2014): 399–410.
7. C. L. Ogden et al., "Prevalence of Childhood and Adult Obesity in the United States, 2011–2012," 2014.
8. A. Go et al., "AHA Statistical Update Heart Disease and Stroke Statistics—2014 Update," 2014.
9. Ibid.
10. World Health Organization, "Obesity and Overweight Fact Sheet," March 2013, www.who.int/mediacentre/factsheets/fs311/en.
11. Ibid.; International Obesity Taskforce, "Obesity—The Global Epidemic," 2014, www.iaso.org/iotf/obesity/obesitytheglobalepidemic.
12. American Diabetes Association, "Statistics About Diabetes," January 2011, www.diabetes.org/diabetes-basics/statistics
13. J. Cawley and C. Meyerhoefer, "The Medical Care Costs of Obesity: An Instrumental Variables Approach," *Journal of Health Economics* 31, no. 1 (2012): 219, DOI: 10.1016/j.jhealeco.2011.10.003; J. P. Moriarty et al., "The Effects of Incremental Costs of Smoking and Obesity on Health Care Costs among Adults," *Journal of Occupational and Environmental Medicine* 54, no. 3 (2012): 286, DOI: 10.1097/JOM.0b013e318246f1f4.
14. C. Murtaugh et al., "Lifetime Risk and Duration of Chronic Diseases and Disability," *Journal of Aging and Health* 23, no. 3 (2011): 554–77.
15. World Health Organization, "Obesity and Overweight Fact Sheet," March 2013.
16. T. Tanaka, J. S. Ngwa, and F. J. van Rooij, "Genome-wide Meta-Analysis of Observational Studies Shows Common Genetic Variants Associated with Macronutrient Intake," *American Journal of Clinical Nutrition* 97, no. 6 (2013): 1395–402; M. M. Hetherington and J. E. Cecil, "Gene-Environment Interactions in Obesity," *Forum Nutrition* 63 (2010): 195–203; M. Graff, J. S. Ngwa, and T. Workalemahu, "Genome-wide Analysis of BMI in Adolescents and Young Adults Reveals Additional Insights into the Effects of the Genetic Loci over the Life Course," *Human Molecular Genetics* 22, no. 17 (2013): 3597–607; K. Silventoinen et al., "The Genetic and Environmental Influences on Childhood Obesity: A Systematic Review of Twin and Adoption Studies," *International Journal of Obesity* 34, no. 1 (2010): 29–40.
17. T. O. Kilpelainen et al., "Physical Activity Attenuates the Influence of *FTO* Variants on Obesity Risk: A Meta-Analysis of 218,166 Adults and 19,268 Children," *PLoS Medicine* 8, no. 11 (2012), e1001116, DOI:10.1371/journal.pmed.1001116; A. S. Richardson et al., "Moderate to Vigorous Physical Activity Interactions with Genetic Variants and Body Mass Index in a Large US Ethnically Diverse Cohort," *Pediatric Obesity* 9, no. 2 (2013): e35n46, DOI: 10.1111/j.2047-6310.2013.00152.
18. J. C. Wells. "The Evolution of Human Adiposity and Obesity: Where Did It All Go Wrong?," *Disease Models and Mechanisms* 5, no. 5 (2012): 595–607, DOI: 10.1242/dmm.009613; J. R. Speakman et al., "Evolutionary Perspectives on the Obesity Epidemic: Adaptive, Maladaptive, and Neutral Viewpoints," *Annual Review of Nutrition* 33 (2013): 289–317.
19. A. Tremblay et al., "Adaptive Thermogenesis Can Make a Difference in the Ability of Obese Individuals to Lose Body Weight," *International Journal of Obesity* 37 (2013): 759–64.
20. A. Tremblay et al., "Adaptive Thermogenesis Can Make a Difference in the Ability of Obese Individuals to Lose Body Weight," 2013.
21. M. Rotondi, F. Magri, and L. Chiovato, "Thyroid and Obesity: Not a One Way Interaction," *The Journal of Clinical Endocrinology and Metabolism* 96, no. 2 (2011): 344–56.
22. D. E. Cummings et al., "Plasma Ghrelin Levels after Diet-Induced Weight Loss or Gastric Bypass Surgery," *New England Journal of Medicine* 346, no. 21 (2002): 1623–30.
23. M. Khatib et al., "Effect of Ghrelin on Regulation of Growth Hormone Release: A Review," *The Health Agenda* 2, no. 1 (2014); C. DeVriese et al., "Focus on the Short- and Long-Term Effects of Ghrelin on Energy Homeostasis," *Nutrition* 26, no. 6 (2010): 579–84; T. Castaneda et al., "Ghrelin in the Regulation of Body Weight and Metabolism," *Frontiers in Neuroendocrinology* 31, no. 1 (2010): 44–60.
24. P. Marzullo et al. "Investigations of Thyroid Hormones and Antibodies in Obesity: Leptin Levels Are Associated with Thyroid Autoimmunity Independent of Bioanthropometric, Hormonal and Weight-Related Determinants," *The Journal of Clinical Endocrinology and Metabolism* 95, no. 8 (2010): 3965–72;. H. Feng et al., "Review: The Role of Leptin in Obesity and the Potential for Leptin Replacement Therapy," *Endocrine* 44 (2013): 33–39.
25. L. K. Mahan and S. Escott-Stump, *Krause's Food, Nutrition, and Diet Therapy,* 13th ed. (New York, NY: W. B. Saunders, 2012).
26. L. Poston, L. F. Harthoorn, and E. M Van Der Beek, "Obesity in Pregnancy: Implications for the Mother and Lifelong Health of the Child–A Consensus Statement," *Pediatric Research* 69, no. 2 (2011): 175–80; K. L. Connor et al., "Nature, Nurture or Nutrition? Impact of Maternal Nutrition on Maternal Care, Offspring Development and Reproductive Function," *Journal of Physiology* 590, no. 9 (2012): 2167–80.
27. M. A. Schuster et al. "Racial and Ethnic Health Disparities among Fifth-Graders in Three Cities," *The New England Journal of Medicine* 367, no. 8 (2012): 735–45; C. L. Odgen et al., "Prevalence of Obesity

and Trends in Body Mass Index among U.S. Children and Adolescents. 1999–2010," *Journal of the American Medical Association* 307 (2012): 483–90.
28. C. Gillespie et al., "The Growing Concern of Poverty in the United States: An Exploration of Food Prices and Poverty on Obesity Rates for Low-Income Citizens," *Undergraduate Economic Review* 8, no. 1 (2012): 1–38.
29. J. F. Sallis et al., "Role of Built Environments in Physical Activity, Obesity and Cardiovascular Disease," *Circulation* 125, no. 5 (2012): 729–737; F. Li et al., "Built Environment, Adiposity, and Physical Activity in Adults Aged 50–75," *American Journal of Preventive Medicine* 35, no. 1 (2008): 38–46.
30. U.S. Department of Health and Human Services, "Summary Health Statistics for U.S. Adults: National Health Interview Survey, 2012," *Vital and Health Statistics* 10, no. 260 (2014), Available at www.cdc.gov/nchs/data/series/sr_10/sr10_260.pdf.
31. Centers for Disease Control and Prevention, "Prevalence of Underweight among Adults Aged 20 years and Over: United States 1960–1962 and 2007–2010," September 2012, www.cdc.gov/nchs/data/hestat/underweight_adult_07_10/underweight_adult_07_10.htm; Centers for Disease Control and Prevention, "Prevalence of Underweight among Children and Adolescents Aged 2–19 Years: United States, 1963–1965 through 2007–2010, www.cdc.gov/nchs/data/hestat/underweight_child_07_10/underweight_child_07_10.htm.
32. Centers for Disease Control and Prevention, "About BMI for Adults," September 2011, www.cdc.gov/healthyweight/assessing/bmi/adult_bmi/index.html.
33. J. I. Mechanick et al., "Clinical Practice Guidelines for the Perioperative Nutritional, Metabolic and Nonsurgical Support of the Bariatric Surgery Patient—2013 Update," *Endocrine Practice* 19, no. 2 (2013): e1–36, www.aace.com/files/publish-ahead-of-print-final-version.pdf.
34. K. M. Flegal et al., "Prevalence and Trends in Obesity among U.S. Adults, 1999–2010," *Journal of the American Medical Association* 307, no. 5 (2012): 491–97.
35. R. Puhl, "Weight Stigmatization toward Youth: A Significant Problem in Need of Societal Solutions," *Childhood Obesity* 7, no. 5 (2011): 359–63; S. A. Mustillo, K. Budd, and K. Hendrix, "Obesity, Labeling, and Psychological Distress in Late-Childhood and Adolescent Black and White Girls: The Distal Effects of Stigma," *Social Psychology Quarterly* 76, no. 3 (2013): 268–89.
36. M. Bombelli et al., "Impact of Body Mass Index and Waist Circumference on the Long Term Risk of Diabetes Mellitus, Hypertension and Cardiac Organ Damage," *Hypertension* 58, no. 6 (2011): 1029–1035; S. Czernichow et al., "Body Mass Index, Waist Circumference and Waist-Hip Ratio: Which Is the Better Discriminator of Cardiovascular Disease Mortality Risk? Evidence from an Individual-Participant Meta-Analysis of 82,864 Participants from Nine Cohort Studies," *Obesity Reviews* 12, no. 9 (2011): 1467–78.
37. National Heart, Lung, and Blood Institute, "Classification of Overweight and Obesity by BMI, Waist Circumference and Associated Disease Risks," 2012, www.nhlbi.nih.gov/health/public/heart/obesity/lose_wt/bmi_dis.htm.
38. University of Maryland Medical Center, Rush University, "Waist to Hip Ratio Calculator," Accessed March 2014, www.healthcalculators.org/calculators/waist_hip.asp
39. World Health Organization, "Waist Circumference and Waist-Hip Ratio: Report of WHO Expert Consultation," 2011, http://whqlibdoc.who.int/publications/2011/9789241501491_eng.pdf.
40. E. Stice et al., "Risk Factors and Prodomal Eating Pathology," *Journal of Child Psychology and Psychiatry* 51, no. 4 (2010): 518–25.
41. S. N. Bleich, J. A. Wolfson, and S. Vine, "Diet-Beverage Consumption and Caloric Intake among US Adults, Overall and by Body Weight," *American Journal of Public Health* 104, no. 3 (2014): e72–78.
42. L. Gray, N. Cooper, A. Dunkley et al., "A Systematic Review and Mixed Treatment Comparison of Pharmacological Interventions for the Treatment of Obesity," *Obesity Reviews* 13, no. 6 (2012): 483–98.
43. Federal Drug Administration, "FDA Consumer Updates: HCG Diet Products are Illegal," March 2014, www.fda.gov/forconsumers/consumerupdates/ucm281333.htm
44. Federal Drug Administration, "Questions and Answers about FDA's Initiative against Contaminated Weight Loss Products," September 2013, www.fda.gov/drugs/resourcesforyou/consumers/questionsanswers/ucm136187.htm; U.S. Food and Drug Administration, "Follow-Up to the November 2009 Early Communication about an Ongoing Safety Review of Sibutramine, Marketed as Meridia," January 2010, www.fda.gov/Drugs/DrugSafety/stmarketDrugSafetyInformationforPatientsandProviders/DrugSafetyInformationforHeathcareProfessionals/ucm198206.htm.
45. ConsumerSearch, "Diet Pills: Reviews," 2012, www.consumersearch.com/diet-pills
46. F. Rubino et al., "Metabolic Surgery to Treat Type 2 Diabetes: Clinical Outcomes and Mechanisms of Action," *Annual Review of Medicine* 61 (2010): 393–411; S. Brethauer et al., "Can Diabetes Be Surgically Cured? Long-term Metabolic Effects of Bariatric Surgery in Obese Patients with Type 2 Diabetes Mellitus," *Annals of Surgery* 258, no. 4 (2013): 628–37.
47. D. E. Arterburn et al., "A Multi-Site Study of Long Term Remission and Relapse of Type 2 Diabetes Mellitus Following Gastric Bypass Obesity Surgery," *Obesity Surgery* 23, no. 1 (2013): 93–102; C. D. Still et al., "Preoperative Prediction of Type 2 Diabetes Remission after Roux-en-Y Gastric Bypass Surgery: A Retrospective Cohort Study," *The Lancet Diabetes & Endocrinology* 2, no. 1 (2014): 38–45.
48. J. S. Blake, *Nutrition and You*, 2nd ed. (San Francisco, CA, Pearson Education, 2011).
49. University of the West of England, "30% of Women Would Trade at Least One Year of Their Life to Achieve Their Ideal Body Weight and Shape," March 2011, http://info.uwe.ac.uk/news/UWENews/news.aspx?id=1949.
50. University of Minnesota Health Talk, "Social Media May Inspire Unhealthy Body Image," May 2013, www.healthtalk.umn.edu/2013/05/15/thigh-gap-and-social-media.
51. Ibid.
52. Centers for Disease Control and Prevention, "FASTSTATS: Obesity and Overweight," November 2013, www.cdc.gov/nchs/fastats/overwt.htm.
53. J. B. Webb et al., "Do You See What I See?: An Exploration of Inter-Ethnic Ideal Body Size Comparisons among College Women," *Body Image* 10, no. 3 (2013): 369–79.
54. Mayo Clinic Staff, "Body Dysmorphic Disorder," May 2013, www.mayoclinic.com/health/body-dysmorphic-disorder/DS00559.
55. J. D. Feusner et al., "Abnormalities of Object Visual Processing in Body Dysmorphic Disorder," *Psychological Medicine* 41, no. 11 (2011): 2385–97, DOI: 10.1017/S0033291711000572.
56. Body Image Health, "The Model for Healthy Body Image and Weight," Accessed May 2014, http://bodyimagehealth.org/model-for-healthy-body-image.
57. I. Ahmed et al., "Body Dysmorphic Disorder," Medscape Reference, Updated January 2014, http://emedicine.medscape.com/article/291182-overview.
58. Mayo Clinic Staff, "Body Dysmorphic Disorder," 2013; KidsHealth, "Body Dysmorphic Disorder," May 2013, http://kidshealth.org/parent/emotions/feelings/bdd.html.
59. I. Ahmed et al., "Body Dysmorphic Disorder," Medscape Reference, Updated January 2014, http://emedicine.medscape.com/article/291182-overview.
60. J. Reel, *Eating Disorders: An Encyclopedia of Causes, Treatment and Prevention*, Portsmouth, NH: Greenwood Publishing, 2013); A. Taheri et al., "The Relationship between Social Physique Anxiety and Anthropometric Characteristics of the Nonathletic Female Students," *Annals of Biological Research* 3, no. 6 (2012): 2727–29; A. Sicilia et al, "Exercise Motivation and Social Physique Anxiety in Adolescents," *Psychologica Belgica* 54, no. 1 (2014): 111–29, DOI: http://dx.doi.org/10.5334/pb.ai.
61. American Psychiatric Association, *Diagnostic and Statistical Manual of Mental Disorders*, 5th ed. (Washington, DC: American Psychiatric Association, 2013).
62. Academy for Eating Disorders, "Prevalence of Eating Disorders," 2014, www.aedweb.org/Prevalence_of_ED.htm.
63. American College Health Association, *National College Health Assessment II: Reference Group Executive Summary, Fall 2013* (Hanover, MD: American College Health Association, 2014), Available at www.acha-ncha.org/reports_ACHA-NCHAII.html.
64. L. M. Gottschlich, "Female Athlete Triad," Medscape Reference, Drugs, Diseases & Procedures, January 25, 2012, http://emedicine.medscape.com/article/89260-overview#a0156.
65. Alliance for Eating Disorders, What Are Eating Disorders?, 2013, www.allianceforeatingdisorders.com/portal/what-are-eating-disorders#.Uycs4_Pn9lY.
66. Ibid.
67. S. A. Swanson, et al., "Prevalence and Correlates of Eating Disorders in Adolescents: Results from the National Comorbidity Survey Replication Adolescent Supplement," *Archives of General Psychiatry* 68, no. 7 (2011): 714–23, DOI: 10.1001/archgenpsychiatry.2011.22.
68. American Psychiatric Association, *Diagnostic and Statistical Manual of Mental Disorders*, 2013.
69. National Eating Disorders Association, "Anorexia Nervosa," www.nationaleatingdisorders.org/anorexia-nervosa.
70. P. Crocker et al., "Body-Related State Shame and Guilt in Women: Do Causal Attributions Mediate the Influence of Physical Self-Concept and Shame and Guilt Proneness," *Body Image* 11, no. 1 (2013): 19–26; A. R. Smith, T. E. Joiner, and D. R. Dodd, "Examining Implicit Attitudes Toward Emaciation and Thinness in Anorexia Nervosa," *International Journal of Eating Disorders* 47, no. 2 (2013): 138–47; R. N. Carey, N. Donaghue, and P. Broderick, "Concern among Australian Adolescent Girls: The Role of Body Comparisons with Models and Peers," *Body Image* 11, no. 1 (2014): 81–84.
71. A.D.A.M. Medical Encyclopedia, U.S. National Library of Medicine, "Anorexia Nervosa," February 2013, www.ncbi.nlm.nih.gov/pubmedhealth/PMH0001401; B. Suchan et al., "Reduced Connec-

tivity between the Left Fusiform Body Area and the Extrastriate Body Area in Anorexia Nervosa Is Associated with Body Image Distortion," *Behavioural Brain Research* 241 (2013): 80–85, DOI: 10.1016/j.bbr.2012.12.002; G. Frank et al., "Altered Temporal Difference Learning in Bulimia Nervosa," *Biological Psychiatry* 70, no. 8 (2011): 728–35, DOI: 10.1016/j.biopsych.2011.05.011.

72. R. Kessler et al., "The Prevalence and Correlates of Binge Eating Disorder in the World Health Organization World Mental Health Surveys," *Biological Psychiatry* 73, no. 9 (2013): 904–14, DOI: 10.1016/j.biopsych.2012.11.020.
73. American Psychiatric Association, "DSM-5 Feeding and Eating Disorders," 2013 www.dsm5.org/documents/eating%20disorders%20fact%20sheet.pdf
74. National Institute of Mental Health, "Eating Disorders," January 2013, www.nimh.nih.gov/health/topics/eating-disorders/index.shtml.
75. T. A. Oberndorfer et al., "Altered Insula Response to Sweet Taste Processing after Recovery from Anorexia and Bulimia Nervosa," *American Journal of Psychiatry* 170, no.10 (2013): 1143–51.
76. Mayo Clinic, "Binge–Eating Disorder," April 2012, www.mayoclinic.com/health/binge-eating-disorder/DS00608.
77. R. Kessler et al., "The Prevalence and Correlates of Binge Eating Disorder in the World Health Organization World Mental Health Surveys," 2013.
78. Castlewood Treatment Center for Eating Disorders, "Binge Eating Disorder DSM-V," January 2012, www.castlewoodtc.com.
79. K. N. Franco, Cleveland Clinic Center for Continuing Education, "Eating Disorders," 2011, www.clevelandclinicmeded.com/medicalpubs/diseasemanagement/psychiatry-psychology/eating-disorders; Mirasol Eating Disorder Recovery Centers, "Eating Disorder Statistics," Accessed March 2014, www.mirasol.net/eating-disorders/information/eating-disorder-statistics.php.
80. H. Goodwin, E. Haycraft, and C. Meyer, "The Relationship between Compulsive Exercise and Emotion Regulation in Adolescents," *British Journal of Health Psychology* 17, no. 4, (2012): 699–10.
81. J. J. Waldron, "When Building Muscle Turns into Muscle Dysmorphia," *Association for Sport Applied Psychology*, Accessed March 2014, www.appliedsportpsych.org/resource-center/health-fitness-resources/when-building-muscle-turns-into-muscle-dysmorphia.
82. M. Silverman, "What Is Muscle Dysmorphia?," Massachusetts General Hospital, February 18, 2011, https://mghocd.org/what-is-muscle-dysmorphia/; J. J. Waldron, "When Building Muscle Turns into Muscle Dysmorphia," 2014.
83. L. M. Gottschlich et al., "Female Athlete Triad," *Medscape Reference*, Accessed March 2014, http://emedicine.medscape.com/article/89260-overview.

Pulled Statistic

page 206, C. D. Fryar and R. B. Ervin, "Caloric Intake from Fast Food among Adults: United States, 2007–2010," NCHS Data Brief, no. 114 (2013), www.cdc.gov

Chapter 3

1. U.S. Department of Agriculture, Economic Research Service, "U.S. Per Capita Loss-Adjusted Food Availability: Total Calories," Updated April 2010, www.ers.usda.gov/Data/FoodConsumption/app/reports/displayCommodities.aspx?reportName=Total+Calories&id=36#startForm; U.S. Department of Agriculture, Economic Research Service, "Summary Findings," *Food Availability (Per Capita) Data System*, updated August 2012, www.ers.usda.gov/data-products/food-availability-%28per-capita%29-data-system/summary-findings.aspx#.UYLNPcphris.
2. D. Grotto and E. Zied, "The Standard American Diet and Its Relationship to the Health Status of Americans," *Nutrition in Clinical Practice* 25, no. 6 (2010): 603–12, DOI: 10.1177/0884533610386234.
3. Institute of Medicine of the National Academies, Food and Nutrition Board, *Dietary Reference Intakes for Water, Potassium, Sodium, Chloride, and Sulfate* (Washington, DC: The National Academies Press, 2004), Available at http://iom.edu/Reports/2004/Dietary-Reference-Intakes-Water-Potassium-Sodium-Chloride-and-Sulfate.aspx.
4. Institute of Medicine of the National Academies, Food and Nutrition Board, *Dietary References for Water, Potassium, Sodium, Chloride, and Sulfate* (Washington, DC: The National Academies Press, 2005), Available at www.nal.usda.gov/fnic/DRI/DRI_Water/water_full_report.pdf.
5. American College of Sports Medicine (ACSM), "Selecting and Effectively Using Hydration for Fitness," 2011, Available at www.acsm.org/docs/brochures/selecting-and-effectively-using-hydration-for-fitness.pdf.
6. U.S. Department of Agriculture, Agricultural Research Service, Beltsville Human Nutrition Research Center, Food Surveys Research Group (Beltsville, MD) and U.S. Department of Health and Human Services, Centers for Disease Control and Prevention, National Center for Health Statistics (Hyattsville, MD), *What We Eat in America, NHANES 2009–2010 Data: Table 1. Nutrient Intakes from Food: Mean Amounts Consumed per Individual by Gender and Age, in the United States, 2009–2010*, www.ars.usda.gov/SP2UserFiles/Place/12355000/pdf/0910/tables_1-40_2009-2010.pdf.
7. Food and Nutrition Board, Institute of Medicine, *Dietary Reference Intakes for Energy, Carbohydrate, Fiber, Fat, Fatty Acids, Cholesterol, Protein, and Amino Acids (Macronutrients)* (Washington, DC: National Academies Press, 2005), Available at www.nap.edu/openbook.php?isbn=0309085373.
8. S. M. Phillips and L. J. C. van Loon, "Dietary Protein for Athletes: From Requirements to Optimum Adaptation," *Journal of Sports Science* 29, S1 (2011): S29–S38.
9. Institute of Medicine of the National Academies, "Dietary, Functional, and Total Fiber," in *Dietary Reference Intakes for Energy, Carbohydrate, Fiber, Fat, Fatty Acids, Cholesterol, Protein, and Amino Acids* (Washington, DC: The National Academies Press, 2005), 339–421, www.nap.edu/openbook.php?isbn=0309085373.
10. Ibid.
11. Q. Ben et al., "Dietary Fiber Intake Reduces Risk for Colorectal Adenoma: A Meta-Analysis," *Gastroenterology* 146, no. 3 (2014): 689–99.
12. K. Maki et al., "Whole-Grain Ready-to-Eat Oat Cereal, as Part of a Dietary Program for Weight Loss, Reduces Low-Density Lipoprotein Cholesterol in Adults with Overweight and Obesity More than a Dietary Program Including Low-Fiber Control Foods," *Journal of the American Dietetic Association* 110, no. 2 (2010): 205–14.
13. B. Yao et al., "Dietary Fiber Intake and Risk of Type 2 Diabetes: A Dose-Response Analysis of Prospective Studies," *European Journal of Epidemioly* 29, no. 2 (2014): 79–78, DOI: 10.1007/s10654-013-9876-x.
14. Institute of Medicine of the National Academies, "Dietary, Functional, and Total Fiber," in *Dietary Reference Intakes for Energy, Carbohydrate, Fiber, Fat, Fatty Acids, Cholesterol, Protein, and Amino Acids* (Washington, DC: The National Academies Press, 2005), 339–421, www.nap.edu/openbook.php?isbn=0309085373.
15. C. E. Ramsden et al., "Use of Dietary Linoleic Acid for Secondary Prevention of Coronary Heart Disease and Death: Evaluation of Recovered Data from the Sydney Diet Heart Study and Updated Meta-Analysis," *British Medical Journal* 346 (2013): e8707, DOI: http://dx.doi.org/10.1136/bmj.e8707; L. Gillingham, S. Harris-Janz, and P. Jones, "Dietary Monounsaturated Fatty Acids Are Protective against Metabolic Syndrome and Cardiovascular Disease Risk Factors," *Lipids* 46, no. 3 (2011): 209–28, DOI: 10.1007/s11745-010-3524-y.
16. W. Willet, "Dietary Fats and Coronary Heart Disease," *Journal of Internal Medicine* 272, no. 1 (2012): 13–24; N. Bendson et al., "Consumption of Industrial and Ruminant Trans Fatty Acids and Risk of CHD: A Systemic Review and Meta-Analysis of Cohort Studies," *European Journal of Clinical Nutrition* 65, no. 7 (2011): 773–83.
17. U.S. Food and Drug Administration, "FDA Targets Trans Fats in Processed Foods," *FDA Consumer Updates*, December 2013, www.fda.gov/ForConsumers/ConsumerUpdates/ucm372915.htm.
18. Ibid.
19. H. J. Silver et al., "Consuming a Balanced High Fat Diet for 16 Weeks Improves Body Composition, Inflammation and Vascular Function Parameters in Obese Premenopausal Women," *Metabolism* 63, no. 4 (2014): 562–73, DOI: 10.1016/j.metabol.2014.01.004; Z. Shadman, "Association of High Carbohydrate versus High Fat Diet with Glycated Hemoglobin in High Calorie Consuming Type 2 Diabetics," *Journal of Diabetes and Metabolic Disorders* 12, no. 1 (2013): 27.
20. Food and Nutrition Board, Institute of Medicine, *Dietary Reference Intakes for Energy*, 2005.
21. National Institutes of Health Office of Dietary Supplements, "Dietary Supplement Fact Sheet: Vitamin D," Reviewed June 2011, http://ods.od.nih.gov/factsheets/VitaminD-HealthProfessional.
22. U.S. Department of Agriculture, *What We Eat in America*, NHANES 2009-2010, Data: Table 1, 2010, www.ars.usda.gov/Services/docs.htm?docid=18349; C. Ayala et al., "Application of Lower Sodium Intake Recommendations to Adults—United States, 1999–2006," *Morbidity and Mortality Weekly* (*MMWR*) 58, no. 11 (2009): 281–83.
23. U.S. Department of Agriculture, *What We Eat in America*, Data: Table 1, 2010.
24. R. L. Bailey et al., "Estimation of Total Usual Calcium and Vitamin D Intakes in the United States," *Journal of Nutrition* 140, no. 4 (2010): 817–22, DOI: 10.3945/jn.109.118539.
25. Academy of Nutrition and Dietetics, "Position of the Academy of Nutrition and Dietetics: Functional Foods." *Journal of the Academy of Nutrition and Dietetics* 113, no. 8 (2013): 1096–103, DOI: 10.1016/j.jand.2013.06.002.
26. Ibid.
27. Ibid.
28. M.E. Obrenovich, et al., "Antioxidants in Health, Disease, and Aging," *CNS Neurol Disord Drug Targets* 10, no. 2 (2011):192–207; V. Ergin, R. E. Hariry, and C. Karasu, "Carbonyl Stress in Aging Process: Role of Vitamins and Phytochemicals as Redox Regulators," *Aging and Disease* 4, no. 5 (2013): 276–94, DOI: 10.14336/AD.2013.0400276.
29. Academy of Nutrition and Dietetics, "Position of the Academy of Nutrition and Dietetics: Functional Foods," 2013; G. M. Cole and S. A. Frautschy, "DHA May Reduce Age-Related

Dementia," *Journal of Nutrition* 140, no. 4 (2010): 869–74; D. Swanson, R. Block, and S. A. Mousa, "Omega-3 Fatty Acids EPA and DHA: Health Benefits Throughout Life," *Advanced Nutrition* 3, no.1 (2012): 1–7.
30. P. Hemarajata and J. Versalovic, "Effects of Probiotics on Gut Microbiota: Mechanisms of Intestinal Immunomodulation and Neuromodulation," *Therapeutic Advances in Gastroenterology* 6, no. 1 (2013): 39–51; R. Krajmalnik-Brown et al., "Effects of Gut Microbes on Nutrient Absorption and Energy Regulation," *Nutrition Clinical Practice* 27, no. 2 (2012): 201–14.
31. L. Hooper et al., "Effects of Chocolate, Cocoa, and Flavan-3-ols on Cardiovascular Health: A Systematic Review and Meta-Analysis of Randomized Trials," *American Journal of Clinical Nutrition* 95, no. 3, (2012): 740–53, DOI: 10.3945/ajcn.111.023457; D. Grassi et al., "Protective Effects of Flavanol-Rich Dark Chocolate on Endothelial Function and Wave Reflection during Acute Hyperglycemia," *Hypertension* 60, no. 3 (2012): 827–32, DOI: 10.1161/HYPERTENSIONAHA.112.193995; S. Ramos-Romero et al., "Effect of a Cocoa Flavonoid-Enriched Diet on Experimental Autoimmune Arthritis," *British Journal of Nutrition* 107, no. 4 (2012): 523–32, DOI: 10.1017/S000711451100328X.
32. U.S. Food and Drug Administration, "Nutrition Facts Label: Proposed Changes Aim to Better Inform Food Choices," February 2014, www.fda.gov/ForConsumers/ConsumerUpdates/ucm387114.htm.
33. U.S. Department of Agriculture and U.S. Department of Health and Human Services, *Dietary Guidelines for Americans, 2010,* 7th ed. (Washington, DC: U.S. Government Printing Office, 2010), www.cnpp.usda.gov/publications/dietaryguidelines/2010/policydoc/policydoc.pdf.
34. U.S. Department of Agriculture, "Empty Calories: How Do I Count the Empty Calories I Eat?," Updated June 4, 2011, www.choosemyplate.gov/foodgroups/emptycalories_count_table.html.
35. U.S. Department of Agriculture, *Eating Healthy on a Budget: The Consumer Economics Perspective,* September 2011, www.choosemyplate.gov/food-groups/downloads/ConsumerEconomicsPerspective.pdf; U.S. Department of Agriculture, *Smart Shopping for Veggies and Fruits,* Center for Nutrition Policy and Promotion, September 2011, www.choosemyplate.gov/food-groups/downloads/TenTips/DGTipsheet9SmartShopping.pdf; U.S. Centers for Disease Control and Prevention, *30 Ways in 30 Days to Stretch Your Fruit and Vegetable Budget,* Fruits and Veggies: More Matters, September 2011, www.fruitsandveggiesmatter.gov/downloads/Stretch_FV_Budget.pdf.
36. The Vegetarian Resource Group, "How Often Do Americans Eat Vegetarian Meals? And How Many Adults in the U.S. Are Vegetarian?," *Vegetarian Resource Group Blog,* May 2012, www.vrg.org/blog/2012/05/18/how-often-do-americans-eat-vegetarian-meals-and-how-many-adults-in-the-u-s-are-vegetarian.
37. C. G. Lee et al., "Vegetarianism as a Protective Factor for Colorectal Adenoma and Advanced Adenoma in Asians," *Digestive Diseases and Science* 59, no. 5 (2013): 1025–35, DOI 10.1007/s10620-013-2974-5.
38. Office of Dietary Supplements, "Frequently Asked Questions," July 2013, http://ods.od.nih.gov/Health_Information/ODS_Frequently_Asked_Questions.aspx#; V. A. Moyer, "Vitamin, Mineral, and Multivitamin Supplements for the Primary Prevention of Cardiovascular Disease and Cancer: U.S. Preventive Services Task Force Recommendation Statement," *Annals of Internal Medicine,* 2014, DOI:10.7326/M14-0198.
39. Office of Dietary Supplements, "Vitamin A Fact Sheet for Consumers," June 2013, http://ods.od.nih.gov/factsheets/VitaminA-QuickFacts/; Office of Dietary Supplements, "Vitamin E Fact Sheet for Consumers," June 2013, http://ods.od.nih.gov/factsheets/list-all/VitaminE-QuickFacts/; Office of Dietary Supplements, "Vitamin D Fact Sheet for Consumers," June 2013, http://ods.od.nih.gov/factsheets/VitaminD-QuickFacts/
40. Academy of Nutrition and Dietetics, "It's About Eating Right: Dietary Supplements," January 2013, www.eatright.org/public/content.aspx?id=7918.
41. The Organic Trade Association, "Eight in Ten U.S. Parents Report They Purchase Organic Products," April 2013, http://www.ota.com/organic-consumers/consumersurvey2013.html.
42. The Organic Trade Organization, "Consumer-Driven U.S. Organic Market Surpasses $31 Billion in 2011," 2012, www.organicnewsroom.com/2012/04/us_consumerdriven_organic_mark.html.
43. Mayo Clinic, "Organic Food: Is It More Nutritious?," September 2012, www.mayoclinic.org/healthy-living/nutrition-and-healthy-eating/in-depth/organic-food/art-20043880?pg=2.
44. K. Brandt et al., "Agroecosystem Management and Nutritional Quality of Plant Foods: The Case of Organic Fruits and Vegetables," *Critical Reviews in Plant Sciences* 30, no. 1–2 (2011): 177–97; C. Smith-Spangler et al., "Are Organic Foods Safer or Healthier Than Conventional Alternatives? A Systematic Review," *Annals of Internal Medicine* 157, no. 5 (2012): 348–66, DOI: 10.7326/0003-4819-157-5-201209040-00007.
45. U.S. Environmental Protection Agency, "Pesticides and Foods: Health Problems Pesticides May Pose," May 2012, www.epa.gov/pesticides/food/risks.htm.
46. U.S. Department of Agriculture, Pesticide Data Program: 21st Annual Summary, Calendar Year 2011, Agricultural Marketing Service, February 2013, from www.ams.usda.gov/AMSv1.0/getfile?dDocName=stelprdc5102692.
47. U.S. Food and Drug Administration, "Food Irradiation: What You Need to Know," March 2014, www.fda.gov/Food/ResourcesForYou/Consumers/ucm261680.htm.
48. U.S. Department of Agriculture, Economic Research Service, "Adoption of Genetically Engineered Crops in the U.S.," July 2013, www.ers.usda.gov/data-products/adoption-of-genetically-engineered-crops-in-the-us.aspx.
49. Center for Food Safety, "About Genetically Engineered Foods," Accessed March 2014, www.centerforfoodsafety.org/issues/311/ge-foods/about-ge-foods.
50. Union of Concerned Scientists, "Genetic Engineering Risks and Impacts," November 2013, www.ucsusa.org/food_and_agriculture/our-failing-food-system/genetic-engineering/risks-of-genetic-engineering.html.
51. L. P. Brower et al., "Decline of Monarch Butterflies Overwintering in Mexico: Is the Migratory Phenomenon at Risk?," *Insect Conservation and Diversity* 5, no. 2 (2012): 95–100.
52. Union of Concerned Scientists, "Genetic Engineering Risks and Impacts," November 2013, www.ucsusa.org/food_and_agriculture/our-failing-food-system/genetic-engineering/risks-of-genetic-engineering.html.
53. G. Pinholster, "AAAS Board of Directors: Legally Mandating GM Food Labels Could 'Mislead and Falsely Alarm Consumers,'" *AAAS News,* October 2012, www.aaas.org/news/aaas-board-directors-legally-mandating-gm-food-labels-could-mislead-and-falsely-alarm; World Health Organization, "20 Questions on Genetically Modified Foods," Accessed March 2014, www.who.int/foodsafety/publications/biotech/20questions/en.
54. National Institute of Allergy and Infectious Diseases, "Food Allergy," August 2013, www.niaid.nih.gov/topics/foodallergy/Pages/default.aspx.
55. R. S. Gupta et al., "The Prevalence, Severity, and Distribution of Childhood Food Allergy in the United States," *Journal of Pediatrics* 128, no. 1 (2011): e9–e17, DOI: 10.1542/peds.2011-0204.
56. National Institute of Allergy and Infectious Diseases, "Food Allergy," 2013.
57. U.S. Food and Drug Administration, "Food Allergies: What You Need to Know," April 2013, www.fda.gov/food/resourcesforyou/consumers/ucm079311.htm.
58. J. N. Keith et al., "The Prevalence of Self-Reported Lactose Intolerance and the Consumption of Dairy Foods among African American Adults Less than Expected," *Journal of the National Medical Association* 103 (2011): 36–45.
59. A. Rubio-Tapia et al., "The Prevalence of Celiac Disease in the United States," *American Journal of Gastroenterology* 107, no. 10 (2012): 1538–44, DOI: 10.1038/ajg.2012.219.
60. U.S. Department of Health and Human Services, "Food Safety Modernization Act (FSMA)," November 2013, www.fda.gov/Food/Guidance-Regulation/FSMA/ucm304045.htm.
61. Centers for Disease Control and Prevention, "Estimates of Food-Borne Illnesses in the United States," January 2014, www.cdc.gov/foodborne-burden/index.html.
62. Centers for Disease Control and Prevention, "Trends in Foodborne Illness in the United States, 2012," April 2013, www.cdc.gov/features/dsfood-net2012.
63. Centers for Disease Control and Prevention, Estimates of Foodborne Illness in the United States, CDC 2011 Estimates: Findings, Updated January 8, 2014, from www.cdc.gov/foodborneburden/2011-foodborne-estimates.html.
64. R. Johnson, "The U.S. Trade Situation for Fruit and Vegetable Products," *Congressional Research Service,* January 2014, Available at www.fas.org/sgp/crs/misc/RL34468.pdf.
65. S. Clark et al., "Frequency of US Emergency Department Visits for Food-Related Acute Allergic Reactions," *Journal of Allergy Clinical Immunology* 127, no. 3 (2011): 682–83, DOI: 10.1016/j.jaci.2010.10.040.

Pulled Statistics

page 59, D. King, A. Mainous, C. Lambourne, "Trends in Dietary Fiber Intake in the United States, 1999–2008," *Journal of the Academy of Nutrition and Dietetics* 112, no. 5 (2012): 642–48, DOI: 10.1016/j.jand.2012.01.019.
page 191, K. Heidal, et al., "Cost and Calorie Analysis of Fast Food Consumption in College Students," Food and Nutrition Sciences 3, no. 7 (2012): 942–46, DOI:10.4236/fns.2012.37124.

Chapter 4

1. American Psychological Association, "Stress in America: Missing the Health Care Connection," February 2013, www.apa.org/news/press/releases/

stress/2012/full-report.pdf; S. Bethune, "Health-care Falls Short on Stress Management," *Monitor on Psychology* 44, no. 4 (2013): 22.
2. American Psychological Association, "Stress in America," 2013; S. Bethune, "Health-care Falls Short on Stress Management," 2013; American Psychological Association, *Stress in America 2010, Key Findings*, 2010, www.apa.org/news/press/releases/stress/key-findings.pdf.
3. B. Vanaelst et al. "The Association between Childhood Stress and Body Composition, and the Role of Stress-Related Lifestyle Factors—Cross-Sectional Findings from the Baseline ChiBS Survey," *International Journal of Behavioral Medicine*, (2013), DOI: 10.1007/s12529-013-9294-1. (Epub ahead of print.); S. M.Wilson and A. F. Sato, "Stress and Paediatric Obesity: What We Know and Where To Go," *Stress and Health* 30, no. 2 (2014):91–102, DOI: 10.1002/smi.2501.
4. B. L. Seaward, *Managing Stress: Principles and Strategies for Health and Well-Being*, 8th ed. (Sudbury, MA: Jones & Bartlett, 2013), 8; National Institute of Mental Health (NIMH), "Stress Fact Sheet," Accessed January 2014, www.nimh.nih.gov/health/publications/stress/stress_factsheet_ln.pdf.
5. American Psychological Association, "Stress in America," 2013.
6. Ibid.
7. S. Cohen and D. Janicki-Deverts, "Who's Stressed? Distributions of Psychological Stress in the United States in Probability Samples from 1983, 2006, and 2009," *Journal of Applied Social Psychology* 42, no. 6 (2012): 1320–34, DOI: 10.1111/j.1559-1816.2012.00900.x.
8. H. Selye, *Stress without Distress* (New York: Lippincott Williams & Wilkins, 1974), 28–29.
9. W. B. Cannon, *The Wisdom of the Body* (New York: Norton, 1932).
10. M. P. Picard and D. M. Turnbull, "Linking the Metabolic State and Mitochonrial DNA in Chronic Disease, Health and Aging," *Diabetes* 62, no. 3 (2013), Available at http://diabetes.diabetesjournals.org/content/62/3/672.full; S. Cohen et al., "Chronic Stress, Glucocorticoid Receptor Resistance, Inflammation and Disease Risk," *Proceedings of the National Academy of Sciences of the United States of America* 109, no. 16 (2012): 5995–99, DOI: 10.1073/pnas.1118355109.
11. S. Taylor, *The Tending Instinct: Women, Men and the Biology of Our Relationships* (New York: Henry Holt and Company, 2002).
12. A. Crum, P. Salovey, and S. Achor, "Rethinking Stress: The Role of Mindsets in Determining the Stress Response," *Journal of Personality and Social Psychology* 104, no. 4 (2013): 716–33.
13. P. Thoits, "Stress and Health: Major Findings and Policy Implications," *Journal of Health and Social Behavior*, no. 51 (2010): 554–55, DOI: 10.1177/0022146510383499; K. M. Scott et al., "Associations between Lifetime Traumatic Events and Subsequent Chronic Physical Conditions: A Cross-National, Cross-Sectional Study," *PLoS One* 8, no. 11 (2013): DOI: 10.1371/journal.pone.0080573.
14. A. Steptoe and M. Kivimaki, "Stress and Cardiovascular Disease: An Update on Current Knowledge," *Annual Review of Public Health* 34 (2013): 337–54; E. Backe et al., "The Role of Psychosocial Stress at Work for the Development of Cardiovascular Disease: A Systematic Review," *International Archives of Occupational and Environmental Health* 85, no. 1 (2011): 67–79; A. Steptoe, A. Rosengren, and P. Hjemdahl, "Introduction to Cardiovascular Disease, Stress, and Adaptation" in *Stress and Cardiovascular Disease*, eds. A. Steptoe, A. Rosengren, and P. Hjemdahl (New York: Springer, 2012), 1–14.
15. A. Steptoe and Mike Kivimaki."Stress and Cardiovascular Disease," 2013; S. Richardson et al., "Meta-Analysis of Perceived Stress and Its Association with Incident Coronary Heart Disease," *American Journal of Cardiology* 110, no. 12 (2012): 1711–17.
16. T. Lang et al. "Social Determinants of Cardiovascular Diseases," *Public Health Reviews* 33, no. 2 (2012): 601–22; M. Kivimaki et al., "Job Strain as a Risk Factor for Coronary Heart Disease: A Collaborative Meta-Analysis of Individual Participants," *The Lancet* 380, no. 9852 (2012): 1491–97; E. Mostofsky et al., "Risk of Acute Myocardial Infarction After the Death of a Significant Person on One's Life. The Determinants of Myocardial Infarction Onset Study," *Circulation* 125, no. 3 (2012): 491–96, DOI: 10.1161/CIRCULATIONAHA.111.061770.
17. K. Scott, S. Melhorn, and R. Sakai, "Effects of Chronic Social Stress on Obesity," *Current Obesity Reports Online First*, Accessed January 12, 2012, DOI: 10.1007/s13679-011-0006-3; F. Ippoliti, N. Canitano, and R. Businare, "Stress and Obesity as Risk Factors in Cardiovascular Diseases: A Neuroimmune Perspective, *Journal of Neuroimmune Pharmacology* 8, no. 1 (2013): 212–26; S. Pagota et al., "Association of Post-Traumatic Stress Disorder and Obesity in a Nationally Representative Sample," *Obesity* 20, no. 1 (2012): 200–205.
18. N. Ribertim et al., "Corticotropin Releasing Factor-Induced Amygdala Gamma Aminobutyric Acid Release Plays a Key Role in Alcohol Dependence," *Biological Psychiatry* 67, no. 9 (2010): 831–39; E. P. Zorrilla et al., "Behavioral, Biological, and Chemical Perspectives on Targeting CRF(1) Receptor Antagonists to Treat Alcoholism," *Drug and Alcohol Dependence* 128, no. 3 (2013): 175–86.
19. Mayo Clinic, "Stress and Hair Loss: Are They Related?," January 2014, www.mayoclinic.com/health/stress-and-hair-loss/AN01442.
20. American Diabetes Association, "How Stress Affects Diabetes," 2013, www.diabetes.org/living-with-diabetes/complications/mental-health/stress.html; A. Pandy et al., "Alternative Therapies Useful in the Management of Diabetes: A Systematic Review," *Journal of Bioallied Science* 3, no. 4 (2011): 504–12.
21. National Digestive Diseases Information Clearinghouse (NDDIC), "Irritable Bowel Syndrome: How Does Stress Affect IBS?," October 2013, http://digestive.niddk.nih.gov/ddiseases/pubs/ibs/#stress.
22. H. F. Herlong, "Digestive Disorders 2013," *The Johns Hopkins White Papers* (2013) www.johnshopkinshealthalerts.com.
23. G. Marshall, ed., "Stress and Immune-Based Diseases," *Immunology and Allergy Clinics of North America* 31, no. 1 (2011): 1–148; L. Christian, "Psychoneuroimmunology in Pregnancy: Immune Pathways Linking Stress with Maternal Health, Adverse Birth Outcomes and Fetal Development," *Neuroscience and Biobehavioral Reviews* 36, no. 1 (2012): 350–61, DOI: 10.1016/j.neubiorev.2011.07.005; A. Pedersen, R. Zachariae, and D. Bovbjerb, "Influence of Psychological Stress on Upper Respiratory Infection: A Meta-Analysis of Prospective Studies," *Psychosomatic Medicine* 7 (2010): 823–32.
24. American College Health Association (ACHA), *American College Health Association–National College Health Assessment II (ACHA-NCHA II): Reference Group Data Report, Fall 2013* (Hanover, MD: American College Health Association, 2014).
25. M. Marin et al., "Chronic Stress, Cognitive Functioning and Mental Health," *Neurobiology of Learning and Memory* 96, no. 4 (2011): 583–95; R. M. Shansky and J. Lipps, "Stress-Induced Cognitive Dysfunction: Hormone-Neurotransmitter Interactions in the Prefrontal Cortex," *Neuroscience and Biobehavioral Reviews* 7 (2013): 123, Available at www.ncbi.nlm.nih.gov/pmc/articles/PMC3617365.
26. E. Dias-Ferreira et al., "Chronic Stress Causes Frontostriatal Reorganization and Affects Decision-Making," *Science* 325, no. 5940 (2009): 621–25; D. de Quervan et al., "Glucocorticoids and the Regulation of Memory in Health and Disease," *Frontiers in Neuroendocrinology* 30, no. 3 (2009): 358–70.
27. L. Johansson, "Can Stress Increase Alzheimer's Disease Risk in Women?," *Expert Review of Neurotherapeutics* 14, no. 2 (2014): 123–25, DOI: 10.1586/14737175.2014.878651.
28. T. Frodi and V. O'Keane, "How Does the Brain Deal with Cumulative Stress? A Review with Focus on Developmental Stress, HPA Axis Function and Hippocampal Structure in Humans," *Neurobiology of Disease* 52 (2013): 24–37; P. S. Nurius, E. Uehara, and D. F. Zatzick, "Intersection of Stress, Social Disadvantage, and Life Course Processes: Reframing Trauma and Mental Health," *American Journal of Psychiatric Rehabilitation* 16 (2013): 91–114; K. Scott et al., "Association of Childhood Adversities and Early-Onset Mental Disorders with Adult-Onset Chronic Physical Conditions," *Archives of General Psychiatry* 68, no. 8 (2011): 833–44.
29. National Headache Foundation, "Press Kits: Categories of Headache," 2013, www.headaches.org/press/NHF_Press_Kits/Press_Kits_-_Categories_Of_Headache
30. Mayo Clinic, "Tension Headache: Symptoms," July 2013, www.mayoclinic.org/diseases-conditions/tension-headache/basics/symptoms/con-20014295.
31. WebMD, "Migraines and Headache Health Center: Tension Headaches," 2013, www.webmd.com.
32. National Headache Foundation, "Migraine," Accessed 2014, www.headaches.org/education/Headache_Topic_Sheets/Migraine.
33. Ibid.
34. Ibid.
35. Ibid.
36. National Headache Foundation, "Cluster Headaches," 2013, www.headaches.org
37. American College Health Association, *National College Health Assessment II: Reference Group Data Report, Fall 2013*, 2014.
38. J. Gaultney, "The Prevalence of Sleep Disorders in College Students: Impact on Academic Performance," *Journal of American College Health* 59, no. 2 (2010): 91–97; K. Ahrberg et al., "Interaction between Sleep Quality and Academic Performance," *Journal of Psychiatric Research* 46, no. 12 (2012): 1618–22.
39. K. M. Orzech et al., "Sleep Patterns Are Associated with Common Illness in Adolescents," *Journal of Sleep Research* (2013), DOI: 10.1111/jsr.12096. (Epub ahead of print.); J. M. Krueger and J. A. Majde, "Sleep and Host Defense," in *Principles and Practice of Sleep Medicine*, eds. M. H. Kryger, T. Roth, and W. C. Dement (St. Louis, MO: Saunders, 2011), 261–90; M. Manzer and M. Hussein, "Sleep-Immune System Interaction: Advantages and Challenges of Human Sleep Loss Model," *Frontiers of Neurology* 3, no. 2 (2012): DOI: 10.3389/fneur.2012.00002.

40. X. Yu et al., "TH17 Cell Differentiation Is Regulated by Circadian Clock," *Science* 342, no. 6159 (2013): 727–30; T. Bollinger et al., "Sleep, Immunity and Circadian Clocks: A Mechanistic Model," *Gerontology* 56, no. 6 (2010): 574–80, DOI: 10.1159/000281827.
41. R. Lanfranchi, F. Prince, D. Filipini, and J. Carrier, "Sleep Deprivation Increases Blood Pressure in Healthy Normotensive Elderly and Attenuates the Blood Pressure Response to Orthostatic Challenges," *Sleep* 34, no. 3 (2010): 335–39; F. Cappucio, D. Cooper, and D. Lanfranco, "Sleep Duration Predicts Cardiovascular Outcomes: A Systematic Review and Meta-Analysis of Prospective Studies," *European Heart Journal* 32 (2011): 1484–92, DOI: 10.1093/eurheartj/ehr007.
42. M. A. Miller and F. P. Cappuccio, "Biomarkers of Cardiovascular Risk in Sleep Deprived People," *Journal of Human Hypertension* 27 (2013): 583–8; F. P. Cappuccio et al., "Sleep Duration Predicts Cardiovascular Outcomes,"2011; S. Agarwal, N. Bajaj, and C. Bae, "Association between Sleep Duration and Cardiovascular Disease: Results from the National Health and Nutrition Examination Survey (NHANES 2005–2008), supplement 1, *Journal of the American College of Cardiology* 59, no. 13 (2012), E1514; F. Sofi et al., "Insomnia and Risk of Cardiovascular Disease: A Meta-analysis," *European Journal of Preventive Cardiology* 21, no. 1 (2014): 51–67.
43. National Institutes of Health, "Information about Sleep," 2011, http://science.education.nih.gov/supplements/nih3/sleep/guide/info-sleep.htm; C. Peri and M. Smith, "What Lack of Sleep Does to Your Mind," WebMD, Accessed January 20, 2012, www.webmd.com/sleep-disorders/excessive-sleepiness-10/emotions-cognitive.
44. E. Fortier-Brochu et al., "Insomnia and Daytime Cognitive Performance: A Meta-Analysis," *Sleep Medicine Reviews* 16, no. 1 (2011), DOI: 10-1016/j.smrv.2011.03.008; W. Klemm, "How Sleep Helps Memory," *Psychology Today*, March 11, 2011, www.psychologytoday.com/blog/memory-medic/201103/how-sleep-helps-memory; M. A. Miller et al., "Chapter: Sleep and Cognition," in *Sleep Disorders* (2014), in press.
45. Z. Terpening et al., "The Contributors of Nocturnal Sleep to the Consolidation of Motor Skill Learning in Healthy Aging and Parkinson's Disease," *Journal of Sleep Research* 22, no. 4 (2013): 398–405; L. Genzel et al., "Complex Motor Sequence Skills Profit from Sleep," *Neuropsychobiology* 66, no. 4 (2012): 237–43, DOI: 10.1159/000341878.
46. Centers for Disease Control and Prevention, "Drowsy Driving: Asleep at the Wheel," January 2014, www.cdc.gov/features/dsdrowsydriving.
47. Centers for Disease Control and Prevention, "Insufficient Sleep Is a Public Health Epidemic," January 2014, www.cdc.gov/features/dssleep/; F. Cappuccio et al. "Sleep Duration and All-Cause Mortality: Systematic Review," *Sleep* 33, no. 5 (2010): 585–92.
48. National Sleep Foundation, "Caffeine and Sleep," 2011, Accessed February, 2014, www.sleepfoundation.org/article/sleep-topics/caffeine-and-sleep.
49. R. Lazarus, "The Trivialization of Distress," in *Preventing Health Risk Behaviors and Promoting Coping with Illness*, eds. J. Rosen and L. Solomon (Hanover, NH: University Press of New England, 1985), 279–98.
50. D. Hellhammer, A. Stone, J. Hellhammer, and J. Broderick, "Measuring Stress," *Encyclopedia of Behavioral Neurosciences* 2 (2010): 186–91.
51. L. D. Rosen et al., "Is Facebook Creating "iDisorders"? The Link between Clinical Symptoms of Psychiatric Disorders and Technology Use, Attitudes and Anxiety," *Computers in Human Behavior* 29, no. 3 (2013): 1243–54, Available at http://dx.doi.org/10.1016/j.chb.2012.11.012.
52. NIH Medline Plus, "Avid Cellphone Use by College Kids Tied to Anxiety, Lower Grades," December 2013, www.nlm.nih.gov/;medlineplus/news/fullstory_143389.html; S. Deatherage et al., "Stress, Coping and the Internet Use of College Students," *Journal of American Health* 62, no. 1 (2014): 40–46, DOI: 10.1080/07448481.2013.843536.
53. S. Schwartz et al., "Acculturation and Well-Being among College Students from Immigrant Families," *Journal of Clinical Psychology* (2012), DOI: 10.1002/jclp21847. (Epub ahead of print.); A. Pieterse, R. Carter, S. Evans, and R. Walter, "An Exploratory Examination of the Associations among Racial and Ethnic Discrimination, Racial Climate, and Trauma-Related Symptoms in a College Student Population," *Journal of Counseling Psychology* 57, no. 3 (2010): 255–63; A. McAleavey, L. Castonguay, and B. Locke, "Sexual Orientation Minorities in College Counseling: Prevalence, Distress, and Symptom Profiles," *Journal of College Counseling* 14, no. 2 (2011): 127–42.
54. K. Cokley et al., "An Examination of the Impact of Minority Status Stress and Imposter Feelings on the Mental Health of Diverse Ethnic Minority College Students," *Journal of Multicultural Counseling and Development* 41, no. 2 (2013): 82–95; D. Iwamoto, L. Kenji, and W. Ming, "The Impact of Racial Identity, Ethnic Identity, Asian Values and Race-Related Stress on Asian Americans and Asian International College Students' Psychological Well-Being," *Journal of Counseling Psychology* 57, no. 1 (2010): 79–91.
55. E. Brondolo et al. "Racism and Hypertension: A Review of the Empirical Evidence and Implications for Clinical Practice," *American Journal of Hypertension* 24, no. 5 (2011): 518–24; F. Fuchs, "Editorial: Why Do Black Americans Have Higher Prevalence of Hypertension?," *Hypertension* 57 (2011): 370–80.
56. P. Hoffman, *Examining Factors of Acculturative Stress on International Students as They Affect Utilization of Campus-Based Health and Counseling Services at Four-Year Public Universities in Ohio*, Doctoral Dissertation, Bowling Green State University, Higher Education Administration, 2010; S. Sumer, *International Students' Psychological and Sociocultural Adaptation in the United States*, Doctoral Dissertation, Georgia State University, 2009.
57. K. Karren et al., *Mind/Body Health: The Effects of Attitudes, Emotions, and Relationships*, 4th ed. (San Francisco: Benjamin Cummings, 2010).
58. B. L. Seaward, *Managing Stress*, 2012.
59. K. Brown, *Predictors of Suicide Ideation and the Moderating Effects of Suicide Attitudes*, masters thesis, University of Ohio, 2011, http://etd.ohiolink.edu/view.cgi?acc_num=tolego1301765761; J. Gomez, R. Miranda, and L. Polanco, "Acculturative Stress, Perceived Discrimination and Vulnerability to Suicide Attempts among Emerging Adults," *Journal of Youth and Adolescence* 40, no. 11 (2011): 1465–76.
60. K. Glanz, B. Rimer, and F. Levis, eds., *Health Behavior and Health Education: Theory, Research, and Practice*, 4th ed. (San Francisco: Jossey-Bass, 2008).
61. S. Abraham, "Relationship between Stress and Perceived Self-Efficacy among Nurses in India," *International Conference on Technology and Business Management*, March 2012, www.icmis.net/ictbm/ictbm12/ICTBM12CD/pdf/D2144-done.pdf; B. L. Seaward, *Managing Stress: Principles and Strategies for Health and Well-Being*, 2012.
62. M. Friedman and R. H. Rosenman, *Type A Behavior and Your Heart* (New York: Knopf, 1974).
63. M. Whooley and J. Wong, "Hostility and Cardiovascular Disease," *Journal of the American College of Cardiology* 58, no. 12 (2011): 1228–30; J. Newman et al. "Observed Hostility and the Risk of Incident Ischemic Heart Disease: A Perspective Population Study from the 1995 Canadian Nova Scotia Health Survey," *Journal of the American College of Cardiology* 58, no. 12 (2011): 1222–28.
64. G. Mate, *When the Body Says No: Understanding the Stress-Disease Connection*, (Hoboken, NJ: John Wiley & Sons, 2011).
65. H. Versteeg, V. Spek, and S. Pedersen, "Type D Personality and Health Status in Cardiovascular Disease Populations: A Meta-Analysis of Prospective Studies," *European Journal of Cardiovascular Prevention and Rehabilitation* (2011), DOI: 10.1177/1741826711425338. (Epub ahead of print.); F. Mols and F. J. Denollet, "Type D Personality in the General Population: A Systematic Review of Health Status, Mechanisms of Disease and Work-Related Problems," *Health and Quality of Life Outcomes* 8, no. 9 (2010): 1–10, Available at www.hqlo.com/content/8/1/9
66. S. Kobasa, "Stressful Life Events, Personality, and Health: An Inquiry into Hardiness," *Journal of Personality and Social Psychology* 37 (1979): 1–11.
67. C. D. Schetter and C. Dolbier, "Resilience in the Context of Chronic Stress and Health in Adults," *Social and Personality Psychology Compass* 5 (2011): 634–52, DOI: 10.1111/j.1751-9004.2011.00379.x.
68. C. Ryff et al., "Psychological Resilience in Adulthood and Later Life: Implications for Health," *Annual Review of Gerontology and Geriatrics* 32, no. 1 (2012): 73–92.
69. E. Chen et al., "Protective Factors for Adults from Low-Childhood Socioeconomic Circumstances: The Benefits of Shift-and-Persist for Allostatic Load," *Psychosomatic Medicine* 74, no. 2 (2012): 178–86, DOI:10.1097/PSY. 0B013e31824206fd.
70. B. L. Seaward, *Managing Stress*," 2012.
71. M. E. P. Seligman, *Flourishing: A Visionary New Understanding of Happiness and Well-Being* (New York: Free Press/Simon and Schuster, 2011); M. E. P. Seligman, *Authentic Happiness: Using the New Positive Psychology to Realize Your Potential for Lasting Fulfillment* (New York: Free Press/Simon and Schuster, 2002).
72. L. Poole et al., "Associations of Objectively Measured Physical Activity with Daily Mood Ratings and Psychophysiological Stress Responses in Women," *Psychophysiology* 48 (2011): 1165–72, DOI: 10.1111/j.1469-8986.2011.01184.x; D. A. Girdano, D. E. Dusek, and G. S. Everly, *Controlling Stress and Tension*, 9th ed. (San Francisco: Benjamin Cummings, 2012), 375.
73. G. Colom et al., "Study of the Effect of Positive Humour as a Variable That Reduces Stress. Relationship of Humour with Personality and Performance Variables," *Psychology in Spain* 15, no. 1 (2011): 9–21.
74. B. L. Seaward, *Managing Stress*, 2012.
75. C. Stern et al. "Effects of Implementation Intention on Anxiety, Perceived Proximity and Motor Performance," *Personality and Social Psychology Bulletin* 39, no. 5 (2013): 623–35; M. A. Adriaanse et al., "Breaking Habits with Implementation Intentions: A Test of Underlying Processes," *Personality and Social Psychology Bulletin* 37, no. 4 (2011): 502–13; A. Dalton and S. Spiller, "Too Much of a Good Thing: The Benefits of Imple-

mentation Intentions Depend on the Number of Specific Goals," *Journal of Consumer Research* 39, no. 3 (2012): 600–614.
76. American College Health Association (ACHA), *National College Health Assessment II: Reference Group Data Report, Fall 2013*, 2014.
77. *Yoga Journal*, "Yoga in America," Accessed February 2014, www.yogajournal.com/press/yoga_in_america?print=1.
78. NIH Medline Plus, "What Yoga Can and Can't Do for You," December 2013, www.nlm.nih.gov/medlineplus/news/fullstory_143813.html; J. Kiecolt-Glaser et al., "Stress, Inflammation, and Yoga Practice," *Psychosomatic Medicine* 72, no. 2 (2010): 113–21.
79. V. Barnes and D. Orme-Johnson, "Prevention and Treatment of Cardiovascular Disease in Adolescents through the Transcendental Meditation Program," *Current Hypertension Reviews* 8, no. 3 (2012): 1573–1621.

Pulled Statistics

page 82, American College Health Association (ACHA), *American College Health Association–National College Health Assessment II (ACHA-NCHA II): Reference Group Data Report, Fall 2013* (Hanover, MD: American College Health Association, 2014).

page 87, American Psychological Association, "Stress in America: Missing the Health Care Connection," February 2013, Available at: http://www.apa.org/news/press/releases/stress/2012/full-report.pdf.

page 89, National Sleep Foundation, "2011 Sleep in America Poll: Communications Technology and Sleep," March 2011. Available at: http://www.sleepfoundation.org/article/sleep-america-polls/2011-communications-technology-use-and-sleep.

Chapter 5

1. A. S. Go et al., "Heart Disease and Stroke Statistics—2014 Update: A Report from the American Heart Association," *Circulation* (2014) 129:e28-e292.
2. The International Diabetes Federation, *Diabetes Atlas*, 6th ed. 2014, Available at www.idf.org/diabetesatlas.
3. American Diabetes Association, "Fast Facts: Data and Statistics about Diabetes," March 2013, http://professional.diabetes.org/admin/UserFiles/0%20-%20Sean/FastFacts%20March%202013.pdf.
4. American Cancer Society, "Cancer Facts and Figures," Accessed May 2014, Available at www.cancer.org/research/cancerfactsstatistics/cancerfactsfigures2014/index.
5. American Cancer Society, "Cancer Facts and Figures," 2014.
6. A .S. Go et al., "Heart Disease and Stroke Statistics—2014 Update, 2014.
7. Ibid.
8. Ibid.
9. Ibid.
10. Ibid.
11. Ibid.
12. Ibid.
13. Ibid.
14. Ibid.
15. Ibid.
16. Ibid.
17. Ibid.
18. Ibid.
19. Ibid.
20. World Health Organization, "Cardiovascular Diseases (CVDs)—Key Facts," Accessed April 2014, www.who.int/mediacentre/factsheets/fs317/en/#.
21. Ibid.
22. A. S. Go et al., "Heart Disease and Stroke Statistics—2014 Update," 2014.
23. Centers for Disease Control and Prevention, Media Relations, *MMWR–Morbidity and Mortality Weekly Report*, News Synopsis for April 4, 2013, April 2013, www.cdc.gov/media/mmwrnews/2013/0404.html.
24. A. S. Go et al., "Heart Disease and Stroke Statistics—2014 Update," 2014.
25. Centers for Disease Control and Prevention, "High Blood Pressure Facts," March 2014, www.cdc.gov/bloodpressure/facts.htm.
26. A. S. Go et al., "Heart Disease and Stroke Statistics—2014 Update," 2014.
27. American Heart Association, "Peripheral Artery Disease: Undertreated and Understudied in Women," 2012, http://newsroom.heart.org/pr/aha/peripheral-artery-disease-undertreated-228645.aspx; A. S. Go et al., "Heart Disease and Stroke Statistics—2014 Update," 2014.
28. American Heart Association, "Peripheral Artery Disease: Undertreated and Understudied in Women," 2012, http://newsroom.heart.org/pr/aha/peripheral-artery-disease-undertreated-228645.aspx.
29. A.S. Go et al., "Heart Disease and Stroke Statistics—2014 Update," 2014.
30. Ibid.
31. Ibid.
32. B. M. Kissela et al., "Age at Stroke: Temporal Trends in Stroke Incidence in a Large, Biracial Population," *Neurology* 79, no. 17 (2012): 1781–87.
33. A. S. Go et al., "Heart Disease and Stroke Statistics—2014 Update," 2014.
34. Ibid.
35. Ibid.
36. Ibid.
37. Ibid.
38. Ibid.
39. C. J. L Murray et al., "The State of US Health, 1990–2010 Burden of Diseases, Injuries, and Risk Factors," *Journal of the American Medical Association* 310, no. 6 (2013): 591–608.
40. S. Gardener et al., "Dietary Patterns Associated with Alzheimer's Disease and Related Chronic Disease Risk: A Review," *Journal of Alzheimer's Disease and Parkinsonism* S10 (2013): 2161–460; S. Sharp et al., "Hypertension Is a Potential Risk Factor for Vascular Dementia: Systematic Review," *International Journal of Geriatric Psychiatry* 26, no. 7 (2011): 661–69; F. Testai and P. Gorelick, "Vascular Cognitive Impairment and Alzheimer's Disease: Are These Disorders Linked to Hypertension and Other Cardiovascular Risk Factors?," *Clinical Hypertension and Vascular Diseases*, Part 4 (2011): 195–210.
41. A. S. Go et al., "Heart Disease and Stroke Statistics—2014 Update," 2014.
42. S. Grundy et al., "Definition of Metabolic Syndrome. Report of the National Heart, Lung, and Blood Institute/American Heart Association Conference on Scientific Issues Related to Definition," *Circulation* 109, no. 2 (2011): 433–39.
43. A. S. Go et al., "Heart Disease and Stroke Statistics—2014 Update," 2014.
44. Ibid.
45. Ibid.
46. Ibid.
47. National Cancer Institute, "Fact Sheet: Harms of Smoking and Benefits of Quitting," January 2011, www.cancer.gov/cancertopics/factsheet/tobacco/cessation.
48. R. Chowdhury et al., "Association of Dietary, Circulating, and Supplement Fatty Acids with Coronary Risk: A Systematic Review and Meta-Analysis," *Annals of Internal Medicine* 160, no. 6 (2014): 398–406.
49. G. Schwarts et al., "Effects of Dalcetrapib in Patients with a Recent Acute Coronary Syndrome," *New England Journal of Medicine* 367, no. 22 (2012): 2089–2099; C. Zheng and M. Aikawa, "High Density Lipoproteins: From Function to Therapy," *American College of Cardiology* 60, no. 23 (2012): 2380–83.
50. K. M. Moon et al., "Lipoprotein-Associated Phospholipase A2 Is Associated with Atherosclerotic Stroke Risk: The Northern Manhattan Study," *PLoS ONE* 9, no. 1 (2014): e83393, DOI:10.1371/journal.pone.0083393; C. A. Garza et al., "The Association between Lipoprotein-Associated Phospholipse A2 and Cardiovascular Disease: A Systematic Review," *Mayo Clinic Proceedings* 82, no. 2 (2007): 159–65.
51. B. M. Sondermeijer et al., "Non-HDL Cholesterol vs. Apo B for Risk of Coronary Heart Disease in Healthy Individuals: The EPIC-Norfolk Prospective Population Study," *European Journal of Clinical Investigation* 43, no. 10 (2013): 1009–1015.
52. A. S. Go et al., "Heart Disease and Stroke Statistics—2014 Update," 2014.
53. Z. Wang et al., "Black and Green Tea Consumption and the Risk of Coronary Artery Disease: A Meta Analysis," *American Journal of Clinical Nutrition* 93, no. 3 (2011): 506–15; L. Hooper et al., "Effects of Chocolate, Cocoa, and Flavan-3-ols on Cardiovascular Health: A Systematic Review and Meta-analysis of Randomized Trials," *American Journal of Clinical Nutrition* 95, no. 3 (2012): 740–51.
54. Mayo Clinic, "Top 5 Lifestyle Changes to Reduce Cholesterol," September 2012, www.mayoclinic.org/diseases-conditions/high-blood-cholesterol/in-depth/reduce-cholesterol/art-20045935.
55. A. S. Go et al., "Heart Disease and Stroke Statistics—2014 Update,"2014.
56. Ibid.
57. A. Steptoe and M. Kivimaki, "Stress and Cardiovascular Disease: An Update on Current Knowledge," *Annual Review of Public Health* 34 (2013): 337–54; R. C. Thurston, M. Rewak, and L. D. Kubzansky, "An Anxious Heart: Anxiety and the Onset of Cardiovascular Diseases," *Progress in Cardiovascular Diseases* 55, no. 6: 524–37.
58. A. S. Go et al., "Heart Disease and Stroke Statistics—2014 Update," 2014.
59. American Heart Association, "Understand Your Risk of Heart Attack," October 2012, www.heart.org/HEARTORG/Conditions/HeartAttack/UnderstandYourRiskofHeartAttack/Understand-Your-Risk-of-Heart-Attack_UCM_002040_Article.jsp.
60. Ibid.
61. The Emerging Risk Factors Collaboration, "C-Reactive Protein, Fibrinogen and CVD Prediction," *New England Journal of Medicine* 367, no. 14 (2012): 1310–20.
62. D. Wald, J. Morris, and N. Wald, "Reconciling the Evidence on Serum Homocysteine and Ischemic Heart Disease: A Meta-Analysis," *PLoS ONE* 6, no. 2 (2011): e16473; J. Abraham and L. Cho, "The Homocysteine Hypothesis: Still Relevant to the Prevention and Treatment of Cardiovascular Disease?," *Cleveland Clinic Journal of Medicine* 77, no. 12 (2010): 911–18.
63. American Heart Association, "Homocysteine, Folic Acid, and Cardiovascular Disease,"

January 2012, www.heart.org/HEARTORG/GettingHealthy/NutritionCenter/Homocysteine-Folic-Acid-and-Cardiovascular-Disease_UCM_305997_article.jsptsite.com/html/stent.html.
64. Heartsite, "Coronary Stents," Available at http://www.heartsite.com/html/stent.html.
65. C. M. Rembold, "Review: Aspirin Does Not Reduce CHD or Cancer Mortality But Increases Bleeding," *Annals of Internal Medicine* 156, no. 12 (2012): JC6–3; C. Ling et al., "Aspirin to Prevent Incident Cardiovascular Disease: Is It Causing More Damage Than It Prevents?," *Clinical Practice* 9, no. 3 (2012): 223–25.
66. American Heart Association, "Prevention and Treatment of Heart Attack," January 2013, www.heart.org/HEARTORG/Conditions/HeartAttack/PreventionTreatmentofHeartAttack/Prevention-and-Treatment-of-Heart-Attack_UCM_002042_Article.jsp .
67. A. S. Go et al., "Heart Disease and Stroke Statistics—2014 Update," 2014.
68. American Cancer Society, "Cancer Facts and Figures 2014," 2014, www.cancer.org/research/cancerfactsstatistics/cancerfactsfigures2014/index.
69. Ibid.
70. Ibid.
71. Ibid.
72. U.S. Surgeon General, "The Health Consequences of Smoking—50 Years of Progress: A Report of the Surgeon General, 2014," 2014, www.surgeongeneral.gov/library/reports/50-years-of-progress/index.html.
73. Ibid; American Cancer Society, "Cancer Facts and Figures 2014," 2014, www.cancer.org/research/cancerfactsstatistics/cancerfactsfigures2014/index; Centers for Disease Control and Prevention, "Tobacco Use: Targeting the Nation's Leading Killer—At-a-Glance 2011," Accessed May 2014, www.cdc.gov/chronicdisease/resources/publications/aag/pdf/2011/tobacco_aag_2011_508.pdf.
74. American Cancer Society, "Cancer Facts and Figures 2014," 2014.
75. W. Chen et al., "Moderate Alcohol Consumption During the Adult Life, Drinking Patterns and Breast Cancer Risk," *Journal of the American Medical Association* 306, no. 17 (2011): 1884–90; S.Y. Park et al., "Alcohol Consumption and Breast Cancer Risk among Women from Five Ethnic Groups with Light to Moderate Intake: The Multiethnic Cohort Study," *International Journal of Cancer* 134, no. 6 (2014): 1504–10.
76. American Cancer Society, "Cancer Facts and Figures 2014," 2014; D. Parkin, "Cancers Attributable to Consumption of Alcohol in the UK in 2010," *British Journal of Cancer* 105 (2011): S14–S18, DOI:10:10.1038/bjc.2011.476; National Cancer Institute, "Alcohol and Cancer Risk Sheet," Accessed May 2014, www.cancer.gov/cancertopics/factsheet/Risk/alcohol; I. Tramacere et al., "A Meta-Analysis on Alcohol Drinking and Gastric Cancer Risk," *Annals of Oncology* 23, no. 1 (2012): 28–36; S. Gupta et al., "Risk of Pancreatic Cancer by Alcohol Dose, Duration, and Pattern of Consumption, Including Binge Drinking: A Population-Based Study," *Cancer Causes & Control* 21, no. 7 (2010): 1047–59.
77. M. Jin et al., "Alcohol Drinking and All Cancer Mortality: A Meta-analysis," *Annals of Oncology* 24, no. 3 (2013): 807–16.
78. American Cancer Society, "Cancer Facts and Figures 2014," 2014.
79. C. Eheman et al., "Annual Report to the Nation on the Status of Cancer, 1975–2008, Featuring Cancers Associated with Excess Weight and Lack of Sufficient Physical Activity," *Cancer* 118, no. 9 (2012): 2338–66, DOI: 10.1002/cncr.27514/full; American Cancer Society, "Cancer Facts and Figures 2014," 2014.
80. H. R. Harris et al., "Body Fat Distribution and Risk of Premenopausal Breast Cancer in the Nurses' Health Study II," Journal of the National Cancer Institute 103, no. 3 (2011): 373–78.
81. American Cancer Society, "The Obesity-Cancer Connection and What We Can Do About it," February 2013, www.cancer.org/cancer/news/expertvoices/post/2013/02/28/the-obesity-cancer-connection-and-what-we-can-do-about-it.aspx; C. Eheman et al., "Annual Report to the Nation on the Status of Cancer, 1975–2008, Featuring Cancers Associated with Excess Weight and Lack of Sufficient Physical Activity," *Cancer* 118, no. 9 (2012): 2338–66, DOI: 10.1002/cncr.27514/full.
82. American Cancer Society, Cancer Facts and Figures 2014, 2014.
83. American Cancer Society, "Breast Cancer Overview: What Causes Breast Cancer?" January 2014, www.cancer.org/Cancer/BreastCancer/DetailedGuide/breast-cancer-what-causes.
84. American Cancer Society, "Cancer Facts and Figures for Hispanic/Latinos, 2012–2014," 2014, Available at www.cancer.org/acs/groups/content/@epidemiologysurveilance/documents/document/acspc-034778.pdf; M. Banegas et al., "The Risk of Developing Invasive Breast Cancer in Hispanic Women," *Cancer* 119, no. 7 (2013): 1373–80.
85. American Cancer Society, "Menopausal Hormone Therapy and Cancer Risk," 2013, www.cancer.org/Cancer/CancerCauses/OtherCarcinogens/MedicalTreatments/menopausal-hormone-replacement-therapy-and-cancer-risk; J. Manson et al., "Menopausal Hormone Therapy and Health Outcomes During the Intervention and Extended Poststopping Phases of the Women's Health Initiative Randomized Trials," *JAMA* 310, no. 13 (2013): 1353–68; A. Pesatori et al., "Reproductive and Hormonal Factors and Risk of Lung Cancer: The EAGLE Study," *International Journal of Cancer* 132, no. 11 (2013): 2630–39.
86. Y. Guo et al., "Association between C-reactive Protein and Risk of Cancer: A Meta-Analysis of Prospective Cohort Studies," *Asian Pacific Journal of Cancer Prevention* 14 (2013), DOI: http://dx.doi.org/10.7314/APJCP.2013.14.1.243.
87. S. Grivennikov, F. Gretan, and M. Karin, "Immunity, Inflammation, and Cancer," *Cell* 140, no. 6 (2010): 883–99, DOI: 10.1016/j.cell.2010.01.025.
88. American Cancer Society, "Infectious Agents and Cancer," March 2014, www.cancer.org/Cancer/CancerCauses/OtherCarcinogens/InfectiousAgents/InfectiousAgentsandCancer/infectious-agents-and-cancer-intro.
89. American Cancer Society, "Expert Voices: Viruses, Bacteria and Cancer, or It's Not All Smoke and Sunlight," March 2012, www.cancer.org/cancer/news/expertvoices/post/2012/03/04/viruses-bacteria-and-cancer-or-ite28099s-not-all-smoke-and-sunlight.aspx; American Cancer Society, "Cancer Facts and Figures," 2014.
90. Centers for Disease Control and Prevention, "Human Papillomavirus Vaccination Coverage among Adolescent Girls, 2007-2012, and Postlicensure Vaccine Safety Monitoring, 2006-2013--United States," July 2013, www.cdc.gov/mmwr/preview/mmwrhtml/mm6229a4.htm; American Cancer Society, "Cancer Facts and Figures," 2014; National Cancer Institute, "Fact Sheet–HPV and Cancer," 2012, www.cancer.gov/cancertopics/factsheet/Risk/HPV.
91. American Cancer Society, "Cancer Facts and Figures," 2014.
92. American Cancer Society, "Infectious Agents and Cancer," Accessed May 2014, www.cancer.org/cancer/cancercauses/othercarcinogens/infectiousagents/infectiousagentsandcancer/infectious-agents-and-cancer-toc.
93. American Cancer Society, "Cancer Facts and Figures," 2014.
94. Ibid.
95. American Cancer Society, "Why Lung Cancer Strikes Nonsmokers," October 2013, www.cancer.org/cancer/news/why-lung-cancer-strikes-nonsmokers.
96. American Cancer Society, "Cancer Facts and Figures," Accessed May 2014, Available at http://www.cancer.org/research/cancerfactsstatistics/cancerfactsfigures2014/index.
97. Centers for Disease Control and Prevention, "Smoking and Tobacco Use: Quitting Smoking," February 2014, www.cdc.gov/tobacco/data_statistics/fact_sheets/cessation/quitting/index.htm?utm_source=feedburner&utm_medium=feed&utm_campaign=Feed%3A+CdcSmokingAndTobaccoUseFactSheets+(CDC+-+Smoking+and+Tobacco+Use+-+Fact+Sheets).
98. American Cancer Society, "Colorectal Cancer Facts and Figures, 2014–2016," Accessed May 2014, Available at www.cancer.org/acs/groups/content/documents/document/acspc-042280.pdf; American Cancer Society, "Cancer Facts and Figures," 2014.
99. American Cancer Society, "Cancer Facts and Figures 2014," 2014.
100. Ibid.
101. American Cancer Society, "Colorectal Cancer Facts and Figures, 2014-2016," 2014, www.cancer.org/acs/groups/content/documents/document/acspc-042280.pdf.
102. Ibid; American Cancer Society, "Cancer Facts and Figures 2014," 2014.
103. American Cancer Society, "Colorectal Cancer Facts and Figures, 2014-2016," 2014, www.cancer.org/acs/groups/content/documents/document/acspc-042280.pdf.
104 S. London. "Colorectal Cancer Incidence rises sharply in younger adults." Oncology Practice. January. 2014. http://www.oncologypractice.com/single-view/colorectal-cancer-incidence-rising-sharply-among-younger-adults/a00ffbf510248b815e386d354d058b4b.html.
105. American Cancer Society, "Colorectal Cancer Facts and Figures, 2014-2016," 2014; American Cancer Society, "Cancer Facts and Figures 2014," 2014.
106. Ibid.
107. American Cancer Society, "Cancer Facts and Figures," 2014.
108. American Cancer Society, "Magnetic Resonance Imaging," January 2014, www.cancer.org/cancer/breastcancer/moreinformation/breastcancerearlydetection/breast-cancer-early-detection-a-c-s-recs-m-r-i.
109. American Cancer Society, "Cancer Facts and Figures," 2014.
110. Ibid.
111. Ibid.
112. Ibid.
113. Breast Cancer.org, "Genetics," April 2014, www.breastcancer.org/risk/factors/genetics.
114. Y. Wu, D. Zhang, and S. Kang, "Physical Activity and Risk of Breast Cancer: A Meta-Analysis of Prospective Studies," *Breast Cancer Research and Treatment* 137, no. 3 (2013): 869–82.

115. J. Dong et al., "Dietary Fiber Intake and Risk of Breast Cancer: A Meta-Analysis of Prospective Cohort Studies," *American Journal of Clinical Nutrition* 94, no. 3 (2011): 900–905; D. Aune et al. "Dietary Fiber and Breast Cancer Risks: A Systematic Review and Meta Analysis of Prospective Studies," *Annals of Oncology*, 2012: DOI:10.1093/annuls/mdr589.
116. American Cancer Society, "Cancer Facts and Figures 2014," 2014.
117. Ibid.
118. Ibid.
119. C. Heckman et al., "Psychiatric and Addictive Symptoms of Young Adult Female Indoor Tanners," *American Journal of Health Promotion* 28, no. 3 (2014): 168–74; C. Harrington et al., "Activation of the Mesostriatal Reward Pathway with Exposure to Ultraviolet Radiation (UVR) vs. Sham UVR in Frequent Tanners: A Pilot Study," *Addictive Biology* 17, no. 3 (2012): 680–86.
120. NCSL, "Indoor Tanning Restrictions for Minors—A State-by-State Comparison," May 2014, www.ncsl.org/research/health/indoor-tanning-restrictions.aspx; American College of Dermatology, "The Dangers of Indoor Tanning Beds," 2014, www.aad.org/spot-skin-cancer/understanding-skin-cancer/dangers-of-indoor-tanning; D. Lazovich et al., "Indoor Tanning and Risk of Melanoma: A Case-Control Study in a Highly Exposed Population," *Cancer Epidemiology Biomarkers and Prevention* 19, no. 6 (2010): 1557–68, DOI:10.1158/1055-9965.EPI-09-1249; National Cancer Institute, "Tanning Bed Study Shows Strongest Evidence Yet of Increased Melanoma Risk," *NCI Cancer Bulletin*, 2010, www.cancer.gov/ncicancerbulletin/060110/page2; Skin Cancer Foundation, "Skin Cancer Facts," 2012, www.skincancer.org/skin-cancer-information/skin-cancer-facts.
121. American Cancer Society, "Cancer Facts and Figures," 2014.
122. Ibid.
123. Ibid.
124. Ibid.
125. K. Zu et al. "Dietary Lycopene, Angiogenesis, and Prostate Cancer: A Prospective Study in the Prostate-Specific Antigen Era," *Journal of the National Cancer Institute* 106, no. 2 (2014): 1093–97.
126. American Cancer Society, "Cancer Facts and Figures 2014," 2014.
127. American Cancer Society, "Cancer Facts and Figures 2014," 2014.
128. Ibid.
129. American Cancer Society, "Testicular Cancer," February 2014, www.cancer.org/cancer/testicularcancer/detailedguide/testicular-cancer-risk-factors; National Cancer Institute, "General Information about Testicular Cancer," December 2013, www.cancer.gov/cancertopics/pdq/treatment/testicular/Patient/page1#Keypoint2.
130. American Cancer Society, "Cancer Facts and Figures 2014," 2014.
131. Ibid.
132. Ibid.
133. Ibid.
134. Ibid.
135. Ibid.
136. National Cancer Institute, "Endometrial Cancer," 2012, www.cancer.gov/cancertopics/types/endometrial.
137. American Cancer Society, "Cancer Facts and Figures 2014," 2014.
138. Ibid.
139. The International Diabetes Federation, *Diabetes Atlas*, 6th ed., 2014.
140. Ibid.
141. E. Selvin et al., "Trends in Prevalence and Control of Diabetes in the United States, 1988–1994 and 1999–2010," *Annals of Internal Medicine* 160, no. 8 (2014): 517–25.
142. Ibid.
143. American Diabetes Association, "Fast Facts: Data and Statistics about Diabetes," 2013.
144. Centers for Disease Control and Prevention, "Summary Health Statistics for U.S. Adults: National Health Interview Survey, 2012," *Vital and Health Statistics* 10, no. 260 (2014), Available at www.cdc.gov/nchs/products/series/series10.htm.
145. American Diabetes Association, "Fast Facts: Data and Statistics about Diabetes," 2013.
146. Ibid.
147. American Diabetes Association, "Diabetes Basics: Type 1," Accessed May 2014, www.diabetes.org/diabetes-basics/type-1.
148. Ibid.
149. The National Diabetes Information Clearinghouse (NDIC), "National Diabetes Statistics: 2011," September 2013, http://diabetes.niddk.nih.gov/dm/pubs/statistics/#fast.
150. Centers for Disease Control and Prevention, "National Diabetes Fact Sheet: 2011," January 2014, www.cdc.gov/diabetes/pubs/factsheet11.htm.
151. D. Dabelea et al., "Is Prevalence of Type 2 Diabetes Increasing in Youth? The SEARCH for Diabetes in Youth Study," American Diabetes Association 72nd Scientific Sessions (Philadelphia, PA: June 8–12, 2012).
152. D. J. Pettitt et al., "Prevalence of Diabetes in U.S. Youth in 2009: The Search for Diabetes in Youth Study," *Diabetes Care* 37, no. 2 (2014): 402–408.
153. Ibid.
154. A. M. Kanaya et al., "Understanding the High Prevalence of Diabetes in U.S. South Asians Compared with Four Racial/Ethnic Groups: The MASALA and MESA Studies," *Diabetes Care* (2014), DOI:10.2337/dc13-2656; American Heart Association, "Statistical Fact Sheet, 2013 Update: Diabetes," 2013, Available at www.heart.org/idc/groups/heart-public/@wcm/@sop/@smd/documents/downloadable/ucm_319585.pdf.
155. R. Mihaescu et al., "Genetic Risk Profiling for Prediction of Type 2 Diabetes," *PLoS Currents* 3 (2011): DOI: 10.1371/currents.RRN1208; E. Ntzani, K. Evangelia, and F. Kavvoura, "Genetic Risk Factors for Type 2 Diabetes: Insights from the Emerging Genomic Evidence," *Current Vascular Pharmacology* 10, no. 2 (2012): 147–55.
156. J. Logue et al., "Association between BMI Measured within a Year After Diagnosis of Type 2 Diabetes and Mortality," *Diabetes Care* 36, no. 4 (2013): 887–93; M. Ashwell, P. Gunn, and S. Gibson, "Waist-to-Height Ratio Is a Better Screening Tool Than Waist Circumference and BMI for Adult Cardiometabolic Risk Factors: Systematic Review and Meta-Analysis," *Obesity Reviews* 13, no. 3 (2012): 275–86.
157. M. Schulze et al., "Body Adiposity Index, Body Fat Content and Incidence of Type 2 Diabetes," *Diabetologia* (2012), DOI. 10.1007/s00125-012-2499-z.
158. L. Bromley et al., "Sleep Restriction Decreases the Physical Activity of Adults at Risk for Type 2 Diabetes," *Sleep* 35, no. 7 (2012): 977–84, DOI:10.5665/sleep.1964.
159. S. Reutrakul and E. V. Cauter, "Interactions between Sleep, Circadian Function, and Glucose Metabolism: Implications for Risk and Severity of Diabetes," *Annals of the New York Academy of Sciences* 1311, no. 1 (2014): 151–73, DOI: 10.1111/nyas.12355A; A. Bonnefond et al., "Rare MTNRIB Variants Impairing Melatonin Receptor 1B Function Contribute to Type 2 Diabetes," *Nature Genetics* (2012), DOI: 10.1038/ng.1053; F. Cappuccio et al., "Quantity and Quality of Sleep and Incidence of Type 2 Diabetes: A Systematic Review and Meta-Analysis," *Diabetes Care* 33, no. 2 (2010): 414–20; R. Hancox and C. Landlus, "Association between Sleep Duration and Haemoglobin A1c in Young Adults," *Journal of Epidemiology & Community Health* (2011), DOI: 10.1136/jech-2011-200217. (Epub ahead of print.)
160. E. Donga et al., "A Single Night of Partial Sleep Deprivation Induces Insulin Resistance in Multiple Metabolic Pathways in Healthy Subjects," *Journal of Clinical Endocrinology and Metabolism* 95, no. 6 (2010): 2963–8, doi: 10.1210/jc.2009-2430; J. P. Chaput et al., "Short Sleep Duration as a Risk Factor for Development of the Metabolic Syndrome in Adults," *Preventive Medicine* 57, no. 6 (2013): 872–77; R. Hancox and C. Landlus, "Associations between Sleep Duration and Haemoglobin," 2011.
161. E. Feracioli-Oda, A Qawasmi, and M. Bloch, "Meta-Analysis: Melatonin for the Treatment of Primary Sleep Disorders." *PLoS ONE* 8 no. 5 (2013): e63773; J. P. Chaput, J. McNeil, and J. P. Despres et al., "Short Sleep Duration," 2013; F. Cappuccio et al., "Quantity and Quality of Sleep," 2010.
162. M. Cosgrove, L. Sargeant, R. Caleyachetty and S. Griffin, "Work Related Stress and Type 2 Diabetes: A Systematic Review and Meta-Analysis," *Occupational Medicine* (2012), DOI: 10.1093/occmed/kqs002. (Epub ahead of print); T. Monk and D. J. Buysse, "Exposure to Shiftwork as a Risk Factor for Diabetes," *Journal of Biological Rhythms* 28, no. 5 (2013): 356–59; M. Novak et al., "Perceived Stress and Incidence of Type 2 Diabetes: A 35 Year Followup Study of Middle Aged Swedish Men," *Diabetic Medicine* 30, no. 1 (2013): e8–e16.
163. E. Puterman, N. Adler, K., Matthews and E. Epel, "Financial Strain and Impaired Fasting Glucose: The Moderating Role of Physical Activity in the Coronary Artery Risk Development in Young Adults Study," *Psychosomatic Medicine* 74, no. 2 (2012): 187–92.
164. P. Puustinen et al., "Psychological Distress Predicts the Development of Metabolic Syndrome: A Prospective Population-Based Study," *Psychosomatic Medicine* 73 (2011): 158–65.
165. Centers for Disease Control and Prevention, "National Diabetes Fact Sheet: 2011," January 2014, Available at www.cdc.gov/diabetes/pubs/factsheet11.htm.
166. National Heart Lung and Blood Institute, "What Is Metabolic Syndrome?," November 2011, www.nhlbi.nih.gov/health/dci/Diseases/ms/ms_whatis.html.
167. American Diabetes Association, "What is Gestational Diabetes?," March 2014, www.diabetes.org/diabetes-basics/gestational/what-is-gestational-diabetes.html.
168. Ibid.; C. Kim et al., "Gestational Diabetes and the Incidence of Type 2 Diabetes: A Systematic Review," *Diabetes Care* 25, no. 10 (2002): 1862–68; G. Chodick et al., "The Risk of Overt Diabetes Mellitus among Women with Gestational Diabetes: A Population-Based Study," *Diabetic Medicine* 27, no. 7 (2010): 779–85.
169. American Diabetes Association, "Fast Facts: Data and Statistics about Diabetes," March 2013, http://professional.diabetes.org/admin/UserFiles/0%20-%20Sean/FastFacts%20March%20

2013.pdf; American Diabetes Association, "Living with Diabetes: Complications," Accessed May 2014, www.diabetes.org/living-with-diabetes/complications/; K. Weinspach et al., "Level of Information about the Relationship between Diabetes Mellitus and Periodontitis—Results from a Nationwide Diabetes Information Program," *European Journal of Medical Research* 18, no. 1 (2013): 6, DOI: 10.1186/2047-783X-18-6.

170. National Kidney Foundation, "Fast Facts," January 2014, www.kidney.org/news/newsroom/factsheets/FastFacts.cfm.
171. American Diabetes Association, "Fast Facts: Data and Statistics about Diabetes," 2013.
172. Prevent Blindness America, "Diabetic Retinopathy Prevalence by Age," Accessed May 2014, www.visionproblemsus.org/diabetic-retinopathy/diabetic-retinopathy-by-age.html.
173. K. Behan, "New ADA Guidelines for Diagnosis, Screening of Diabetes," *Advance Laboratory* 20, no. 1 (2011): 22, Available at http://laboratory-manager.advanceweb.com.
174. American Diabetes Association, "Diagnosing Diabetes and Learning about Prediabetes," March 2014, www.diabetes.org/diabetes-basics/diagnosis.
175. Diabetes Prevention Program Research Group, "Reduction in the Incidence of Type 2 Diabetes in the Incidence of Type 2 Diabetes with Lifestyle Intervention or Metformin," *New England Journal of Medicine* 345 (2002): 393–403.
176. S. Jonnalagadda et al., "Putting the Whole Grain Puzzle Together: Health Benefits Associated with Whole Grains—Summary of American Society for Nutrition 2010 Satellite Symposium," *Journal of Nutrition* 41, no. 5 (2011): 10115–25.
177. R. Post et al., "Dietary Fiber for the Treatment of Type 2 Diabetes Mellitus: A Meta-Analysis," *Journal of the American Board of Family Medicine* 25, no. 1 (2012): 16–23; S. Bhupathiraju et al., "Glycemic Index, Glycemic Load and Risk of Type 2 Diabetes: Results from 3 Large US Cohorts and an Updated Meta-Analysis," *Circulation* 129, Supplement 1 (2014): AP140-AP140; A. Olubukola, P. English, and J. Pinkney, "Systematic Review and Meta-Analysis of Different Dietary Approaches to the Management of Type 2 Diabetes," *The American Journal of Clinical Nutrition* 97, no. 3 (2013): 505–16.
178. A. Wallin et al. "Fish Consumption, Dietary Long-Chain N-3 Fatty Acids, and the Risk of Type 2 Diabetes: Systematic Review and Meta Analysis of Prospective Studies," *Diabetes Care* 35, no. 4 (2012): 918–29; L. Djousse et al., "Dietary Omega-3 Fatty Acids and Fish Consumption and Risk of Type 2 Diabetes," *American Journal of Clinical Nutrition* 93, no. 1 (2011): 113–50.
179. American Diabetes Association, "What We Recommend," December 2013, www.diabetes.org/food-and-fitness/fitness/types-of-activity/what-we-recommend.html; National Diabetes Information Clearing House, "Diabetes Prevention Program," September 2013, http://diabetes.niddk.nih.gov/dm/pubs/preventionprogram/index.aspx.
180. S. R. Kashyap et al., "Metabolic Effects of Bariatric Surgery in Patients with Moderate Obesity and Type 2 Diabetes," *Diabetes Care* 36, no. 8 (2013): 2175–82.
181. P. R. Schauer et al., "Bariatric Surgery versus Intensive Medical Therapy for Diabetes-3 Year Outcomes," *New England Journal of Medicine* 2014, DOI:10.1056/NEJMoa1401329.
182. P. Poirier et al. on Behalf of the American Heart Association Obesity Committee of the Council on Nutrition, Physical Activity, and Metabolism, "Bariatric Surgery and Cardiovascular Risk Factors: A Scientific Statement from the American Heart Association," *Circulation* (March 2011), DOI:10.1161/CIR.0b013e3182149099. (Epub ahead of print.)

Pulled Statistics

page 106, A. S. Go et al., "Heart Disease and Stroke Statistics.—2014 Update: A Report from the American Heart Association," *Circulation*, (2014) 129:e28-e292.
page 120 , Centers for Disease Control and Prevention, "Lung Cancer Risk Factors," February 2013, www.cdc.gov.
page 128, American Cancer Society, "Cancer Facts and Figures 2014," May 2014, Available at http://www.cancer.org/research/cancerfactsstatistics/cancerfactsfigures2014/index.
page 130, American Diabetes Association, "Diabetes Fast facts," 2013, http://www.diabetes.org/diabetes-basics/diabetes-statistics.
page 131, Centers for Disease Control and Prevention. National Diabetes Statistics Report: Estimates of Diabetes and Its Burden in the United States, 2014. Atlanta, GA: U.S. Department of Health and Human Services; 2014.
page 285, Diabetes Prevention Program Research Group, "Reduction in the Incidence of Type 2 Diabetes in the Incidence of Type 2 Diabetes with Lifestyle Intervention or Metformin," New England Journal of Medicine 345 (2002): 393–403.

Chapter 6

1. L. Colloca and C. Grillon, "Understanding Placebo and Nocebo Responses for Pain Management," *Current Pain and Headache Reports* 18, no. 6 (2014): 419, DOI: 10.1007/s11916-014-0419-2.
2. A. Keitel et al., "Expectation Modulates the Effect of Deep Brain Stimulation on Motor and Cognitive Function in Tremor-Dominant Parkinson's Disease," *PLoS One* 8, no. 12 (2013): e81878, DOI: 10.1371/journal.pone.0081878.
3. J. Sarris, M. Fava, I. Schweitzer, and D. Mischoulon, "St John's Wort (Hypericum perforatum) versus Sertraline and Placebo in Major Depressive Disorder: Continuation Data from a 26-Week RCT," *Pharmacopsychiatry* 45, no. 7 (2012): 275–8, DOI: 10.1055/s-0032-1306348; R. A. Litten et al., "The Placebo Effect in Clinical Trials for Alcohol Dependence: An Exploratory Analysis of 51 Naltrexone and Acamprosate Studies," *Alcoholism, Clinical and Experimental Research* 37, no. 12 (2013): 2128–37, DOI: 10.1111/acer.12197; G. L. Petersen et al., "The Magnitude of Nocebo Effects in Pain: A Meta-Analysis," *Pain* (2014), pii: S0304-3959(14)00195-X, DOI: 10.1016/j.pain.2014.04.016. (E-pub ahead of publication.)
4. M. A. Hillen et al., " How Can Communication by Oncologists Enhance Patients' Trust? An Experimental Study," *Annals of Oncology* 25, no. 4 (2014): 896–901.
5. J. Commins, "Defensive Medicine," *Health Leaders Media*, April 13, 2012, www.healthleadersmedia.com/page-4/MAG-278899/Defensive-Medicine.
6. A. T. Chien and M. B. Rosenthal, "Waste Not, Want Not: Promoting Efficient Use of Health Care Resources," *Annals of Internal Medicine* 158, no. 1 (2013): 67–68.
7. Consumer Health, "Patient Rights: Informed Consent," March 2013, www.emedicinehealth.com/patient_rights/article_em.htm#patient_rights.
8. Centers for Disease Control and Prevention, "Therapeutic Drug Use," May 2014, www.cdc.gov/nchs/fastats/drug-use-therapeutic.htm.
9. W. Zhong et al., "Age and Sex Patterns of Drug Prescribing in a Defined American Population," *Mayo Clinic Proceedings* 88, no. 7 (2013): 697–707.
10. L. Gallelli et al., "Safety and Efficacy of Generic Drugs with Respect to Brand Formulation," *Journal of Pharmacology and Pharmacotherapeutics* 4, Supplement 1 (2013): S110–14.
11. U.S. Food and Drug Administration, "The Possible Dangers of Buying Medicine over the Internet," 2014, www.fda.gov/forconsumers/consumerupdates/ucm048396.htm.
12. National Center for Complementary and Alternative Medicine, "Complementary, Alternative, or Integrative Health: What's in a Name?," May 2013, http://nccam.nih.gov/health/whatiscam.
13. Ibid.
14. National Center for Complementary and Alternative Medicine, "Health Topics A to Z," 2014, http://nccam.nih.gov/health/atoz.htm.
15. National Center for Complementary and Alternative Medicine, "Traditional Chinese Medicine: An Introduction," October 2013, http://nccam.nih.gov/health/whatiscam/chinesemed.htm.
16. National Center for Complementary and Alternative Medicine, "Ayurvedic Medicine: An Introduction," NCCAM Publication no. D287, August 2013, http://nccam.nih.gov/health/ayurveda/introduction.htm.
17. Ibid.
18. National Center for Complementary and Alternative Medicine, "Homeopathy: An Introduction," May 2013, http://nccam.nih.gov/health/homeopathy.
19. Ibid.
20. National Center for Complementary and Alternative Medicine, "Chiropractic: An Introduction," NCCAM Publication no. D403, Modified February 2012. http://nccam.nih.gov/health/chiropractic/introduction.htm.
21. Ibid.
22. Bureau of Labor Statistics, U.S. Department of Labor, "Chiropractors," *Occupational Outlook Handbook, 2012–2013 Edition*, March 29, 2012. http://www.bls.gov/ooh/healthcare/chiropractors.htm.
23. Bureau of Labor Statistics, U.S. Department of Labor, "Massage Therapists," *Occupational Outlook Handbook, 2012–2013 Edition*, January 2014, www.bls.gov/ooh/Healthcare/Massage-therapists.htm.
24. Ibid.
25. National Center for Complementary and Alternative Medicine, "Complementary, Alternative, or Integrative Health: What's in a Name?," May 2013, http://nccam.nih.gov/health/whatiscam.
26. National Center for Complementary and Alternative Medicine, "Acupuncture: An Introduction," September 2012, http://nccam.nih.gov/health/acupuncture/introduction.htm.
27. A. J. Vickers et al., "Acupuncture for Chronic Pain: Individual Patient Data Meta-Analysis," *Archives of Internal Medicine* 172, no. 19 (2012): 1444–53.
28. National Center for Complementary and Alternative Medicine, "Acupuncture: An Introduction," 2012.
29. R. Jahnke et al., "A Comprehensive Review of Health Benefits of Qigong and Tai Chi," *American Journal of Health Promotion* 24, no. 6 (2010): e1–e25.
30. D. L. Fazzino et al., "Energy Healing and Pain: A Review of the Literature," *Holistic Nursing Practice* 24, no. 2 (2010): 79–88; National Center for Complementary and Alternative Medicine, "Reiki: An Introduction," April 2013, http://nccam.nih.gov/health/reiki/introduction.htm.
31. Psychoneuroimmunology Research Society, "Mission Statement," November 17, 2010, www.pnirs.org/society/index.cfm.

32. E. Broadbent and H. E. Koschwanez, "The Psychology of Wound Healing," *Current Opinions in Psychiatry* 25, no 2 (2012): 135–40.
33. M. R. Irwin and R. Olmstead, "Mitigating Cellular Inflammation in Older Adults: A Randomized Controlled Trial of Tai Chi," *American Journal of Geriatric Psychiatry* 20, no. 9 (2012): 764–72.
34. Academy of Nutrition and Dietetics, "Position of the Academy of Nutrition and Dietetics: Functional Foods," *Journal of the Academy of Nutrition and Dietetics* 113, no. 8 (2013): 1096–1103.
35. K. Ried et al., "Effect of Cocoa on Blood Pressure," *Cochrane Database of Systematic Reviews* 8, no. CD008893 (2012), DOI: 10.1002/14651858.CD008893.pub2.
36. National Center for Complementary and Alternative Medicine, "Oral Probiotics: An Introduction," December 2012, http://nccam.nih.gov/health/probiotics/introduction.htm
37. National Center for Complementary and Alternative Medicine, "Kava," April 2012, http://nccam.nih.gov/health/kava.
38. Mayo Clinic Staff, "Herbal Supplements: What to Know before You Buy," November 2011, www.mayoclinic.com/health/herbal-supplements/SA00044.
39. U.S. Pharmacopeial Convention, "USP & Patients/Consumers," 2012, www.usp.org/usp-consumers.
40. K. G. Carman and C. Eibner, "Survey Estimates Net Gain of 9.3 Million American Adults with Health Insurance," April 8, 2014, www.rand.org/blog/2014/04/survey-estimates-net-gain-of-9-3-million-american-adults.html.
41. American College Health Association. *American College Health Association–National College Health Assessment II: Reference Group Executive Summary, Fall 2013* (Hanover, MD: American College Health Association, 2014).
42. U.S. Centers for Disease Control and Prevention/National Center for Health Statistics, "Health Insurance Coverage, January–June, 2012," Updated November, 2012, www.cdc.gov/nchs/health_policy/health_insurance_selected_characteristics_jan_jun_2012.htm.
43. Kaiser Family Foundation, "Total HMO Enrollment, July 2012," May 2014, http://kff.org/other/state-indicator/total-hmo-enrollment.
44. Centers for Medicare & Medicaid Services, "National Health Expenditure Projections 2012–2022: Forecast Summary," November, 2013, www.cms.gov/Research-Statistics-Data-and-Systems/Statistics-Trends-and-Reports/NationalHealthExpendData/Downloads/proj2012.pdf.
45. Ibid.
46. Bureau of Labor Statistics, U.S. Department of Labor, "Physicians and Surgeons," *Occupational Outlook Handbook, 2014–2015*, Modified January 2014, www.bls.gov/ooh/healthcare/physicians-and-surgeons.htm.
47. American Hospital Association, "Fast Facts on U.S. Hospitals," January 2014, www.aha.org/research/rc/stat-studies/fast-facts.shtml.
48. O. W. Brawley, *How We Do Harm: A Doctor Breaks Ranks about Being Sick in America* (New York, NY: St. Martin's Press, 2011).
49. Centers for Medicare and Medicaid Services, "National Health Expenditure Projections 2012–2022: Forecast Summary," 2013.
50. Ibid.
51. America's Health Insurance Plans, "Fast Check: Administrative Costs," November 2012, www.ahip.org/ACA-Toolbox/Documents/Communications-Toolkit/Fact-Check–Administrative-Costs.aspx.
52. P. Krugman, "The Medicaid Cure," January 10, 2014, *The New York Times*; Right to Health Care ProCon.org, "Should All Americans Have the Right (Be Entitled) to Health Care?" Updated January 2014, http://healthcare.procon.org.
53. United Nations, "The Universal Declaration of Human Rights," 1948, www.un.org/en/documents/udhr.
54. P. Krugman, "The Medicaid Cure," 2014.
55. Department of Health and Human Services, "Report to Congress: National Strategy for Quality Improvement in Health Care," 2011, www.ahrq.gov/workingforquality/nqs/nqs2011annlrpt.htm.

Pulled Statistics

page 146, Centers for Disease Control and Prevention, "Therapeutic Drug Use," May 2014, www.cdc.gov/nchs/fastats/drug-use-therapeutic.htm.
page 148, P. M. Barnes, B. Bloom, and R. L. Nahin, "Complementary and Alternative Medicine Use among Adults and Children: United States, 2007," *National Health Statistics Reports*, no. 12 (Hyattsville, MD: National Center for Health Statistics, 2008), Available at www.cdc.gov.
page 158, Robert Wood Johnson Foundation, "Survey: Physicians Are Aware that Many Medical Tests and Procedures Are Unnecessary, See Themselves as Solution," May 2014, www.rwjf.org/en/about-rwjf/newsroom/newsroom-content/2014/04/survey--physicians-are-aware-that-many-medical-tests-and-procedu.html.

Photo Credits

Chapter 1 1: Image Source/Alamy; 3: Anton Gvozdikov/Getty Images; 3: Graham Mitchell/Exactostock/Superstock; 3: Pearson Education; 3: Photodisc/Getty Images; 3: Teo Lannie/PhotoAlto Agency RF Collections/Getty Images; 3: Teo Lannie/PhotoAlto Agency/Getty Images; 5: Miroslav Georgijevic/Vetta/Getty Images; 7: Rolf Adlercreutz/Alamy; 8: Ali Ender Birer/iStock/360/Getty Images; 8: Ali Ender Birer/Shutterstock; 8: Bob Jacobson/keepsake/Corbis; 8: Craig Veltri/iStock / 360/Getty Images; 8: Dandanian/Getty Images; 8: Deymos/Shutterstock; 8: GVictoria/Shutterstock; 8: Kirsty Pargeter/iStock/360/Getty Images; 8: PaulMaguire/iStock/360/Getty Images; 8: Rod Ferris/Shutterstock; 8: Stephen VanHorn/Alamy; 8: Tatuasha/Shutterstock; 8: Walter Cruz/MCT/Newscom; 9: Dan Dalton/Digital Vision/Getty Images; 9: Daniel Grill/Alamy; 9: MIXA/Getty Images; 10: Karl Weatherly/Photodisc/Getty Images; 10: Pearson Education; 11: Moodboard/Corbis; 12: Wavebreakmedia Ltd/Getty Images; 13: Blue Jean Images/Alamy; 13: Pearson Education; 14: Pearson Education; 16: Nenad Aksic/E+/Getty Images; 16: Nenad Aksic/Getty Images; 17: Mark Cowan/UPI/Newscom; 18: Alamy; 18: Pearson Education; 18: Pearson Education; 18: Thomas Smith Photography/Alamy; 20: Daniel Hurst/Getty Images; 20: Daniel Hurst/iStock/360/Getty Images; 20: windu/Shutterstock; 21: Dennis Welsh/AGE Fotostock; 21: Dennis Welsh/UpperCut Image/AGE Fotostock; 22: Image Source/Getty Images; 23: Index Stock Imagery/PhotoLibrary/Getty Images; 24: Aleksandr Lobanov/Getty Images; 24: Aleksandr Lobanov/iStock/360/Getty Images; 24: Pearson Education; 24: Pearson Education

Chapter 2 27: Ted Foxx/Alamy; 29: Big Cheese Photo LLC / Alamy; 30: Wavebreakmedia/Shutterstock; 31: Brand X Pictures/Getty Image; 31: Brand X Pictures/Getty Images; 31: Brand X Pictures/Stockbyte/Getty Images; 32: John Anthony Rizzo/Getty Images; 35: David Madison/Photographer's Choice/Getty Images; 35: JGI/Jamie Grill/Blend Images/Getty Images; 35: Julie Brown/Custom Medical Stock; 35: Life Measurement, Inc.; 35: May/Science Source; 35: Phanie/Science Source; 37: David C. Rehner/Shutterstock; 38: Luis Louro/Shutterstock; 39: Asia Images Group Pte Ltd / Alamy; 40: Bobby Bank/Getty Images; 41: Howard Shooter/DK Images; 42: Custom Medical Stock Photo/Alamy; 42: Sakala/Shutterstock; 44: Brand X Pictures/Stockbyte/Getty Images; 44: Li Kim Goh/E+/Getty Images; 45: Favakeh/Custom Medical Stock Photo/Newscom; 46: Barry Gregg/keepsake/Corbis; 47: Nicholas Monu/Getty Images; 47: Photodisc/Getty Images; 48: LeventeGyori/Shutterstock; 49: WavebreakmediaMicro/Fotolia; 50: Micha Klootwijk/Shutterstock; 51: Gustavo Andrade/Gos Photo Design/Getty Images

Chapter 3 53: Golden Pixels LLC/Alamy; 54: webphotographeer/Getty Images; 55: JR Trice/Shutterstock; 55: Westmacott Photograph/Shutterstock; 56: George Muresan/Shutterstock; 57: Shutterstock; 58: Mike Flippo/Shutterstock; 58: Pearson Learning Photo Studio; 61: David R. Frazier Photolibrary, Inc./Alamy; 62: Barry Gregg/keepsake/Corbis; 62: Barry Gregg/Spirit/Corbis; 63: Barry Gregg/keepsake/Corbis; 63: Barry Gregg/Spirit/Corbis; 63: C Squared Studios/Photodisc/Getty Images; 63: VL@D/Fotolia; 64: Bluefern/Fotolia; 64: Brand Pictures/ AGE Fotostock; 64: Martin Darley /Shutterstock; 65: Barry Gregg/keepsake/Corbis; 65: Barry Gregg/Spirit/Corbis; 66: Matka_Wariatka/iStock/360/Getty Images; 69: Pearson Education; 70: Stockbyte/Getty Images; 72: Brian Hagiwara/Photolibrary/Getty Images; 73: ML Harris/Getty Images; 75: MorePixels/iStock /360/Getty Images; 76: Vladimir Voronin/Fotolia; 78: Dkapp12/iStock/360/Getty Images; 79: Alxpin/E+/Getty Images

Chapter 4 81: 68 altrendo images/Ocean/Corbis; 82: Creatista/Shutterstock; 83: Ariel Skelley/Blend Images/Getty images; 83: Pendygraft/John/St. Petersburg Times/PSG/Newscom; 83: Scott Griessel/Getty Images; 85: Oliver Furrer/Alamy; 86: Getty Images; 87: Getty images; 88: Gladskikh Tatiana/Shutterstock; 89: Radius Images/Getty Images; 90: Radius Images/Corbis; 91: Robert Churchill/Getty Images; 92: Imagerymajestic/Alamy; 93: Kate Sept 2004/E+/Getty Images; 94: Susan Montgomery/Fotolia; 96: SuperStock; 97: Getty Images; 98: DK Images; 99: Uniquely india/Getty Images; 100: iStock/Getty images; 101: Getty Images

Chapter 5 103: B Boissonnet/ Ramble/Corbis; 106: Irina Iglina/Getty Images; 106: Irina Iglina/iStock/360/Getty Images; 111: Radius Images/Alamy; 113: Jupiterimages/Brand X Pictures/Thinkstock/Getty Images; 113: Moodboard/Alamy; 114: Moodboard/Getty Images; 115: Levent Konuk/Shutterstock; 118: Index Stock/Getty Images; 118: PhotoLibrary/Index Stock/Science Source; 119: Dawn Poland/E+/Getty Images; 119: Dawn Poland/Getty Images; 120: dnberty/Getty Images; 121: AfriPics.com/Alamy; 122: Darryl Bush/Modesto Bee/ZumaPress.com/ZUMA Wire Service/Alamy; 124: Digital Vision/Getty Images; 125: Dr. P. Marazzi / Science Source; 125: Dr. P. Marazzi/Science Source; 125: Dr. P. Marazzi/Science Source; 125: James Stevenson/Science Source; 125: James Stevenson/Science Source; 130: Kamdyn R Switzer/Cal Sport Media/Newscom; 132: William Perugini/Shutterstock; 136: Ioana Drutu/Getty Images; 136: Loana Drutu/iStock/360/Getty Images; 137: Getty Images; 137: Sebastian Kaulitzki/Getty Images; 137: vm/Getty Images; 139: Martin Shields/Alamy

Chapter 6 141: ableimages/Alamy; 142: Adrian Sherratt/Alamy; 143: Tatiana Popova/Shutterstock; 145: Jiang Jin/SuperStock; 146: Steve Snowden/Shutterstock; 149: Design Pics Inc/Alamy; 150: Thomas Boehm/Alamy; 151: Monkey Business Images/Shutterstock; 152: Illie Hill, Jr./The Image Works; 153: Jeffrey Blackler/Alamy; 154: eAlisa/Shutterstock; 154: Elena Elisseeva/Shutterstock; 154: joanna wnuk/Shutterstock; 154: Shapiso/Shutterstock; 154: WEKWEK/iStock/Getty Images; 156: Jochen Tack/Alamy; 157: Blend Images/Alamy; **158:**; 160: DNY59/iStockphoto/Getty Images; 160: jo unruh/iStockphoto/Getty Images

Cover Tetra Images/Corbis

Index

Note: Page references followed by *fig* indicate an illustrated figure; by *t* a table; and by *p* a photograph.

D

E

F

G

H

I

J

K

L

M

N

O

P